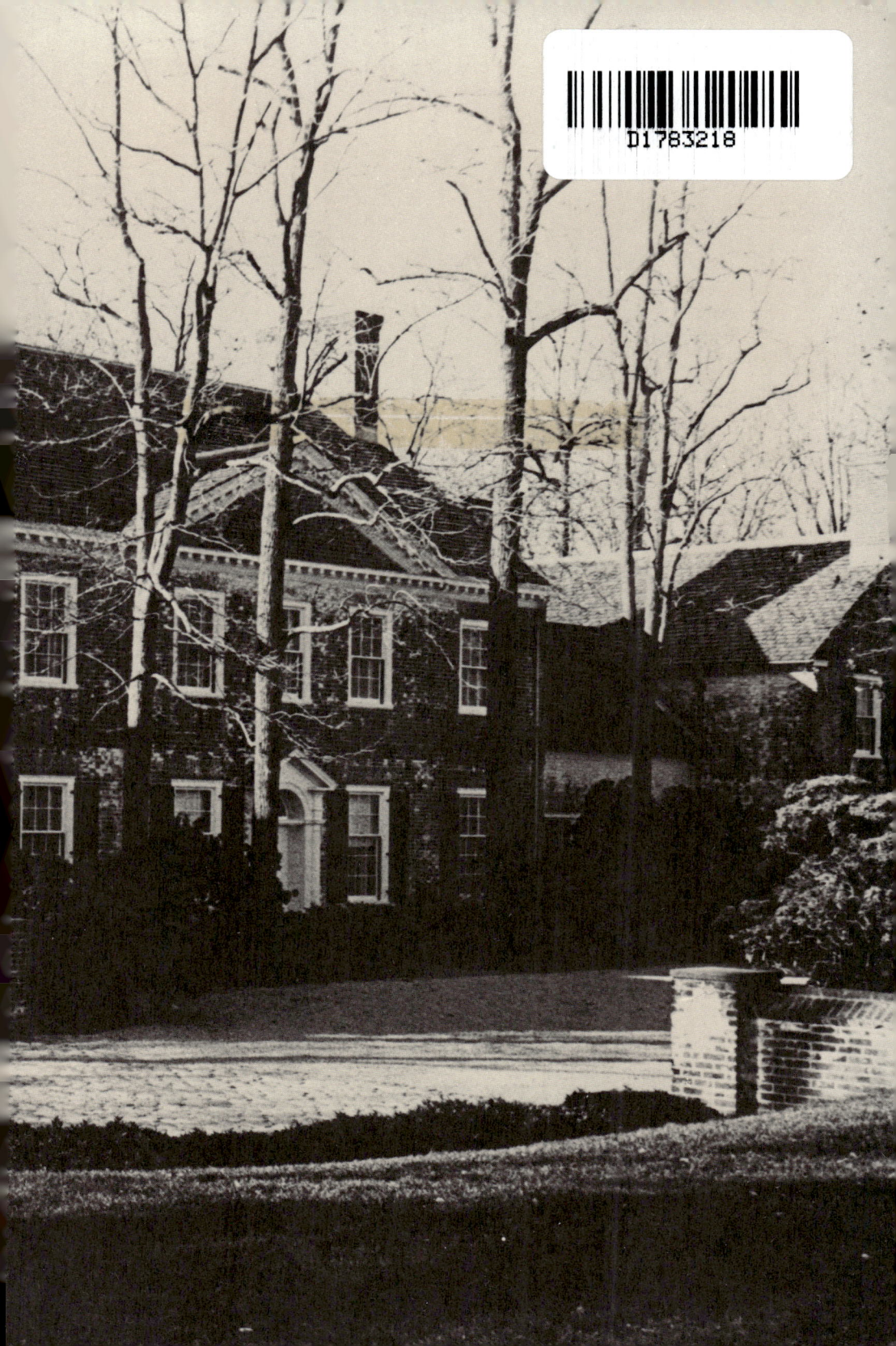

Mechanisms in Tobacco Carcinogenesis

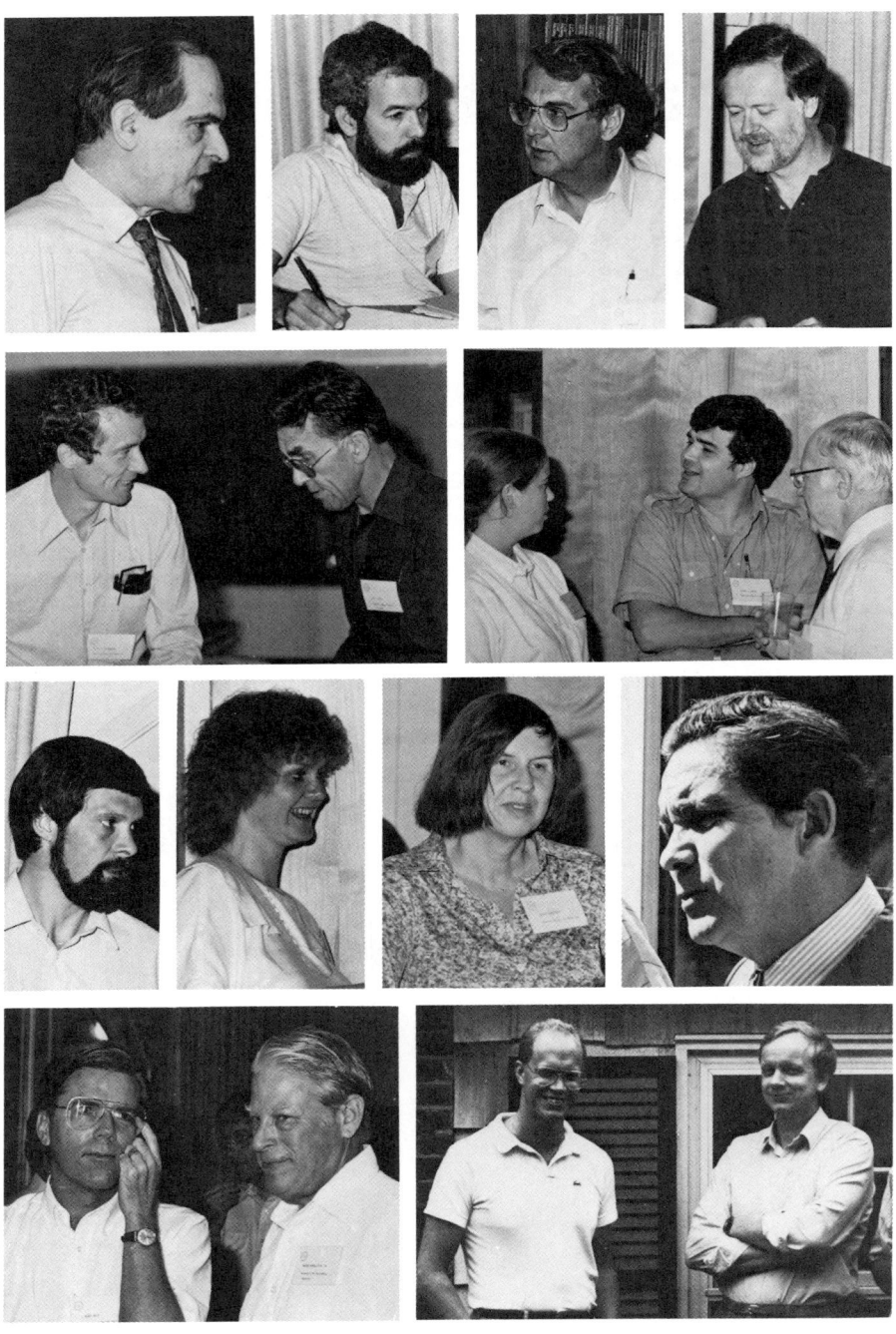

Row 1: D. Hoffmann; G.H. Yoakum; K.Randerath; C.C. Harris.
Row 2: K.D. Brunnemann, C.R. Enzell; N.J. Haley, E.J. LaVoie, P.N. Magee.
Row 3: H.N. Autrup; M.Rosin; E. Randerath; P. Correa.
Row 4: H.d'A. Heck, W. Winkelstein, Jr.; R.C. Grafstrom, H.Tjälve.

Mechanisms in Tobacco Carcinogenesis

Edited by

DIETRICH HOFFMANN
Naylor Dana Institute for Disease Prevention
American Health Foundation

CURTIS C. HARRIS
Laboratory of Human Carcinogenesis
National Cancer Institute

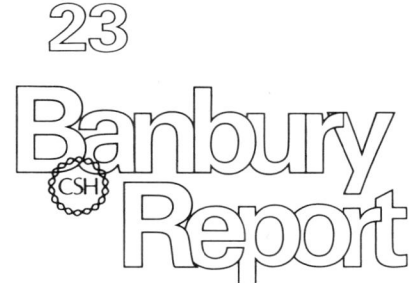

**COLD SPRING HARBOR LABORATORY
1986**

Banbury Report 23: Mechanisms in Tobacco Carcinogenesis

© 1986 by Cold Spring Harbor Laboratory
All rights reserved
Printed in the United States of America
Cover and book design by Emily Harste

Library of Congress Cataloging-in-Publication Data

Mechanisms in tobacco carcinogenesis.

(Banbury report, ISSN 0198-0068 ; 23)
Proceedings of the September 1985 Banbury Center conference on "New Aspects of Tobacco Carcinogenesis."
Includes bibliographies and index.
1. Tobacco—Toxicology—Congresses. 2. Carcinogenesis—Congresses. I. Hoffmann, Dietrich, 1924- II. Harris, Curtis C., 1943-   . III. Banbury Center. IV. Series.
RC268.7.T62M43   1986   616.99'4071   86-12956
ISBN 0-87969-223-5

Authorization to photocopy items for internal or personal use, or the internal or personal use of specific clients, is granted by Cold Spring Harbor Laboratory for libraries and other users registered with the Copyright Clearance Center (CCC) Transactional Reporting Service, provided that the base fee of $1.00 per article is paid directly to CCC, 27 Congress St., Salem, MA 01970. [0-87969-223-5-8/86 $1.00 + .00] This consent does not extend to other kinds of copying, such as copying for general distribution, for advertising or promotional purposes, for creating new collective works, or for resale.

All Cold Spring Harbor Laboratory publications may be ordered directly from Cold Spring Harbor Laboratory, Box 100, Cold Spring Harbor, New York 11724. (Phone: 1-800-843-4388) In New York State (516) 367-8425.

BANBURY REPORT SERIES

Banbury Report	1:	Assessing Chemical Mutagens
Banbury Report	2:	Mammalian Cell Mutagenesis
Banbury Report	3:	A Safe Cigarette?
Banbury Report	4:	Cancer Incidence in Defined Populations
Banbury Report	5:	Ethylene Dichloride: A Potential Health Risk?
Banbury Report	6:	Product Labeling and Health Risks
Banbury Report	7:	Gastrointestinal Cancer: Endogenous Factors
Banbury Report	8:	Hormones and Breast Cancer
Banbury Report	9:	Quantification of Occupational Cancer
Banbury Report	10:	Patenting of Life Forms
Banbury Report	11:	Environmental Factors in Human Growth and Development
Banbury Report	12:	Nitrosamines and Human Cancer
Banbury Report	13:	Indicators of Genotoxic Exposure
Banbury Report	14:	Recombinant DNA Applications to Human Disease
Banbury Report	15:	Biological Aspects of Alzheimer's Disease
Banbury Report	16:	Genetic Variability in Responses to Chemical Exposure
Banbury Report	17:	Coffee and Health
Banbury Report	18:	Biological Mechanisms of Dioxin Action
Banbury Report	19:	Risk Quantitation and Regulatory Policy
Banbury Report	20:	Genetic Manipulation of the Early Mammalian Embryo
Banbury Report	21:	Viral Etiology of Cervical Cancer
Banbury Report	22:	Genetically Altered Viruses and the Environment
Banbury Report	23:	New Mechanisms in Tobacco Carcinogenesis

CORPORATE SPONSORS

Agrigenetics Corporation
American Cyanamid Company
Amersham International plc
Becton Dickinson and Company
Biogen S.A.
Cetus Corporation
Ciba-Geigy Corporation
CPC International, Inc.
E.I. du Pont de Nemours & Company
Genentech, Inc.
Genetics Institute
Hoffmann-La Roche Inc.
Johnson & Johnson
Eli Lilly and Company
Mitsui Toatsu Chemicals, Inc.
Monsanto Company
Pall Corporation
Pfizer Inc.
Schering-Plough Corporation
Smith Kline & French Laboratories
The Upjohn Company

CORE SUPPORTERS

The Bristol-Myers Fund, Inc.
The Dow Chemical Company
Exxon Corporation
Grace Foundation Inc.
International Business Machines Corporation
Phillips Petroleum Foundation, Inc.
The Procter & Gamble Company
Rockwell International Corporation Trust
The Chevron Fund
Texaco Philanthropic Foundation Inc.

Participants

Herman N. Autrup, Laboratory of Environmental Carcinogenesis, Fibiger Institute, Copenhagen, Denmark

Helmut Bartsch, International Agency for Research on Cancer, Division of Environmental Carcinogenesis, Lyon, France

Georg Becher, Toxicological Department, National Institute of Public Health, Oslo, Norway

Frederick A. Beland, National Center for Toxicological Research

Klaus D. Brunnemann, Naylor Dana Institute for Disease Prevention, American Health Foundation

Allan H. Conney, Laboratory of Experimental Carcinogenesis and Metabolism, Roche Institute of Molecular Biology

Pelayo Correa, Department of Pathology, Louisiana State University Medical Center

Margareta Curvall, Swedish Tobacco Company, Stockholm, Sweden

Curt R. Enzell, Swedish Tobacco Company, Stockholm, Sweden

Roland C. Grafstrom, Department of Toxicology, Karolinska Institute, Stockholm, Sweden

Nancy Jean Haley, Naylor Dana Institute for Disease Prevention, American Health Foundation

Curtis C. Harris, Laboratory of Human Carcinogenesis, National Cancer Institute

Stephen S. Hecht, Naylor Dana Institute for Disease Prevention, American Health Foundation

Henry d'A. Heck, Chemical Industry Institute of Toxicology

Dietrich Hoffmann, Naylor Dana Institute for Disease Prevention, American Health Foundation

Edmond J. LaVoie, Division of Environmental Carcinogenesis, American Health Foundation

Peter N. Magee, Fels Research Institute, Temple University School of Medicine

Thomas B. Owen, Division of Cancer Etiology, National Cancer Institute

Ismail Parsa, Department of Pathology, State University of New York, Downstate Medical Center

Anthony E. Pegg, Department of Physiology and Cancer Research Center, Pennsylvania State University College of Medicine

Miriam Poirier, National Cancer Institute

Erika Randerath, Department of Pharmacology, Baylor College of Medicine

Kurt Randerath, Department of Pharmacology, Baylor College of Medicine

Gerhard Scherer, Council on Smoking and Health, Hamburg, Federal Republic of Germany

Steven D. Stellman, American Cancer Society

Miriam Rosin, British Columbia Cancer Research Centre, Vancouver, British Columbia, Canada

Steven R. Tannenbaum, Department of Applied Biological Sciences, Massachusetts Institute of Technology

Hans Tjälve, Department of Pharmacology and Toxicology, Swedish University of Agricultural Sciences

Warren Winkelstein, Jr., Department of Biomedical and Environmental Health Sciences, School of Public Health, University of California, Berkeley

Deborah M. Winn, Biostatistics Branch, National Cancer Institute

Marcus B. Wise, Analytical Chemistry Division, Oak Ridge National Laboratory

George Yoakum, National Cancer Institute

Preface

Epidemiological investigations and animal studies over several decades have delineated the major impacts of tobacco usage on human health. It is now recognized that the single most important etiological factor in human cancer in developed nations is the use of tobacco. One of the next major challenges is to use the techniques and theories of molecular and cell biology to refine our understanding of tobacco's role in human carcinogenesis.

The Banbury Center conference on New Aspects of Tobacco Carcinogenesis, held in September 1985, brought together key workers from the long-established facets of tobacco carcinogenesis research with experts in molecular biology, cell biology, and biochemistry. The result of this interaction was to develop new insights into the mechanisms of carcinogenesis. The value of this approach to the complex and vitally important issue of tobacco carcinogenesis is clear in the presentations published in this volume and is particularly apparent in the discussions following each paper.

Examples of the new approaches toward understanding tobacco carcinogenesis include the recent advances in analytical techniques, such as postlabeling of metabolites and radioimmunoassays for DNA adducts, which should allow the specific effects of tobacco carcinogens to be directly assessed. Such evidence could be of great significance in verifying long-standing descriptive epidemiological and animal studies assessing tobacco and its carcinogens. These data should also help us understand the molecular and cellular mechanisms that underlie the neoplastic process and the determinations of cancer risk in tobacco chewers and smokers.

The success of this Banbury meeting was due in large part to the enthusiasm and unstinting efforts of the organizers, Curtis C. Harris of the National Cancer Institute and Dietrich Hoffmann of the American Health Foundation. I should also like to take this opportunity to thank my predecessor as director of the Banbury Center, Michael Shodell, for the skill and enthusiasm which he showed in developing this and many previous meetings during his four years at the Banbury Center. During this time he was greatly assisted by Bea Toliver, who has been administrative assistant to the Center since its inception, and Judith Blum, the Banbury Center editor, who has been responsible for the efficient translation of the conference proceedings into printed form. The characteristic environment of a Banbury Center meeting owes much to their dedication and that of Katya Davey, the hostess at Robertson House.

Financial support for the Banbury meeting on tobacco carcinogenesis was provided by the James S. McDonnell Foundation, the National Cancer Institute, the Office on Smoking and Health, and the American Cancer Society. Without their support this meeting could not have taken place.

Steve Prentis
Director
Banbury Center

Introduction

DIETRICH HOFFMANN* AND CURTIS C. HARRIS†
*Naylor Dana Institute for Disease Prevention
American Health Foundation
Valhalla, New York 10595
†Laboratory of Human Carcinogenesis
National Cancer Institute
Bethesda, Maryland 20892

An earlier Banbury Conference focused on the state-of-the-art of the less harmful cigarette so as to examine whether a major environmental cancer risk factor could be effectively reduced through concerted efforts of scientists from various scientific disciplines (Gori and Bock 1980). Reduction of exposure achieved by the wide availability of cigarettes with lower smoke yields was indeed reflected in a somewhat lower incidence of lung cancer (International Agency for Research on Cancer 1985); yet it was clear on the basis of epidemiological evidence that health education programs had to be stepped up to discourage onset of smoking among future generations if we were to effectively practice prevention of premature deaths from tobacco-released diseases.

The review of epidemiological and experimental evidence also pointed to the fact that cigarette smoke contains tumor-enhancing substances that increase cancer risk through chronic exposure. However, tobacco smoke also contains sufficient levels of tumor initiators that may render cells susceptible to cancer development by tumor-enhancing substances. Both acquired and inherited host factors may also influence one's susceptibility to tobacco carcinogens.

The recent advances in molecular biology and chemical carcinogenesis prompted us to organize a second Banbury Conference in this field entitled, "New Aspects of Tobacco Carcinogenesis," for the purpose of exchanging information and enhancing communication between epidemiologists and experts in these special laboratory sciences. The outcome of such dialogue should advance our understanding of the association between tobacco usage and cancer, provide better insight into the host factors and mechanisms involved in the induction and propagation of neoplasms by tobacco products, and help to design new research strategies in cancer prevention.

The urgency of interdisciplinary communication and advancement of knowledge in this area of cancer prevention is underscored by a recent position paper of the American Association for Cancer Research, which states that 30-40% of all deaths from cancer are associated with smoking and chewing of tobacco (Loeb et al. 1984).

Beyond the immediate goals of the conference, it is hoped that the publication of its proceedings in this volume will provide updated information on the advances in tobacco carcinogenesis and will stimulate scientists engaged in chemical and environmental carcinogenesis.

REFERENCES

Gori, G.B. and F.G. Bock (ed.). 1980. *Banbury Report 3: A safe cigarette?* Cold Spring Harbor Laboratory, Cold Spring Harbor, New York.

International Agency for Research on Cancer. 1985. *Monographs on the evaluation of the carcinogenic risk of chemicals to humans: Tobacco smoking*, vol. 38. Lyon, France. (In press).

Loeb, L.A., V.L. Vernster, K.E. Warner, J. Abbots, and J. Laszlo. 1984. Smoking and lung cancer: An overview. *Cancer Res.* **44**: 5940.

Contents

Preface / Steve Prentis
Introduction / Dietrich Hoffmann and Curtis C. Harris

SESSION 1: LABORATORY-EPIDEMIOLOGY STUDIES

Uptake of Tobacco Smoke Components / Nancy Jean Haley, Dietrich Hoffmann, and Ernst L. Wynder — 3

Factors Influencing the Urinary Excretion of Nitrosodimethylamine and Nitrosoproline in Human Beings / Allan H. Conney, William A. Garland, Felix Rubio, Halyna Kornychuk, Edward P. Norkus, and Wolfgang Kuenzig — 21

Determination of Exposure to PAH by Analysis of Urine Samples / Georg Becher — 33

Modifiers of Endogenous Carcinogen Formation: Studies on In Vivo Nitrosation in Tobacco Users / Jagadeesan Nair, Hiroshi Ohshima, Brigitte Pignatelli, Marlin Friesen, Christian Malaveille, Sylvie Calmels, and Helmut Bartsch — 45

Hemoglobin Adducts of Tobacco-related Aromatic Amines: Application to Molecular Epidemiology / Steven R. Tannenbaum, Matthew S. Bryant, Paul L. Skipper, and Malcolm Maclure — 63

Analysis of Aniline and o-Toluidine in Human Urine / Karam El-Bayoumy, Jean Donahue, Stephen S. Hecht, and Dietrich Hoffmann — 77

^{32}P-Postlabeling Test for Smoking-related DNA Adducts in Animal and Human Tissues / Kurt Randerath, M. Vijayaraj Reddy, Tommie A. Avitts, Robert H. Miller, Richard B. Everson, and Erika Randerath — 85

The Use of Micronuclei in Tracing the Genotoxic Damage in the Oral Mucosa of Tobacco Users / Hans F. Stich — 99

Validation of Smoking History with the Micronuclei Test / Elizabeth Fontham, Pelayo Correa, Elsie Rodriquez, and Youping Lin — 113

Mutagens in the Urine of Cigarette Smokers / Edmond J. LaVoie, Isaac M. Sasson, and Dietrich Hoffmann — 121

Endogenous Formation of N-Nitrosoproline in Smokers and Nonsmokers / Gerhard Scherer and Franz Adlkofer — 137

SESSION 2: NEW ASPECTS OF TOBACCO CARCINOGENESIS

Chemical Analysis of the Major Constituents in Clove Cigarette Smoke / Marcus B. Wise and Michael R. Guerin   151

Isoprenoid Flavor Components of Tobacco and Their Formation / Curt R. Enzell   163

Perinatal Disposition and Metabolism in Mice and Hamsters of Some N-Nitrosamines Present in Tobacco and Tobacco Smoke / Hans Tjälve, Böel Löfberg, Andre Castonguay, Neil Trushin, and Stephen S. Hecht   179

Laboratory Studies on Oral Cancer and Smokeless Tobacco / Klaus D. Brunnemann, Bogdan Prokopczyk, Dietrich Hoffmann, Jagadeesan Nair, Hiroshi Ohshima, and Helmut Bartsch   197

The Formation of DNA-Protein Cross-links by Aldehydes Present in Tobacco Smoke / Henry d'A. Heck, Mercedes Casanova, Chiu-Wing Lam, and James A. Swenberg   215

SESSION 3: BIOCHEMICAL, CELLULAR, AND MOLECULAR STUDIES ON HUMAN TISSUES AND CELLS

Differences in Metabolism and Biological Effects of NNK in Human Target Cells / Ismail Parsa, Clarence A. Foye, Cathleen M. Cleary, and Dietrich Hoffmann   233

Recent Studies on the Metabolic Activation of Tobacco-specific Nitrosamines: Prospects for Dosimetry in Humans / Stephen S. Hecht, Peter G. Foiles, Steven G. Carmella, Neil Trushin, Abraham Rivenson, and Dietrich Hoffmann   245

Metabolism of Polycyclic Aromatic Hydrocarbons in Human Target Tissues / Herman Autrup   259

Pathobiological Effects of Tobacco Smoke-related Aldehydes in Cultured Human Bronchial Epithelial Cells / Roland C. Grafstrom, James C. Willey, Kristina Sundqvist, and Curtis C. Harris   273

Factors Affecting O^6-Alkylguanine-DNA-alkyltransferase Activity / Anthony E. Pegg   287

In Vitro Carcinogenesis Studies of Human Bronchial Epithelial Cells / Tohru Masui, George H. Yoakum, John F. Lechner, James C. Willey, Paul Amstad, Benjamin F. Trump, and Curtis C. Harris   299

Factors Involved in the Induction of Urinary Bladder Cancer by
   Aromatic Amines / Frederick A. Beland and Fred F. Kadlubar   315

SESSION 4: NEW ASSOCIATIONS OF TOBACCO USE AND CANCER
   RISK

Cigarette Smoking and Cancer of the Uterine Cervix / Warren
   Winkelstein, Jr.   329

The Passive Smoking-Cancer Controversy / Pelayo Correa   343

Smokeless Tobacco and Oral/Pharynx Cancer: The Role of Cofactors /
   Deborah M. Winn   361

Interactions between Smoking and Other Exposures: Occupation and
   Diet / Steven D. Stellman   377

Concluding Remarks / Curtis C. Harris and Dietrich Hoffmann   397

Name Index   403

Subject Index   417

Session 1: Laboratory-Epidemiology Studies

Uptake of Tobacco Smoke Components

NANCY JEAN HALEY, DIETRICH HOFFMANN, AND ERNST L. WYNDER
Naylor Dana Institute for Disease Prevention
American Health Foundation
Valhalla, New York 10595

OVERVIEW

Exposure to tobacco smoke constituents can occur through the active intake of mainstream smoke, the passive intake of sidestream smoke, or the transfer of tobacco smoke constituents by the maternal bloodstream to a developing fetus. Exposure can be evaluated by physiological or biochemical means as well as self-reported daily consumption of tobacco products in active smokers. The actual uptake and body burden of tobacco components can, however, only be quantitated by direct measurements of the constituents or metabolites. Since tobacco smoke is such a complex mixture of gases and particulate matter, a variety of biochemical measures have been developed to assess the uptake of individual constituents.

Nicotine is specific for tobacco and although limited by a short biological half-life, measurement of its major metabolite, cotinine, has proven useful in appraising active and passive uptake as well as transplacental exposure to tobacco smoke constituents.

INTRODUCTION

Smoke uptake during cigarette use has been assessed by a variety of procedures based on the amount of smoke or smoke constituent presented to an individual's mouth, a physiologic change in response to smoking, or the quantification of a smoke component or metabolite present in blood, urine, saliva or exhaled air (Hopkins et al. 1984). Although cigarette smoke is a complex mixture of chemicals (Hoffmann et al. 1983a), only a few components exhibit the selectivity to be associated with only tobacco or are present in biological samples in concentrations measurable by current methodologies. The most common laboratory measures of tobacco smoke absorption include quantitation of thiocyanate or nicotine, and its metabolite, cotinine, in plasma, urine, or saliva (Haley et al. 1983; Hill et al. 1983), as well as carboxyhemoglobin in blood or carbon monoxide in expired air (Wald et al. 1981). Each measure has its particular usefulness as well as its limitations in assessing uptake and absorption of tobacco smoke.

Physiological responses to smoking have also been utilized to estimate the absorption of tobacco smoke (Ashton et al. 1981), but such responses are quite varied from individual to individual and generally must be measured during the actual smoking period. Some of the physiological effects of smoking that have been used to indicate uptake of smoke include a rise in blood pressure and heart rate, a fall in fingertip temperature, toe temperature, and foot blood flow (Ashton et al. 1981). These changes are mainly due to nicotine and occur with a concomitant rise in catecholamine levels (Hill and Wynder 1974). As the major active alkaloid in tobacco smoke, nicotine has been the subject of research studies to determine the mode of action of cigarette smoking on neuropharmacological responses (Benowitz et al. 1982). As a marker of chronic tobacco smoke uptake, however, its usefulness is limited by a short biological half-life (Isaac and Rand 1972). The measurement of cotinine in body fluids provides much more information on the chronic uptake of nicotine and habitual smoking patterns (Hill and Marquardt 1980; Haley et al. 1983); Sepkovic and Haley 1985). Concommitant measures of thiocyanate in body fluids implicate smoking as the mode of nicotine administration, rather than such behaviors as the chewing of tobacco (Palladino et al. 1985).

Exposure to sidestream smoke through passive smoking (Greenberg et al. 1984; Hoffmann et al. 1984), as well as the transfer of tobacco smoke constituents by the maternal bloodstream to the developing fetus (Etzel et al. 1985), can also be evaluated biochemically by the measurement of specific tobacco-related compounds such as nicotine and cotinine. The routes of uptake and the relative absorption of tobacco smoke constituents by active, passive, or secondary exposures can provide indicators of dosage.

RESULTS

Validation of Self-reported Smoking Behavior

Smoking control research has previously relied upon self-report for information concerning smoking status, but the validity of this measure is severely limited as use of tobacco becomes perceived with less public favor. Denial and minimizing the extent of smoking are common practices among youth and announced quitters (Gillies et al. 1982). Biochemical validation presents a more objective alternative to questionnaire data. Plasma and saliva thiocyanate as well as blood carboxyhemoglobin can successfully differentiate smokers from nonsmokers when daily consumption is at least 4-5 cigarettes. However, more sensitive measures are required to validate cigarette use by adolescents or light smokers. Saliva and plasma levels of cotinine have been evaluated for their ability to detect smoking behavior by adolescents. Figure 1 presents the results of one such experiment in which cotinine and thiocyanate were measured in body fluids of adolescents to validate smoking status. Cotinine is quantitated in our laboratory by radioimmunoassay (Langone et al. 1973) and thiocyanate by the method described by Butts et al. (1974). In both plasma and saliva, cotinine analyses could distinguish between smokers and nonsmokers with a high degree of accuracy, whereas thiocyanate determinations provide a less clean-cut answer. Thiocyanate levels in physiological fluids are in-

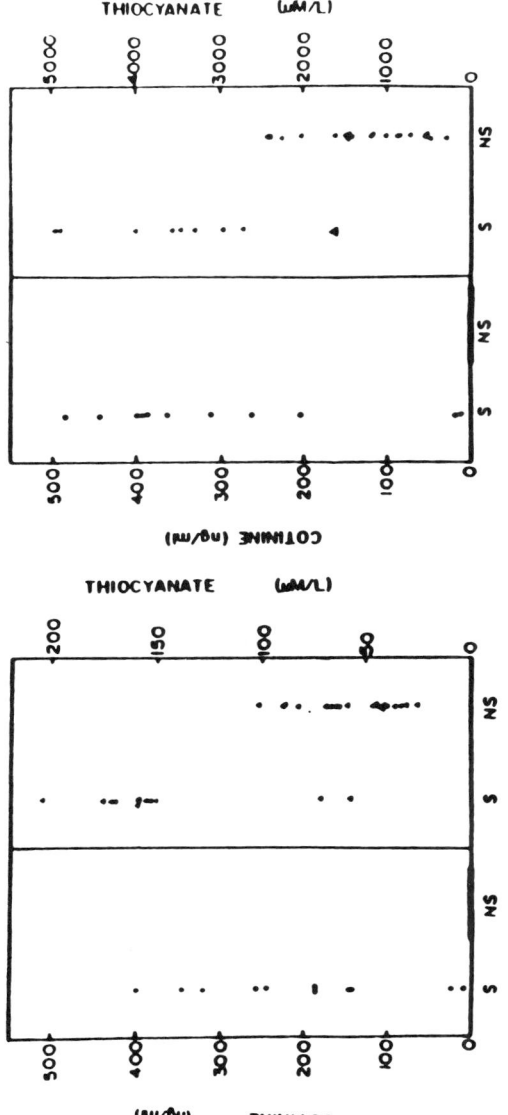

Figure 1
Distribution of cotinine and thiocyanate in the plasma (*left*) and in the saliva (*right*) of smokers and nonsmokers. (*S*) Smokers; (*NS*) nonsmokers. Cotinine was not detected in the plasma or saliva of any of the nonsmokers.

fluenced by the dietary intake of a variety of vegetables and consumption of beer. Cotinine in plasma and saliva is highly correlated (0.90) while the correlation for thiocyanate in these body fluids is less than 0.40.

Recently, we have evaluated the utility of hair samples to validate smoking behavior by measurements of nicotine and cotinine (Haley and Hoffmann 1985). Nicotine was found on the exterior of the hair shaft in both active and passive smokers whereas cotinine, the hepatic metabolite, was found only within the hair shaft of smokers.

Measurement of cotinine in body fluids is now being widely used to measure active smoking behavior. However, the increasing use of oral snuff or chewing tobacco limits the utility of this nicotine-specific measure. The presence of high levels of cotinine in the saliva, urine, or plasma of adolescents ($>$ 200 ng/ml) suggests the use of smokeless tobacco since to achieve such levels with cigarettes, the smoker would typically use at least 15 cigarettes each day and inhale the smoke. Such smoking behavior would result in greatly elevated thiocyanate levels from the inhalation of gas phase of tobacco smoke. High cotinine in the presence of low thiocyanate, therefore, is associated with the use of chewing tobacco or oral snuff (Palladino et al. 1985).

Cigarette Smoking Behavior: Compensation and Nicotine Tolerance

It is generally believed that cigarette smoking and tobacco use revolve around the stimulation received from nicotine and in heavily habituated smokers, the lack of withdrawal symptoms imposed by smoking cessation. The desire by smokers to regulate nicotine levels in the circulation has been shown by several investigators (Russell 1978; Schachter 1978; Moss and Prue 1982) with compensation for changes in nicotine availability emerging as a recognized phenomenon (Sepkovic et al. 1983). The consumption of low yield (i.e., low tar, low nicotine) cigarettes has increased in the United States in the 1970s and early 1980s, due primarily to changes in product marketing and an increased public perception that low yield products mean less hazardous products (Folsom et al. 1984). Considerable evidence has been gathered that smokers compensate for reduced nicotine yield when they switch to low tar/low nicotine cigarettes (Moss and Prue 1982). They appear to self-titrate nicotine by a variety of mechanisms including increasing cigarettes smoked per day or by changing the topographical parameters of smoking behavior, such as depth of inhalation or puff frequency in order to compensate for the lower nicotine yield per cigarette (Russell 1978; Sepkovic et al. 1983, 1984; Haley et al. 1985).

These changes result in greater nicotine delivery per cigarette than is generated by machine smoking under standard conditions (Pillsbury and Bright 1969). It is important to recognize that more intense smoking results not only in higher nicotine yield, but produces higher absorption of carbon monoxide and of the carcinogenic smoke factors including tar and tobacco-specific N-nitrosamines (Hoffmann et al. 1983b).

In a cross-sectional study of cigarette smokers, Hill and coworkers showed that plasma nicotine and cotinine increased with increasing daily consumption of cigarettes (Figure 2). When they were separated into groups of users smoking cigarettes containing more or less than 1 mg nicotine, no differences between the groups were noted in the absorption of carbon monoxide or level of plasma thiocyanate.

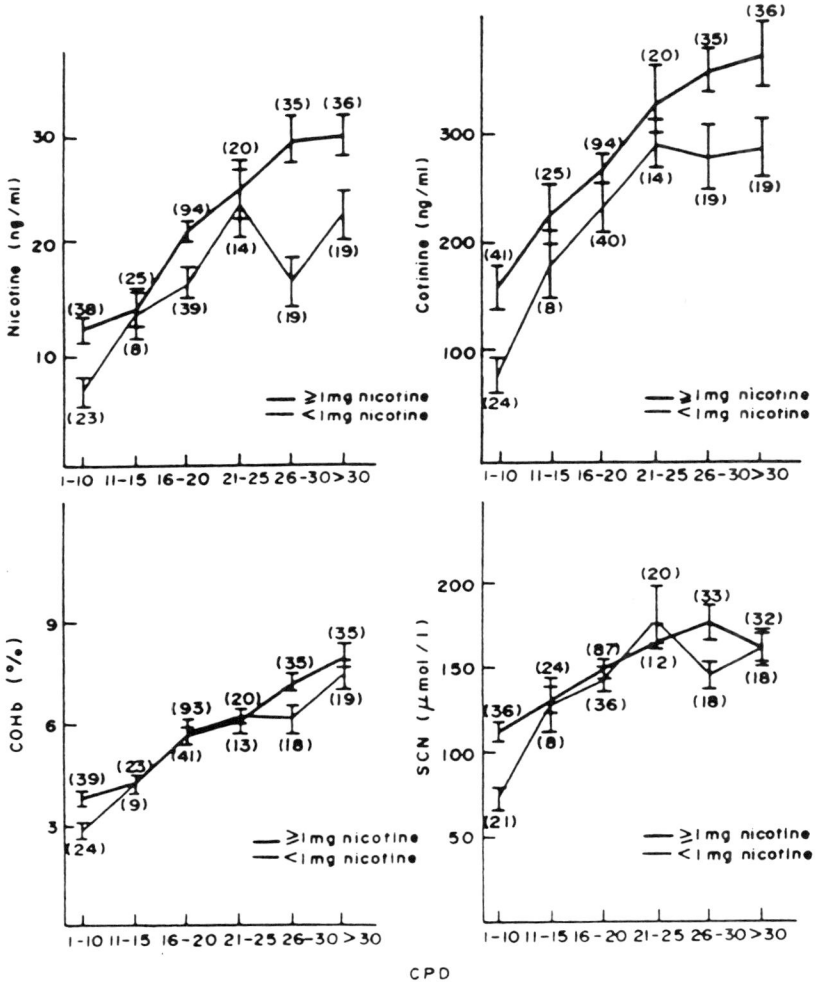

Figure 2
Plasma parameters of cigarette smoke absorption as a function of daily consumption of cigarettes. The average nicotine yield of cigarettes > 1 mg nicotine was 1.28 mg (n = 245); the average yield of cigarettes < 1 mg nicotine was 0.66 mg (n = 125).

Smoker compensation mechanisms may explain the failure of low yield products to result in the reduction of coronary heart disease in men (Aronow 1981) although introduction of filter cigarettes has assisted in reducing the delivery of carcinogenic compounds to levels far below those in nonfiltered products.

Compensation for nicotine can be complete or incomplete depending on the magnitude of reduction in the effective yield of nicotine (Sepkovic et al. 1984). Because complete compensation is not possible when nicotine availability is greatly reduced, attempts to compensate may be more forceful resulting in a greater body burden of gas phase constituents since the latter are not received to the same extent as nicotine according to machine smoking data. Figure 3 compares smokers who received increased or decreased nicotine-containing cigarettes over a period of 8 weeks. Individuals receiving increases in nicotine delivery reached higher levels of plasma cotinine and did not alter smoking behavior as evidenced by cigarettes used per day or inhalation patterns (COHb and SCN). In those smokers receiving reduced nicotine delivery, plasma cotinine dropped with nicotine availability despite increases in cigarettes per day or increased inhalation of gas phase constituents. When these subjects returned to their customary brand, blood levels of cigarette smoke metabolites increased dramatically as the smokers inhaled with their newly acquired smoking patterns.

In other studies where nicotine content was held constant and filter construction varied (Hoffmann et al. 1983b) (Table 1), smokers absorbed increased nicotine relative to carbon monoxide and maintained elevated cotinine levels during use of products with longitudinal air channel filters. Thus, even cigarettes with the same reported yield can present varying amounts of tobacco constituents to the consumer.

Passive Smoking

There has been increasing concern in recent years that nonsmokers exposed to the sidestream smoke of active smokers might be at increased risk for development of respiratory disease and certain cancers (Hirayama 1981; Correa et al. 1983; Garfinkel and Auerbach 1985). The association with cancer risk has not been demonstrated in a dose-response fashion for all tobacco-related cancers (Kabat and Wynder 1984; Koo et al. 1985). However, weak associations have also been reported for passive smoke exposure and childhood brain tumors in the offspring of women passively exposed to environmental tobacco smoke during pregnancy (Preston-Martin et al. 1982).

Quantitative estimates of the risks associated with passive smoking can be attempted after confirmation of actual uptake and absorption of sidestream smoke by exposed nonsmokers. To begin such investigations, we have conducted chamber studies in which nonsmoking volunteers have been exposed to measured doses of sidestream smoke (Hoffmann et al. 1984). The development of sensitive biochemical methodologies enables us to obtain more definitive measurements of exposure

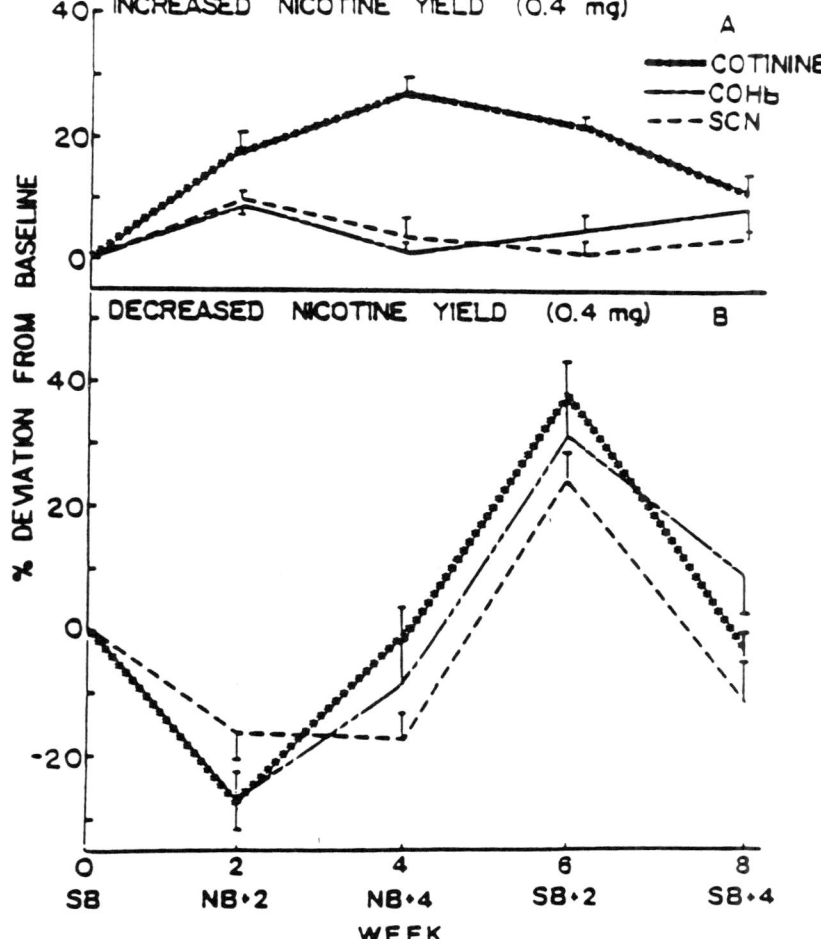

Figure 3
Plasma cotinine, thiocyanate (−*SCN*) and blood carboxyhemoglobin (*COHb*) in smokers who have shifted from their standard brands to either higher nicotine yield cigarettes (*A*) or lower nicotine yield cigarettes (*B*) and then returned to their standard brands. Each point represents the mean ± the standard error of the mean. (*SB*) Standard brand; (*NB*) new brand.

Table 1
Biochemical Measurements of Cigarette Smoke Constituent Absorption

	Perforated filter		Longitudinal air channel filter	
Cigarettes per day	24.5 ± 1.2		21.7 ± 1.3	
Plasma cotinine (ng/ml)	151 ± 17		256 ± 27	
	Baseline	+ 1 Min[a]	Baseline	+ 1 min[a]
First cigarette				
Plasma nicotine (ng/ml)	0.35 ± 0.25	2.6 ± 0.8	0.40 ± 0.20	21.2 ± 6.1
COHb (%)	2.5 ± 0.3	2.9 ± 0.4	1.4 ± 0.3	1.8 ± 0.1
After 2 weeks				
Plasma nicotine (ng/ml)	1.0 ± 0.3	7.6 ± 1.8	1.0 ± 0.3	27.1 ± 7.9
COHb (%)	2.6 ± 0.2	3.3 ± 0.3	2.8 ± 0.3	3.4 ± 0.2

[a] + 1 min samples were drawn 1 min after completion of the cigarette and generally reflect the point of maximum nicotine absorption.

to tobacco smoke by determining the uptake of specific components into body fluids and to calculate the risk factors relative to those inherent in active smoke exposure.

Table 2 shows the average values of markers for exposure in saliva, urine, and plasma of nonsmoking volunteers who spent 80 minutes in a room polluted with the sidestream smoke of 2, 3, or 4 concurrently machine-smoked cigarettes. Biological fluids were collected before and during exposure as well as for 5 hours following exposure.

The most salient points of these studies can be summarized as follows: Neither thiocyanate in saliva, serum, or urine, nor carboxyhemoglobin in blood was significantly elevated. The nicotine levels in saliva increased significantly (maxima of 430, 840, and 880 ng/ml) after 60 minutes of exposure to the three levels of pollution. After the volunteers left the room, salivary nicotine levels decreased rapidly and cotinine rose up to 5 ng/ml during the next 2-hour period. Nicotine in blood did not increase during or after exposure. The most significant results for indicators of tobacco-specific uptake were found in the urine analysis. A dose-response relationship for nicotine uptake was indicated within 2 hours and for cotinine within 2–4 hours after exposure. Table 2 presents these data which could be derived only from controlled research studies where free-living exposures to tobacco smoke were virtually eliminated.

Currently, we are investigating the exposures to and absorption of sidestream smoke in free-living populations, including neonates and infants. These studies are being carried out in collaboration with the Department of Community Pediatrics

Table 2
Nicotine and Cotinine Levels in Saliva, Serum, and Urine of Volunteers[a] (Summary of Average Values)

Time[b] (min)	Saliva (ng/ml)						Serum (ng/ml)				Urine (ng/mg creatinine)					
	Nicotine			Cotinine				Cotinine			Nicotine			Cotinine		
	2[a]	3[a]	4[a]		2[a]	3[a]	4[a]		2[a]	3[a]	4[a]	2[a]	3[a]	4[a]	2[a]	3[a]	4[a]
Baseline	8	1	3														
I 40	350	719	830		1.0	1.1			0.9								
I 60	430	830	880		2.1	1.7			0.9								
O 30	76	157	148						1.2								
O 120	6	17	23		2.5				1.8			24	20	17	14	14	14
O 240	8	2	3		2.0				2.9			26	34	84	16	21	28
O 300	7	7	7		3.5				3.3			40	94	100	21	34	46
									3.4			51	58	48	21	38	55

[a] Numbers represent room pollution by smoke of 2, 3, or 4 cigarettes.
[b] I = Inside exposure room during pollution; O = outside exposure room after leaving the room

at the University of North Carolina, Chapel Hill. In the initial study, saliva and urine were collected from infants whose homes had at least one cigarette smoker and controls whose parents reported no exposure. The findings of the study are summarized in Table 3 with the dose-response relationship between maternal smoking and urinary cotinine levels illustrated in Figure 4.

These studies suggest that biochemical measurements provide good indicators of passive smoking among young children and infants. The noninvasive methodology for evaluating urinary cotinine is especially applicable to very young children.

Studies in adults propose that the majority of nonsmokers in the United Kingdom may have measurable amounts of tobacco-specific compounds circulating in their blood (Jarvis et al. 1984). The results of these studies showed increasing saliva-nicotine concentrations with increasing self-reported exposure, and body fluid cotinine levels which were about 1% of those noted for active smokers. This work did not, however, use creatinine clearance data. A similar study in Japan that measured urine cotinine/mg creatinine reported much higher levels relative to the numbers of cigarettes smoked near nonsmokers (Matsukura et al. 1984) and suggested that exposure to environmental tobacco smoke may result in significant levels of uptake of tobacco constituents. Even this study, however, reports quantitation of nicotine metabolites in body fluids at levels far below those found in active smokers.

Table 3
Urinary and Salivary Concentrations of Nicotine and Cotinine in Infants Exposed and Not Exposed to Tobacco Smoke

Exposure (parental report)	Urine[a]		Saliva[b]	
	Nicotine:Creatinine (ng/mg)	Cotinine:Creatinine (ng/mg)	Nicotine (ng/ml)	Cotinine (ng/ml)
Not exposed				
Median	0	4	0	0
Range	0–59	0–125	0–17.6	0–3
	(n = 18)	(n = 18)	(n = 13)	(n = 13)
Exposed				
Median	53	351	12.7	9
Range	0–370	41–1885	0–166	0–25
	(n = 28)	(n = 28)	(n = 29)	(n = 27)
Significance of difference	$P < 0.0001$	$P < 0.0001$	$P = 0.0003$	$P < 0.0001$

[a] To convert values for nicotine:creatinine and cotinine:creatinine to nmoles per mmole, multiple by 0.698 and 0.642, respectively.
[b] To convert values for nicotine and cotinine to nmoles per liter, multiply by 6.173 and 5.682, respectively.

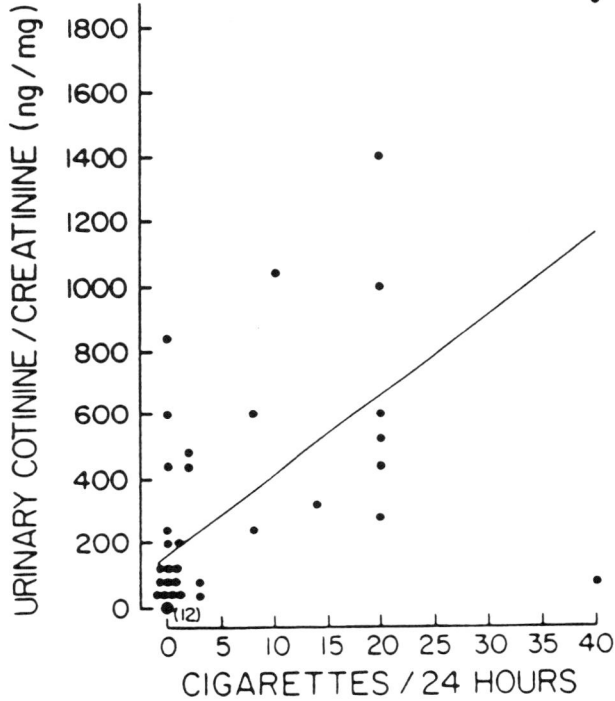

Figure 4
Relation between the number of cigarettes smoked by mothers in the previous 24 hrs and the urinary concentrations of cotinine in their infants (r = 0.67; P = 0.0001; n = 44).

Transplacental Exposure and Fetal Uptake

Maternal smoking is a hazard to the fetus. Babies born to women who smoke during pregnancy weigh about 200 g less than babies born to nonsmoking mothers and have an increased risk of perinatal death, abruptio placenta, and placenta previa (Abel 1980). Little is known, however, about the dose-response relationship between uptake of tobacco smoke constituents and transfer to the developing fetus. Lower respiratory illnesses are more numerous during the first 3 years of life in children of smokers (Fergusson et al. 1981), but the relative importance of smoke exposure before or after birth remains to be evaluated.

In a study of infants born at Memorial Hospital in Chapel Hill, North Carolina, Etzel and colleagues collected urine samples during the first day of life from infants of smoking and nonsmoking mothers. Additional urine samples were collected from the infants of smoking mothers approximately every 12 hours for the first 6 days of life (Etzel et al. 1985). All infants were isolated from exposure to tobacco smoke after birth and were not breast-fed to avoid contamination by the active or passive exposure of the mother to tobacco smoke.

Figure 5 illustrates the cotinine : creatinine ratios found in the urine of exposed and nonexposed babies. Urine cotinine excretion was significantly greater in neonates of smoking mothers. However, among neonates of smokers, there was no clear relationship between newborn urine cotinine : creatinine ratio and maternal cigarette consumption during the 24 hours before delivery ($r = 0.46$). Numerous factors including gestational age, birth weight, and changes in maternal smoking habits during labor and delivery could explain this lack of accord.

The elimination of cotinine from the urine of newborn infants appeared to follow exponential kinetics. The average half-elimination time was 68 hours. This is

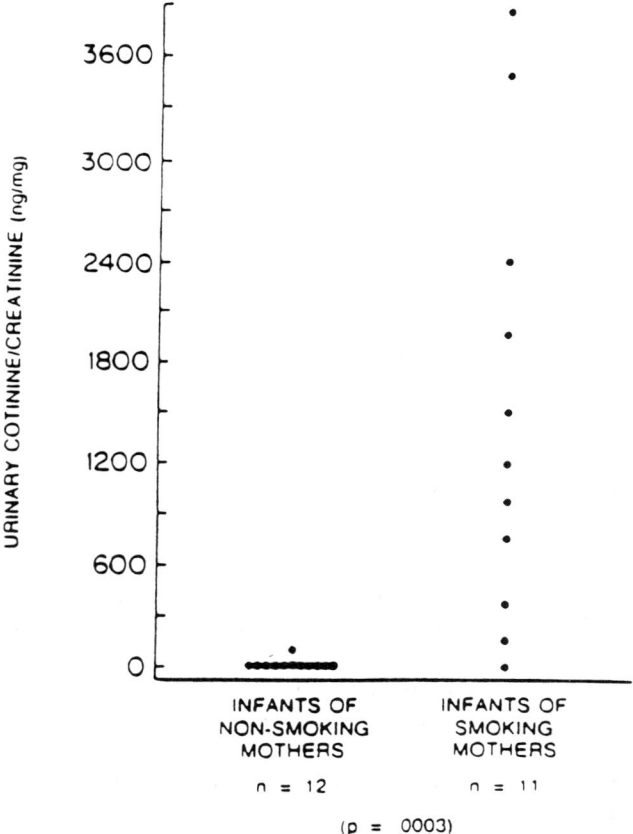

Figure 5
Urinary concentrations of cotinine during first day of life in neonates of smoking and non-smoking mothers. P = 0.0003.

markedly different from that of adults (Table 4). Active smokers have a median $t\ 1/2$ for cotinine elimination of 18 hours and the same parameter has been shown to be 32 hours in individuals passively exposed under controlled conditions (N. Haley and D. Sepkovic, in prep.).

The use of urine cotinine excretion as a measure of in utero exposure to tobacco smoke products should enable us to study more accurately the effects of such exposure during the perinatal period. The long elimination time of cotinine in infants is surprising, and further studies of nicotine metabolism in neonates are being conducted.

DISCUSSION

The uptake and absorption of tobacco smoke constituents can be evaluated by several techniques, both biochemical and physiological. Questionnaire data are becoming restricted in value as the popularity of cigarette smoking declines and public awareness of the health risks of smoking increase. Actual validation of exposure is becoming more necessary than it was in previous years before low yield cigarettes were introduced and concern with sidestream smoke exposure became a public health issue.

The actual uptake of cigarette smoke by smokers can be quantitated by biochemical measures that are sensitive, selective, and responsive to changes in smoking behavior. The quantitation of cotinine, the major metabolite of nicotine, has proven quite useful in validating smoking behavior, especially in adolescents and announced quitters where daily use might be low and in investigating mechanisms of smoker compensation. The Federal Trade Commission's reported tar and nicotine yields provide a guideline for nicotine availability; however, the ability of smokers to obtain levels of nicotine and other smoke constituents varies considerably from smoking machine estimates.

Biochemical markers of smoke intake, such as cotinine in urine, are sufficiently sensitive and specific to identify passive smokers. Those individuals who have been

Table 4

Cotinine Elimination Time in the Plasma and Urine of Smokers and Passively Exposed Nonsmokers

	Plasma (hr)	Urine (hr)
Smokers	18.5 (15.6–27.8)	21.86 (12.6–31.0)
Nonsmokers	49.7 (45–60)	32.7 (23.9–42.6)
Neonates	—	68 (37–160)

evaluated under controlled conditions and in free-living situations generally have cotinine levels between 0.1% and 2% of those observed in cigarette smokers. The precise quantitative relationship between the measured levels of these markers and the intake of carcinogenic compounds in tobacco smoke is not known.

Nicotine is generally regarded as a tobacco-specific compound, and quantitation of this alkaloid and its metabolites provides reliable measures of uptake of the particulate phase of tobacco smoke. With the increasing use of smokeless tobacco, however, measurements of gas phase constituents, such as carbon monoxide or thiocyanate, or the detoxification product of hydrogen cyanide, confirm the source of elevated body levels of nicotine metabolites.

Current research in our laboratory is exploring the fuller spectrum of nicotine metabolites including nicotine-N'-oxides and nicotine dioxides. These compounds can back-convert to the parent alkaloid or be easily nitrosated during circulation. The relative detoxification pathways are important in determining the risk for tobacco-related diseases.

Such work is also important to the issue of passive smoking. Uptake of environmental tobacco smoke by children is an area of concern and active research. Our findings on the relatively long elimination time of cotinine by neonates is now being extended to infants and older children to allow investigations of relative susceptibility to childhood disease versus detoxification and elimination rates. Such work can later be applied to both active and passive smokers.

ACKNOWLEDGMENTS

These studies were supported in part by CA-32617 and CA-29580.

REFERENCES

Abel, E.L. 1980. Smoking during pregnancy: A review of effects on growth and development of offspring. *Hum. Biol.* **52**: 593.

Aronow, W.S.A. 1981. Effect of cigarette smoking and of carbon monoxide on coronary heart disease. In *Smoking and arterial disease* (ed. R.M. Greenhalgh). Pitman Biomedical, Bath, England.

Ashton, H., T. Stepney, R. Telford, and J.W. Thompson. 1981. Cardiovascular and behavioral responses to smoking. In *Smoking and arterial disease* (ed. R.M. Greenhalgh), p. 258. Pitman Medical Press, London.

Benowitz, N.L., P. Jacob, R.T. Jones, and J. Rosenberg. 1982. Interindividual variability in the metabolism and cardiovascular effects of nicotine in man. *J. Pharmacol. Exp. Ther.* **221**: 368.

Butts, W.C., M. Kuehneman, and G.M. Widdowson. 1974. Automated method for determining serum thiocyanate to distinguish smokers from non-smokers. *Clin. Chem.* **20**: 1344.

Correa, P., L.W. Pickle, E. Fontham, Y. Lin, and W. Haenzel. 1983. Passive smoking and lung cancer. *Lancet* **2**: 595.

Etzel, R.A., R.A. Greenberg, N.J. Haley, and F.A. Loda. 1985. Urinary cotinine excretion in neonates exposed to tobacco smoke products *in utero*. *J. Pediatr.* **107**: 146.

Fergusson, D.M., L.J. Horwood, F.T. Shannon, and B. Taylor. 1981. Parental smoking and lower respiratory illness in the first three years of life. *J. Epidemiol. Community Health* **35**: 180.

Folsom, A.R., T. Pechacek, R. DeGaudemaris, R. Luepker, D. Jacobs, and R. Gillum. 1984. Consumption of low yield cigarettes: Its frequency and relationship to serum thiocyanate. *Am. J. Public Health* **74**: 564.

Garfinkel, L., O. Auerbach, L. Joubert. 1985. Involuntary smoking and lung cancer: A case control study. *J. Natl. Cancer Inst.* **75(3)**: 463.

Gillies, P.A., B. Wilcox, C. Coates, F. Kristmundsdotir, and D.J. Reid. 1982. Use of objective measurement in the validation of self-reported smoking in children aged 10 and 11 years: Saliva thiocyanate. *J. Epidemiol. Community Health* **36**: 205.

Greenberg, R.A., N.J. Haley, R.A. Etzel, and F.A. Loda. 1984. Nicotine and cotinine in urine and saliva. *New Engl. J. Med.* **310**: 1075.

Haley, N.J. and D. Hoffmann. 1985. Analysis for nicotine and cotinine in hair to determine cigarette smoker status. *Clin. Chem.* **31**: 1598.

Haley, N.J., C.M. Axelrad, and K.A. Tilton. 1983. Validation of self-reported smoking behavior: Biochemical analyses of cotinine and thiocyanate. *Am. J. Public Health* **73**: 1204.

Haley, N.J., D.W. Sepkovic, D. Hoffmann, and E.L. Wynder. 1985. Cigarette smoking as a risk for cardiovascular disease VI. Compensation with nicotine availability as a single variable. *Clin. Pharmacol. Ther.* **38**: 168.

Hill, P. and E.L. Wynder. 1974. Smoking and cardiovascular disease. Effect of nicotine on serum epinephrine and corticoids. *Am. Heart J.* **87**: 491.

Hill, P. and H. Marquardt. 1980. Plasma and urine changes after smoking different brands of cigarettes. *Clin. Pharmacol. Ther.* **27**: 652.

Hill, P., N.J. Haley, and E.L. Wynder. 1983. Cigarette smoking as a risk for cardiovascular disease I. Biochemical analyses of carboxyhemoglobin, plasma nicotine, cotinine and thiocyanate versus self-reported smoking data. *J. Chronic Dis.* **36**: 439.

Hirayama, T. 1981. Non-smoking wives of heavy smokers have a higher risk for lung cancer: A study from Japan. *Br. Med. J.* **282**: 183.

Hoffmann, D., N.J. Haley, K.D. Brunnemann, J.D. Adams, and E.L. Wynder. 1983a. Cigarette sidestream smoke: Formation, analyses and model studies on uptake by non-smokers. Paper presented at the U.S.-Japan meeting on *New Etiology of Lung Cancer*, p. 13, Hawaii, March 21–23.

Hoffmann, D., S.S. Hecht, N.J. Haley, K.D. Brunnemann, J.D. Adams, and E.L. Wynder. 1983b. Tobacco carcinogenesis: Metabolic studies in humans. In *Human carcinogenesis* (ed. H. Astrup). Academic Press, New York.

Hoffmann, D., J.D. Adams, and N.J. Haley. 1983c. Reported cigarette smoke values: A closer look. *Am. J. Public Health* **73**: 105.

Hoffmann, D., N.J. Haley, J.D. Adams, and K.D. Brunnemann. 1984. Tobacco sidestream smoke: Uptake by nonsmokers. *Prev. Med.* **13**: 608.

Hopkins, R., L.W. Wood, and N.M. Sinclair. 1984. Evaluation of methods to estimate cigarette smoke uptake. *Clin. Pharmacol. Ther.* **36**: 788.

Isaac, P.F. and M.J. Rand. 1972. Cigarette smoking and plasma levels of nicotine. *Nature* **236**: 308.

Jarvis, M., H. Tunstall-Pedoe, C. Feyerabend, C. Vesey, and Y. Salloojee. 1984. Biochemical markers of smoke absorption and self-reported exposure to passive smoking. *J. Epidemiol. and Community Health* **38**: 335.

Kabat, G.C. and E.L. Wynder. 1984. Lung cancer in non-smokers. *Cancer* **53**: 1214.

Koo, L.C., J.H. Ho, and N. Lee. 1985. An analysis of some risk factors for lung cancer in Hong Kong. *Inst. J. Cancer* **35**: 149.

Langone, J., H.B. Gjika, and H. Van Vunakis. 1973. Nicotine and its metabolites: Radioimmunoassay for nicotine and cotinine. *Biochemistry* **12**: 5015.

Matsukura, S., T. Taminato, N. Kitano, Y. Sieno, H. Hamada, M. Uchikashe, H. Nakajima, and Y. Hirata. 1984. Effects of environmental tobacco smoke on urinary cotinine excretion in non-smokers. *New Engl. J. Med.* **311**: 828.

Moss, R.A. and D.M. Prue. 1982. Research on nicotine regulation. *Behav. Ther.* **13**: 31.

Palladino, G., J.D. Adams, K.D. Brunnemann, N.J. Haley, and D. Hoffmann. 1985. Snuff dipping in college students: A clinical profile. *J. Military Med.* (in press).

Pillsbury, H.C. and C.C. Bright. 1972. Comparison of aliquot and complete sample procedure for the determination of nicotine in cigarette smoke. *J. Assoc. Off. Anal. Chem.* **55**: 636.

Preston-Martin, S., M.C. Yee, B. Benton, and B.E. Henderson. 1982. N-nitroso compounds and childhood brain tumors: A case-control study. *Cancer Res.* **42**: 5240.

Russell, M.A.H. 1978. Self-regulation of nicotine intake by smokers. In *Behavioral effects of nicotine* (ed. K. Batlig). Karger, Basal, Switzerland.

Schachter, S. 1978. Pharmacological and psychological determinants of smoking. *Ann. Intern. Med.* **88**: 104.

Sepkovic, D.W. and N.J. Haley. 1985. Biomedical applications of cotinine concentrations in biological fluids. *Am. J. Public Health* **75**: 663.

Sepkovic, D.W., N.J. Haley, C.M. Axelrad, and E.L. Wynder. 1983. Cigarette smoking as a risk for cardiovascular disease III. Biochemical effects with higher nicotine yield cigarettes. *Addict. Behav.* **8**: 59.

Sepkovic, D.W., K. Parker, C. Axelrad, N.J. Haley, and E.L. Wynder. 1984. Cigarette smoking as a risk for cardiovascular disease V. Biochemical parameters with increased and decreased nicotine content cigarettes. *Addict. Behav.* **9**: 255.

COMMENTS

HARRIS: Are there any biochemical predictors of who will compensate the most in terms of trying to raise their nicotine levels?

HALEY: Those individuals who have a higher cotinine level seem to compensate more completely. This might be important to their daily need for nicotine and relief of withdrawal symptoms. It might also have to do with various metabolic pathways for nicotine detoxification. Cotinine is a terminal metabolite while nicotine N'-oxide can back-convert to the parent compound. Body reservoirs of nicotine-N'-oxide might respond to changes in nicotine intake or demand.

TANNENBAUM: Do you have any idea why cotinine is less precise as an indicator of daily dose above 20 cigarettes per day?

HALEY: Probably because of elimination or differences in metabolic pathways of detoxification in heavy smokers. Urinary pH affects the excretion of nicotine and might play a role in some individuals. We are currently looking at users of smokeless tobacco who have cotinine levels of up to 1.2 μg/ml in their serum to see what daily intake of nicotine can result in these high cotinine levels.

CONNEY: Your data indicate that smokers metabolize cotinine more rapidly than nonsmokers. Do you have data on outlyers who have unexpectedly low or high plasma levels of cotinine? It is possible that people who are ingesting alcoholic beverages or are being treated with phenobarbital, diphenylhydantoin, or other inducing drugs may have unusually low levels of cotinine. What are the effects of genetic factors, dietary factors, and environmental chemicals on the metabolism of cotinine?

HALEY: No, we do not have such data. In this small group of subjects, the ranges were tight. We have enlarged the data base to over 2000 subjects and are finding more outlyers. It would be interesting to look at medications taken by this group. We have not done this yet.

HARRIS: It would also be worthwhile doing a twin study, i.e., looking at monozygic versus dizygic twins.

HALEY: Yes, that would be worthwhile.

Factors Influencing the Urinary Excretion of Nitrosodimethylamine and Nitrosoproline in Human Beings

ALLAN H. CONNEY,* WILLIAM A. GARLAND,† FELIX RUBIO,† HALYNA KORNYCHUK,† EDWARD P. NORKUS,†‡ AND WOLFGANG KUENZIG†
*Roche Institute of Molecular Biology
†The Roche Research Laboratories
Roche Research Center
Nutley, New Jersey 07110

OVERVIEW

Quantification of the amounts of carcinogenic N-nitroso compounds in human beings and studies on factors that influence the concentrations of these chemicals in human beings may help in assessing the risk from these chemicals. This paper describes person-to-person and day-to-day differences in the urinary excretion of nitrosodimethylamine (NDMA) and nitrosoproline (NPRO) in healthy volunteers who were allowed to eat their customary home diets and to pursue their normal life-styles. The effects of vitamins C and E administration, the effects of changes in the atmospheric concentration of NO_2, and the effects of smoking and the ingestion of alcoholic beverages on the urinary excretion of NDMA and NPRO are also described.

INTRODUCTION

The presence of carcinogenic N-nitroso compounds in tobacco smoke and elsewhere in the human environment (Bartsch and Montesano 1984; Hoffmann and Hecht 1985) suggests a need to quantify the concentrations of these chemicals in human blood and urine and to use this information to help in the assessment of human risk. In 1982, we described a gas chromatography-high resolution mass spectrometry assay for quantifying nitrosodimethylamine (NDMA) in plasma (Garland et al. 1982). This method utilized many precautions to prevent the measurement of artifacts. In these earlier studies, we reported that the analysis of five human plasma samples by a commonly used vacuum distillation-gas chromatography-thermal energy assay (TEA method) resulted in finding 448 ± 185 pg of apparent NDMA per ml of plasma, but the analysis of the same plasma samples by the high resolution mass spectrometry method revealed less than 31 pg of NDMA

‡*Present address*: Department of Biomedical Research, Our Lady of Mercy Medical Center, Bronx, New York 10466

per ml of plasma (Garland et al. 1982). In our earlier report with the high resolution-mass spectrometry assay, we indicated that only nine of 128 plasma samples from 64 healthy volunteers had quantifiable concentrations of NDMA.

Because of our desire to quantify the concentrations of NDMA in human beings, we have modified the original high resolution mass spectrometry assay so that it can accurately quantify NDMA in urine samples from normal volunteers, and we have also developed a new high resolution mass spectrometry assay for nitrosoproline (NPRO). Although the assays will be described in detail elsewhere, their main features are summarized in Table 1. Each urine sample was collected in the presence of azide to prevent artifactual postcollection nitrosation and in the presence of morpholine so that we could check for postcollection nitrosation by the measurement of nitrosomorpholine at the end of the project. In these studies, no nitrosomorpholine was found. In addition, a bottle containing water, azide and morpholine was opened by each subject during the voiding of urine, and these environmental water blanks were analyzed side-by-side with the urine samples as a check on environmental contamination and on the possible introduction of artifacts during the work-up of the samples. Only six of the 480 environmental water blanks analyzed had a concentration of apparent NDMA greater than 5 pg per ml, which is the limit of quantitation of the assay. This paper describes the urinary excretion of NDMA and NPRO by 24 healthy volunteers who were allowed to eat their customary home diets and to pursue their normal life-styles. We have assessed day-to-day and person-to-person variations in the urinary excretion of NDMA and NPRO by these subjects, and we have also studied the effects of administration of vitamins C and E and of smoking and alcohol ingestion on the urinary excretion of NDMA and NPRO by these subjects.

Table 1
Assays for Urinary Nitrosamines

Parameter	Nitrosamine measured	
	NDMA	NPRO
Internal standard	$[^{15}N_2]$-NDMA	$[^2H_7]$-NPRO
Volume analyzed	20 ml	2 ml
Extraction pH	pH 10	pH 2
Extraction solvent	Methylene dichloride	Ethyl acetate
Derivative	—	Pentafluorobenzyl
"Clean-up"	Preextraction with hexane	TLC of derivative on silica
Gas chromatography	10% SP-1000 packed column	DB-1701 capillary column
Ionization	Positive CI (isobutane)	Negative CI (methane)
Mass spectrometry	m/z 75.0558 and 77.0499	m/z 143.0457 and 150.0896
Calibration standards	0, 10, 20, 40, and 80 pg/ml	0, 1, 5, 10, and 20 ng/ml
Limit of quantitation	5 pg/ml	0.14 ng/ml

RESULTS

Urine samples (complete 24-hour collections) were obtained from 24 normal volunteers from Roche four times a week for 5 weeks. The subjects did not take supplemental vitamins before the start of the study or during weeks 1 and 2 of the study, but they were given 600 mg of vitamin C (ascorbic acid) and 100 international units (iu) of vitamin E (d,1-alpha-tocopherol) four times daily during weeks 3, 4, and 5 of the study. Administration of vitamins C and E did not influence the urinary excretion of NDMA or NPRO (Table 2). Three of the subjects described in Table 2 were smokers, and when the data from these subjects were analyzed separately, there were still no significant effects of the administration of vitamins C and E on the urinary excretion of NDMA or NPRO (Table 3).

Considerable interindividual differences occurred for the urinary excretion of NPRO and somewhat smaller interindividual differences were found for the urinary excretion of NDMA during the 5-week study (Fig. 1). The mean urinary excretion of NPRO (20 measurements for each subject) varied from 0.76 ± 0.63 µg/day for subject number 2 to 9.04 ± 7.41 µg/day for subject number 14. The mean urinary excretion of NDMA varied from 22.4 ± 10.9 ng/day for subject 21 to 75.4 ± 35.0 ng/day for subject 16. Day-to-day variations for each subject during the course of the 20 measurements were considerable as indicated by the SD bars in Figure 1. Day-to-day variations for the urinary excretion of NPRO for the 24 subjects were somewhat greater than the day-to-day variations for the urinary excretion of NDMA. The mean relative SD for day-to-day variations for the 24 subjects was 84% for NPRO and 51% for NDMA. Examination of the 480 urine samples from the 24 subjects revealed that the urinary excretion of NPRO was not correlated with the urinary excretion of NDMA ($r = 0.05$).

It was of considerable interest that the mean urinary excretion of NDMA for the 24 subjects varied as much as fivefold on the different days of the study whereas the mean urinary excretion of NPRO was much more uniform on the different days (Fig. 2). These observations suggested that our entire population of 24 subjects may have been exposed to an environmental source of NDMA or to precursors of NDMA and that the amount of exposure varied on the different days of the study. The possibility was explored that daily changes in the concentration of atmospheric NO_2 may have influenced the urinary excretion of NDMA. We contacted the Bureau of Air Pollution Control of the New Jersey Department of Environmental Protection, and we were able to obtain records of the concentrations of atmospheric NO_2 in Newark, New Jersey and in East Orange, New Jersey (about 10 miles south of Nutley) for 15 days of the study; this data is presented in Figure 2. Plotting the urinary excretion of NDMA (ng/day) versus the average concentration of NO_2 in the atmosphere (ppm) at the two locations indicated a positive relationship ($r = 0.69$; $P < 0.005$) between the urinary excretion of NDMA and the atmospheric concentration of NO_2.

Table 2
Lack of Effect of Supplemental Vitamins C and E on the Urinary Excretion of NDMA and NPRO in Normal Volunteers

Treatment	Duration (weeks)	No. urine samples analyzed	Urinary excretion of		
			NDMA (ng/day)	NPRO (µg/day)	Vitamin C (mg/day)
Control	2	192	38.4 ± 28.8	3.31 ± 4.06	72 ± 107
Vitamins C and E	3	288	38.1 ± 21.2	3.22 ± 4.00	1644 ± 783

Twenty-four subjects not taking supplemental vitamins ate their customary home diets and provided 24-hour urine samples four times a week for 5 weeks. Vitamin C (600 mg) and vitamin E (100 iu) were administered four times a day during weeks 3, 4, and 5. Means ± SD are indicated.

Table 3
Lack of Effect of Supplemental Vitamins C and E on the Urinary Excretion of NDMA and NPRO in Three Smokers

Subject no.	Treatment	Duration (weeks)	No. urine samples analyzed	NDMA (ng/day)	NPRO (μg/day)	Vitamin C (mg/day)
3	Control	2	8	56 ± 22	2.3 ± 0.9	26 ± 11
	Vitamins C and E	3	12	48 ± 16	3.9 ± 2.3	2031 ± 784
16	Control	2	8	84 ± 45	3.9 ± 1.6	32 ± 8
	Vitamins C and E	3	12	70 ± 27	3.7 ± 2.1	1658 ± 749
19	Control	2	8	65 ± 38	1.7 ± 0.6	25 ± 6
	Vitamins C and E	3	12	71 ± 33	1.0 ± 1.1	1317 ± 854

Three smokers not taking supplemental vitamins ate their customary home diets and gave 24-hour urine samples four times a week for 5 weeks. Vitamin C (600 mg) and vitamin E (100 iu) were administered four times a day during weeks 3, 4, and 5. Means ± SD are indicated.

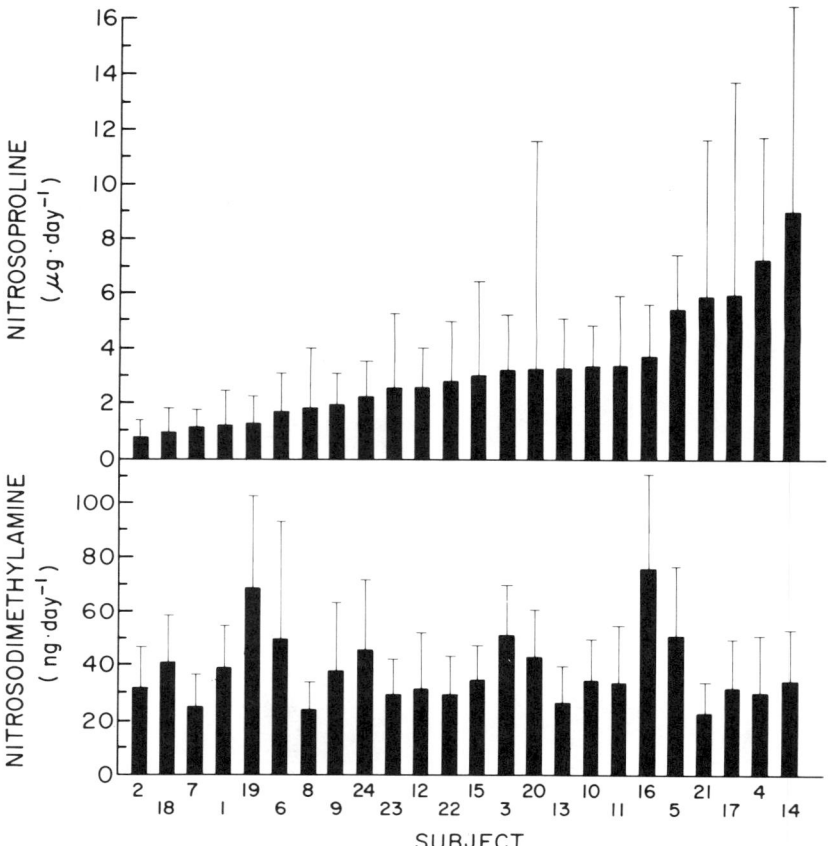

Figure 1
Person-to-person differences in the urinary excretion of nitrosodimethylamine (NDMA) and nitrosoproline (NPRO). Each value is the mean ± SD of 20 measurements with each subject.

Since three of the subjects in our study were smokers and several of the subjects also ingested alcoholic beverages, we evaluated our data to determine whether smoking and/or alcohol ingestion influenced the urinary excretion of NDMA and NPRO. The mean daily urinary excretion of NDMA during the 5-week study was about 100% higher for the three smoking drinkers and about 30% higher for the three nonsmoking drinkers who participated in the study than for the eight control subjects who did not smoke or drink alcoholic beverages (Table 4). The urinary excretion of NPRO by the smoking drinkers was not significantly different from that of the subjects who did not drink or smoke. To obtain further information on the effects of cigarette smoking on the urinary excretion of NDMA, we recruited four

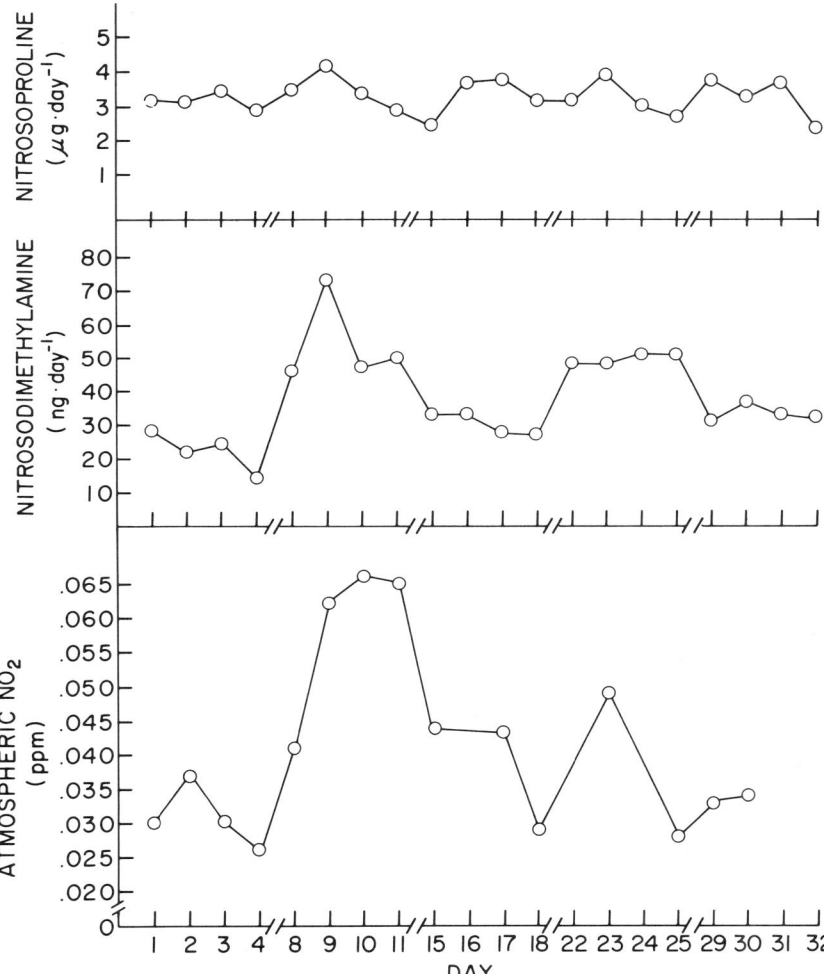

Figure 2
Day-to-day variations in the urinary excretion of nitrosodimethylamine (NDMA) and nitrosoproline (NPRO). Each value for the urinary excretion of N-nitroso compound represents the mean of 24 subjects. The mean atmospheric concentrations of NO_2 on the different days of the study were obtained from the Bureau of Air Pollution Control of the New Jersey Department of Environmental Protection. NO_2 was measured by the standard EPA method described in *Fed. Register 40*: 7049 (1975) as amended in *Fed. Register 41*: 52688 (1976).

Table 4

Urinary Excretion of NDMA in Control Subjects and in Subjects Who Smoked Tobacco and Drank Alcoholic Beverages

Group	No. of subjects	No. of samples	NDMA (ng/day)
Controls	8	160	32.2 ± 21.8
Nonsmoking occasional drinkers	10	200	34.0 ± 19.2
Nonsmoking drinkers	3	60	41.3 ± 21.2[a]
Smoking drinkers	3	60	65.0 ± 31.6[b]

Healthy volunteers gave 24-hour urine samples four times a week for 5 weeks. Control subjects did not smoke or drink alcoholic beverages. Occasional drinkers ingested 0.5–3 alcoholic drinks per week. Drinkers ingested one or more alcoholic beverage each day. Two of the smokers smoked cigarettes and one smoked a pipe. Means ± SD are indicated.

[a] $P < 0.01$ for a comparison with controls (nonsmoking nondrinkers) and $P < 0.02$ for a comparison with occasional drinkers

[b] $P < 0.001$ for a comparison with controls, nonsmoking occasional drinkers, or nonsmoking drinkers

additional cigarette smokers during weeks 3 and 4 of the study, and we compared the urinary excretion of NDMA for the seven smokers and the 21 nonsmokers during the same 2-week interval (eight urine samples during weeks 3 and 4 of the study from each subject). For this comparison, the urinary excretion of NDMA was 46% higher for the smokers than for the nonsmokers (Table 5). It should be noted that three of the nonsmokers were daily drinkers and ten were occasional drinkers of alcohol. In addition, four of the smokers were daily drinkers and the other smokers were occasional drinkers of alcohol. In spite of these considerations, the results of the studies described in Tables 4 and 5 suggest that the daily ingestion of alcoholic beverages as well as smoking is associated with an increased urinary excretion of NDMA in normal volunteers.

Table 5

Urinary Excretion of NDMA in Smokers and Nonsmokers

Group	No. of subjects	No. of samples	Urinary NDMA (ng/day)
Nonsmokers[a]	21	168	36.4 ± 18.6
Smokers[b]	7	56	53.3 ± 26.8[c]

Healthy volunteers gave 24-hour urine samples four times a week for 2 weeks. Six of the smokers smoked cigarettes and one smoked a pipe. Means ± SD are indicated.

[a] Three of the nonsmokers were daily drinkers of alcohol and ten were occasional drinkers.

[b] Four of the smokers were daily drinkers and the other smokers were occasional drinkers.

[c] $P < 0.001$ for nonsmokers versus smokers

DISCUSSION

The results of our studies demonstrated substantial person-to-person and day-to-day differences in the urinary excretion of NDMA and NPRO in normal volunteers who ate their customary home diets and pursued their normal life styles. Although the urinary excretion of endogenous NPRO and the urinary excretion of NPRO after the administration of an exogenous dose of proline and nitrate have been proposed as indices for the formation of carcinogenic N-nitroso compounds in human beings (Bartsch and Montesano 1984), the results of our studies indicate that the urinary excretion of endogenous NPRO is not correlated with the urinary excretion of endogenous NDMA. In addition, although the administration of high doses of vitamins C and E blocks the increased urinary excretion of NPRO that occurs after the administration of high exogenous doses of proline and nitrate (Bartsch and Montesano 1984), the results of the present study indicate that administration of 600 mg of vitamin C and 100 iu of vitamin E four times daily for 3 weeks does not decrease the urinary excretion of endogenous NPRO or NDMA in normal volunteers. Additional studies are needed to determine whether or not the administration of vitamins C and E to individuals who are deficient in vitamins C and E or to individuals who are normally exposed to unusually high levels of precursors of carcinogenic N-nitroso compounds results in a lowering in the amounts of carcinogenic N-nitroso compounds in these individuals.

It was of considerable interest that day-to-day variations in the urinary excretion of NDMA were correlated with day-to-day changes in the atmospheric concentration of NO_2. The results of studies in mice have shown that administration of dimethylamine or other nitrosatable amines followed by exposure of these animals to a high concentration of atmospheric NO_2 resulted in the nitrosation of the amines (Iqbal et al. 1981; Mirvish et al. 1983; Norkus et al. 1984). Additional studies on the possible relationship between atmospheric NO_2 and the urinary excretion of carcinogenic nitrosamines are needed.

The results of the present study suggest that smokers and daily drinkers of alcoholic beverages have a 45-100% increase in the urinary excretion of NDMA. The increased urinary excretion of NDMA may have occurred because of substantial concentrations of both NDMA and nitrosating gases in the tobacco smoke (Hoffmann and Hecht 1985) and because of the inhibitory effect of alcohol on the metabolism of NDMA (Spiegelhalder and Preussmann 1985). The results of earlier studies have indicated that smokers who are given exogenous proline or proline and nitrate excrete larger amounts of NPRO than do nonsmokers who are administered exogenous proline or proline and nitrate (Hoffmann and Brunnemann 1983; Ladd et al. 1984). In one of these studies, smokers and nonsmokers did not differ in their formation of NPRO after a dose of proline, but they did differ when both proline and nitrate were administered (Ladd et al. 1984). The later investigators suggested that elevated levels of thiocyanate in the smokers may have been responsible for the enhanced nitrosation reaction.

SUMMARY

Large person-to-person and day-to-day differences were observed for the urinary excretion of NDMA and NPRO in 24 normal volunteers who were studied on 20 separate occasions. The urinary excretion of NDMA was not correlated with the urinary excretion of NPRO. Administration of 600 mg of vitamin C and 100 iu of vitamin E four times a day for 3 weeks did not influence the urinary excretion of NDMA or NPRO. Day-to-day changes in the urinary excretion of NDMA, but not NPRO, were correlated with changes in the atmospheric concentration of NO_2. Smokers and people who ingested alcoholic beverages daily had an increased urinary excretion of NDMA.

ACKNOWLEDGMENT

We thank Ms. Linda Gregg for her excellent help in the preparation of this manuscript.

REFERENCES

Bartsch, H. and R. Montesano. 1984. Relevance of nitrosamines to human cancer. *Carcinogenesis* **5**: 1381.

Garland, W.A., H. Holowaschenko, W. Kuenzig, E.P. Norkus, and A.H. Conney. 1982. A high resolution mass spectrometry assay for N-nitrosodimethylamine in human plasma. In *Banbury Report 12: Nitrosamines and human cancer* (ed. P.N. Magee), p. 183. Cold Spring Harbor Laboratory, Cold Spring Harbor, New York.

Hoffmann, D. and K.D. Brunnemann. 1983. Endogenous formation of N-nitrosoproline in cigarette smokers. *Cancer Res.* **43**: 5570.

Hoffmann, D. and S.S. Hecht. 1985. Nicotine-derived N-nitrosamines and tobacco-related cancer: Current status and future directions. *Cancer Res.* **45**: 935.

Iqbal, Z.M., K. Dahl, and S.S. Epstein. 1981. Biosynthesis of dimethylnitrosamine in dimethylamine-treated mice after exposure to nitrogen dioxide. *J. Natl. Cancer Inst.* **67**: 137.

Ladd, K.F., H.L. Newmark, and M.C. Archer. 1984. N-nitrosation of proline in smokers and nonsmokers. *J. Natl. Cancer Inst.* **73**: 83.

Mirvish, S.S., J.P. Sams, and P. Issenberg. 1983. The nitrosating agent in mice exposed to nitrogen dioxide: Improved extraction method and localization in the skin. *Cancer Res.* **43**: 2550.

Norkus, E.P., S. Boyle, W. Kuenzig, and W.J. Mergens. 1984. Formation of N-nitrosomorpholine in mice treated with morpholine and exposed to nitrogen dioxide. *Carcinogenesis* **5**: 549.

Spiegelhalder, B. and R. Preussmann. 1985. *In vivo* nitrosation of amidopyrine in humans: Use of "ethanol effect" for biological monitoring of N-nitrosodimethylamine in urine. *Carcinogenesis* **6**: 545.

COMMENTS

CONNEY: The three smokers who drank alcoholic beverages did not have a higher urinary excretion of nitrosoproline than the control subjects who did not drink or smoke.

HOFFMANN: Were they on the same diet or a different one?

CONNEY: All of the subjects were allowed to pursue their normal life styles and to select their own diets and beverages. It would have been interesting to have looked at the blood or urinary levels of dimethylamine, but we did not do this. We did take diet histories from each subject and paid particular attention to the ingestion of fish which may have been a source of dimethylamine. We found no correlation between the intake of fish and the urinary excretion of dimethylnitrosamine. We have not been able to correlate the urinary excretion of dimethylnitrosamine or nitrosoproline with dietary histories.

TANNENBAUM: We have looked at the concentrations of dimethylamine in both blood and gastric juice, as well as saliva; and there's so much of it that you don't have to worry about whether it comes from the diet. The concentration of dimethylamine in fasting gastric juice is about 12mM.

CONNEY: How variable are the dimethylamine levels between different subjects and on different days?

TANNENBAUM: I don't have enough data to say how variable it is, but there are differences between people. It's an interesting question. Nevertheless, I think there is so much dimethylamine present that the limiting reactant is the nitrous acid.

HARRIS: What time of year were these samples collected?

CONNEY: The samples were collected in the fall.

HARRIS: The reason I bring that up is that there are other sources of NO_2, including gas stoves, and in homes that use gas stoves you can get fairly high levels of ambient NO_2. It's another possibility.

HOFFMANN: You did not see any inhibition of the nitrosoproline formation? This would be indicated by urinary excretion. It is interesting that your values are pretty much in agreement with ours.

CONNEY: Our data with nitrosoproline are in very good agreement with your data.

HOFFMANN: Doesn't it mean that these levels come from the diet? I am surprised then that in the case of smokers, you do not see any change when you give ascorbic acid. We have not seen any change when we give ascorbic acid to nonsmokers. We have analyzed the whole dietary intake of proline and therefore know that a high percentage of nitrosoproline already comes from the diet.

TANNENBAUM: That's not necessarily true. We have data indicating that there is an endogenous component of nitrosoproline that does not come from a conventional nitrosating agent. So some of it could come from the diet and some of it could come from just a different compartment. But there are obviously many different sources of nitrosoproline.

HOFFMANN: Yes, but you did not see an inhibition or reduction of nitrosoproline in your smokers when they had been given ascorbic acid.

CONNEY: No, but we studied only three smokers. Two of them were cigarette smokers and one smoked a pipe. Your population was much larger than ours. All of our subjects ingested a relatively high amount of ascorbic acid during the control part of the study as indicated by the urinary excretion of about 75 mg of ascorbic acid per day. If we did our study in a population of subjects who were deficient in vitamins C and E, we may have seen an effect of these vitamins on the urinary excretion of dimethylnitrosamine and nitrosoproline.

Determination of Exposure to PAH by Analysis of Urine Samples

GEORG BECHER
Department of Toxicology
National Institute of Public Health
Geitmyrsveien 75, 0462 OSLO 4, Norway

OVERVIEW

Polycyclic aromatic hydrocarbons (PAH), formed by incomplete combustion of organic material, are ubiquitous in the environment. Epidemiological data suggest that the inhalation of PAH may be associated with an increased risk of urban- and industry-related cancers in man. However, estimation of human exposure to PAH may be very crude because of the lack of reliable analytical data. In order to understand better the health hazard connected with PAH, it seems necessary to monitor the uptake of PAH by analyzing body fluids. This paper describes a method for the determination of PAH and PAH metabolites in urine. The method is applied to urine samples from an occupationally nonexposed control group and from aluminum workers with high exposure to PAH. In the control group, urine extracts from smokers show a significantly higher level of PAH than from nonsmokers. This is attributed to the PAH content in tobacco smoke. However, the high concentrations of PAH found in the working atmosphere of aluminum plants are not reflected to a corresponding extent in the excretion of PAH in urine. This may be correlated with the low excess of lung cancer found in epidemiological studies of workers in the aluminum industry. Nevertheless, determination of PAH and PAH metabolites in urine may serve as an indicator for the human exposures to PAH.

INTRODUCTION

Polycyclic aromatic hydrocarbons (PAH), resulting from incomplete combustion of organic materials, are ubiquitous in our environment (Grimmer 1983). Several of these compounds have been shown to be carcinogenic in animal experiments and are therefore associated with occurrence of various types of cancer in man (IARC 1983). Human exposure to PAH occurs principally by direct inhalation of tobacco smoke and polluted air, by ingestion of contaminated and processed food and water, or by dermal contact with soots, tars, and oils.

Several epidemiological studies have demonstrated an increased risk of lung cancer among workers exposed to coal tar pitch volatiles (IARC 1984). Epidemiological evidence, though inconclusive, points to air pollution as a possible contributory agent in respiratory cancer in urban areas (Anonymous 1972). Tobacco smoking is causally associated with cancer of the lung and other sites (Doll and Peto 1976).

There are, however, several problems in relating the incidence of lung cancer with the exposure to PAH. All the materials mentioned contain PAH in addition to a great number of other agents showing carcinogenic, cocarcinogenic, or promoting effects. Thus, the question arises: What portion of carcinogenicity may arise from PAH? Furthermore, it is often difficult to estimate the actual exposure to PAH from analytical data of the various environmental media alone.

Frequently the concentration of PAH in workplace atmospheres exceeds more than 1000 times the concentration found in urban atmospheres, suggesting that workers exposed to such atmospheres might be at a greatly increased risk of cancer of the respiratory tract. Somewhat surprisingly, the high exposure is not reflected to a great extent in the epidemiological evidence presently available from several industries. This is the case for the aluminum industry in particular (Doll 1984). One reason might be that only a small fraction of the airborne PAH is taken up by the organism and is biologically active.

Because of low vapor pressure, most carcinogenic PAH in the environment are adsorbed onto particles. It is now well recognized that the nature of the particle may influence the biological effect of PAH (Stenbäck et al. 1976; Sun et al. 1982).

With respect to lung cancer, there seem to be several essential processes:

1. The inhaled carcinogen must be retained by the respiratory tract. Adsorption of PAH on particles that are themselves efficiently retained, can increase the PAH dose received.
2. The carcinogens must enter the cells where they are subsequently transformed to reactive metabolites. Transport of carcinogens into the cells can be altered by particles in several ways.

Therefore, determination of PAH concentrations in air samples may not give a good measure of the effective dose of PAH received by the individual. In order to obtain a better understanding of the hazard connected with PAH exposure, we have recently proposed to monitor PAH uptake in the organism by analysis of body fluids, e.g., urine samples (Becher and Bjørseth 1985; Haugen et al. 1986).

PAH, once adsorbed in the organism, are readily metabolized by microsomal enzyme systems to oxygenated, water soluble metabolites (Young et al. 1978). Hepatobiliary excretion and elimination through the feces is the major route by which PAH are removed from the organism. Animal experiments showed that about 10% of a subcutaneously injected dose of benzo[a]pyrene was eliminated in the urine within 6 days after injection (Kotin et al. 1959). The majority of metabolites in the urine appear as water soluble metabolites.

In this paper, we report on the determination of urinary PAH and PAH metabolites in exposed humans using a method based on the reduction of oxygenated PAH metabolites to the parent hydrocarbons (Becher and Bjørseth 1983; Becher et al. 1984).

RESULTS

The analytical procedure to evaluate PAH uptake included the extraction of PAH and PAH metabolites from urine using cartridges containing C_{18}-modified silica, reduction of the metabolites back to PAH by refluxing with hydriodic acid (reversed metabolism), and subsequent analysis of prominant PAH by high-performance liquid chromatography (HPLC) with fluorimetric detection (Becher and Bjørseth 1983).

The reduction of oxygenated PAH metabolites was performed according to Konieczny and Harvey (1979) who reported the efficient reduction of polycyclic aromatic quinones, phenols, phenol ethers and phenol esters to PAH by refluxing with hydriodic acid in acetic acid. Table 1 shows the results for two parallel analyses of a urine sample from an exposed worker. One analysis included the reduction of metabolites yielding the sum of unmetabolized and metabolized PAH. For the other part of the sample, the reduction step was omitted resulting in the unmetabolized PAH in the sample. The table shows that after reduction PAH has increased approximately fivefold.

Figure 1 shows a typical HPLC/fluorescence chromatogram of PAH isolated from an exposed worker's urine. Apart from being remarkably sensitive, HPLC with fluorescence detection also allows for the selective determination of PAH in the presence of nonfluorescing interferences.

Figure 2 shows the urinary PAH profile of occupationally nonexposed smokers and nonsmokers. Ten representative PAH, ranging from fluorene to benzo[a]-pyrene, are selected for profile analysis. Correction has been made for varying dilu-

Table 1
PAH in an Exposed Worker's Urine without and with Reduction of Metabolites (µg/liters)

PAH	Without reduction	With reduction
1. Fluorene	ND	4.2
2. Phenanthrene	6.85	9.8
3. Authracene	ND	4.4
4. Fluoranthene	1.12	9.8
5. Pyrene	0.37	5.5
6. Benzo(a)fluorene	ND	3.1
7. Benz(a)anthracene	0.17	2.0
8. Chrysene	0.18	Obscured
9. Benzo(e)pyrene	ND	0.7
10. Benzo[a]pyrene	0.01	0.13
11. Dibenz(a,h)anthracene	ND	0.57
Total	8.7	40.2

ND = not detected
Reprinted, with permission, from Becher and Bjørseth (1983).

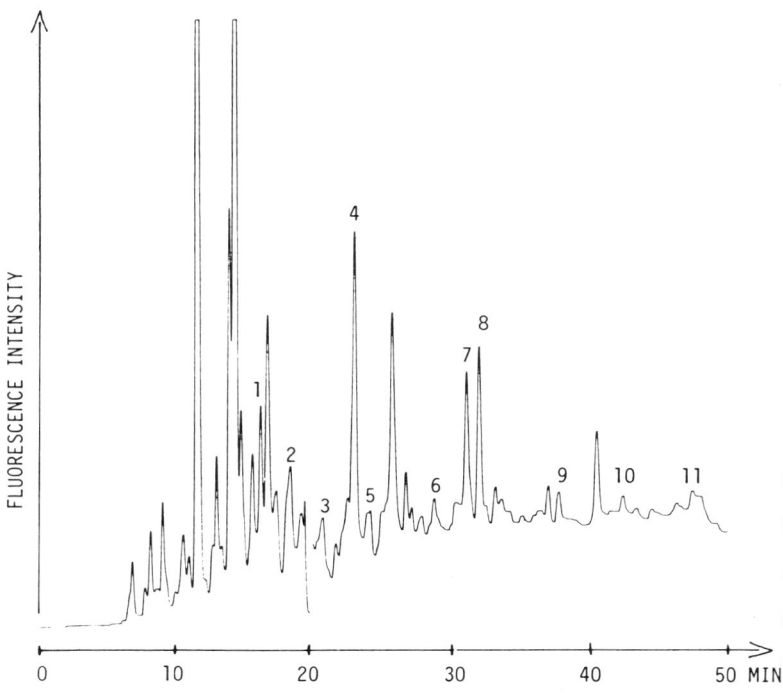

Figure 1
Reversed phase HPLC chromatogram of PAH in urine from an exposed worker. For peak identities, see Table 1. Reprinted, with permission, from Becher and Bjørseth (1983).

tions of the urine samples by expressing the results in µg PAH/mmole creatinine. The creatinine values varied from 3.7 to 24 mmole/liter with an average of 10.8 mmole/liter. The mean value for the sum of the ten PAH in smokers' urine was 3.62 µg/mmole creatinine as compared to 0.52 µg/mmole for nonsmokers' urine.

The PAH exposure levels of workers from the potroom of an aluminum plant using vertical pin Söderberg technology were determined by personal sampling of airborne particulate PAH. A typical capillary gas chromatogram of a filter extract from a personal sample is shown in Figure 3. More than 20 PAH compounds were identified in all samples. The sum of particulate PAH in the personal samples varied from 52 to 268 µg/m^3 (1-9.8 µg BaP/m^3) with an average of 126 µg/m^3 (3.4 µg BaP/m^3). In Norway an administrative norm of 40 µg total particulate PAH per m^3 has been established, determined as time-weighed average for a normal 8-hour work day.

Figure 4 shows the concentration of ten PAH in 15 urine samples from smoking and nonsmoking aluminum workers. The sum of the ten PAH in the different samples varied from 1.12 to 6.48 µg/mmole creatinine.

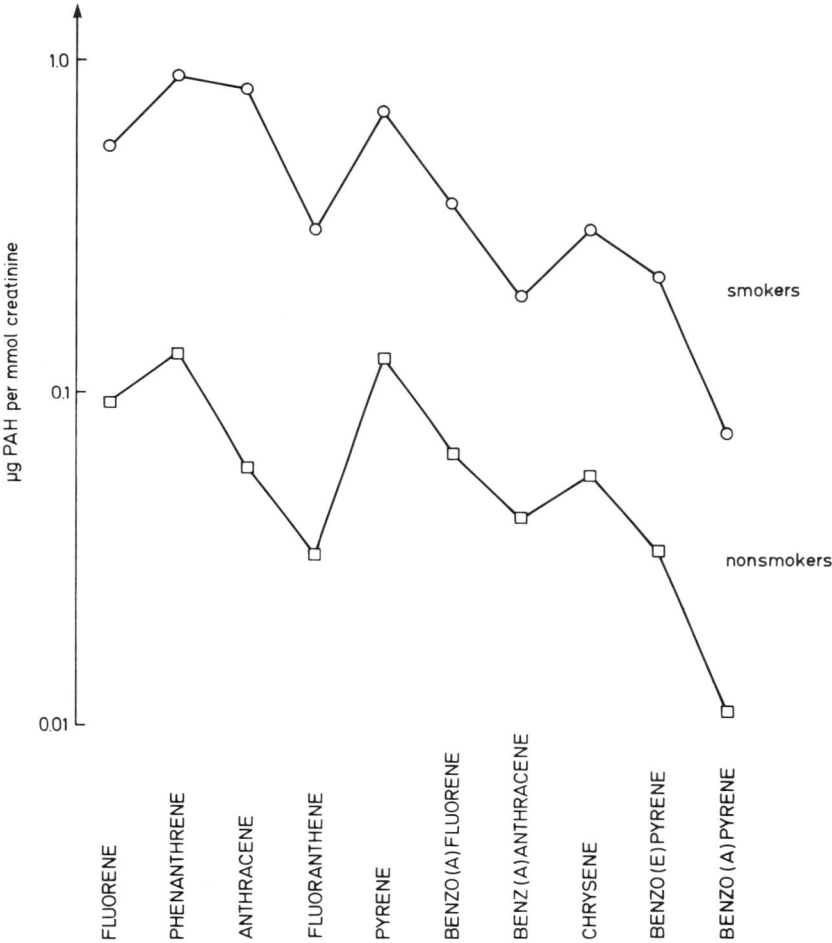

Figure 2
PAH profile of urine samples from occupationally nonexposed smokers (N = 4) and nonsmokers (N = 5).

For comparison the average PAH concentrations found in the workplace atmosphere are also given in Figure 4. The profile of urinary excreted PAH seems to correspond well to the air concentrations. However, it should be taken into account that the air sampling efficiency for three-ring PAH is low due to their volatility. Fluorene is not retained at all on the filter and only about 3% of the

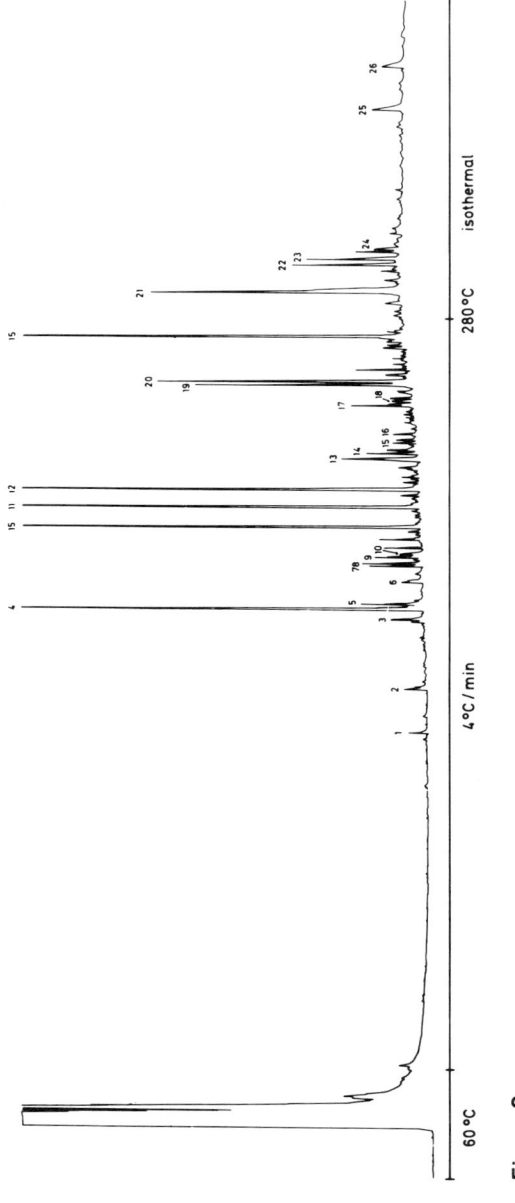

Figure 3
Typical capillary gas chromatogram of particulate PAH from personal sampling in the pot-room of an aluminum plant. Main components: (4) Phenanthrene; (11) fluoranthrene; (12) pyrene; (13) Benzo(a)fluorene; (19) benzo(a)anthracene; (20) chrysene/triphenylene; (21) benzo(b/j/k)fluoranthene; (22) benzo(e)pyrene; (23) benzo(a)pyrene; (25) indeno(1,2,3-cd)-pyrene; (26) benzo(ghi)perylene. Reprinted, with permission, from Becher et al. (1984).

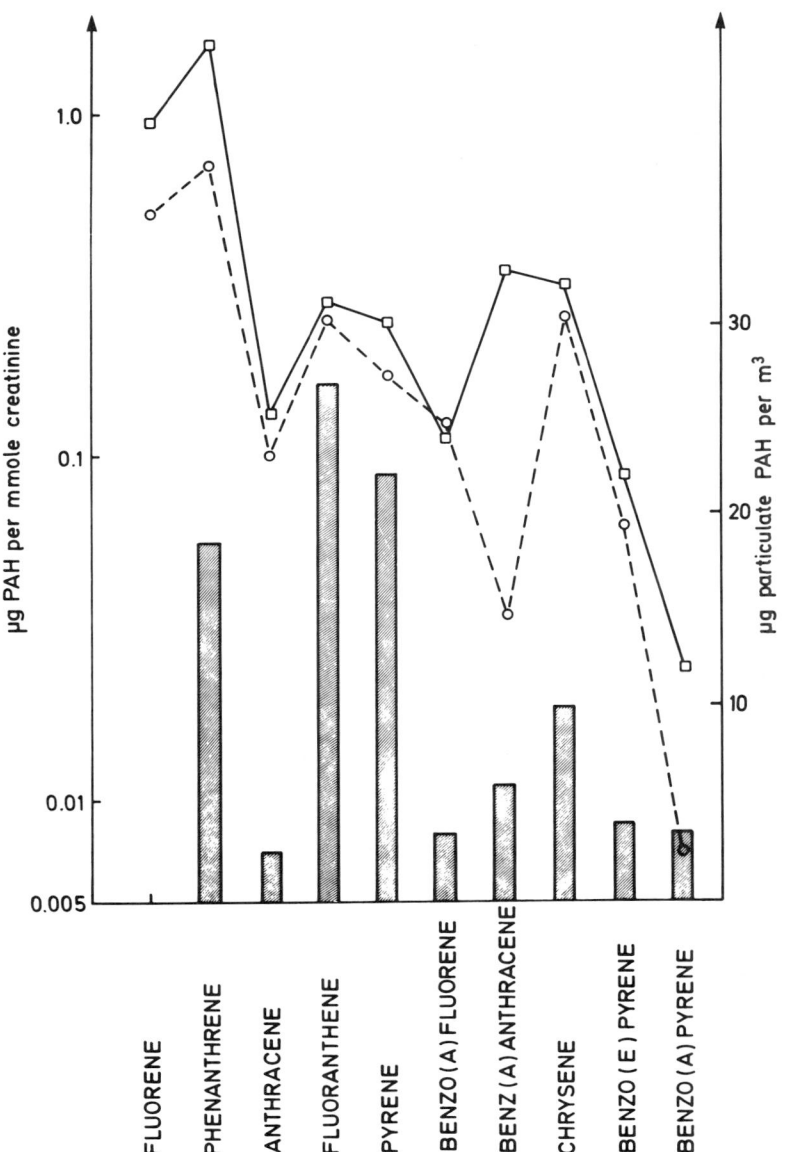

Figure 4
Mean values for concentrations of individual PAH in worker's urine and particulate PAH in work atmosphere (bars). Reprinted, with permission, from Becher et al. (1984).

total airborne phenanthrene and anthracene is found in the particulate phase. The figure demonstrates further that there is no significant difference in PAH profiles in urine from smoking and nonsmoking aluminum workers.

A comparison of the mean PAH concentrations in the urine samples from the four different categories of persons studied is given in Figure 5. A significant increase in PAH excretion is observed for nonsmokers among exposed workers compared to the nonsmoking control group. However, for smoking workers the high level of PAH in work atmosphere is not reflected in a significant increase in PAH excretion.

DISCUSSION

Human exposure to PAH from various media have been estimated by Santodonato et al. (1980). Using the available monitoring data, they calculated the daily intake

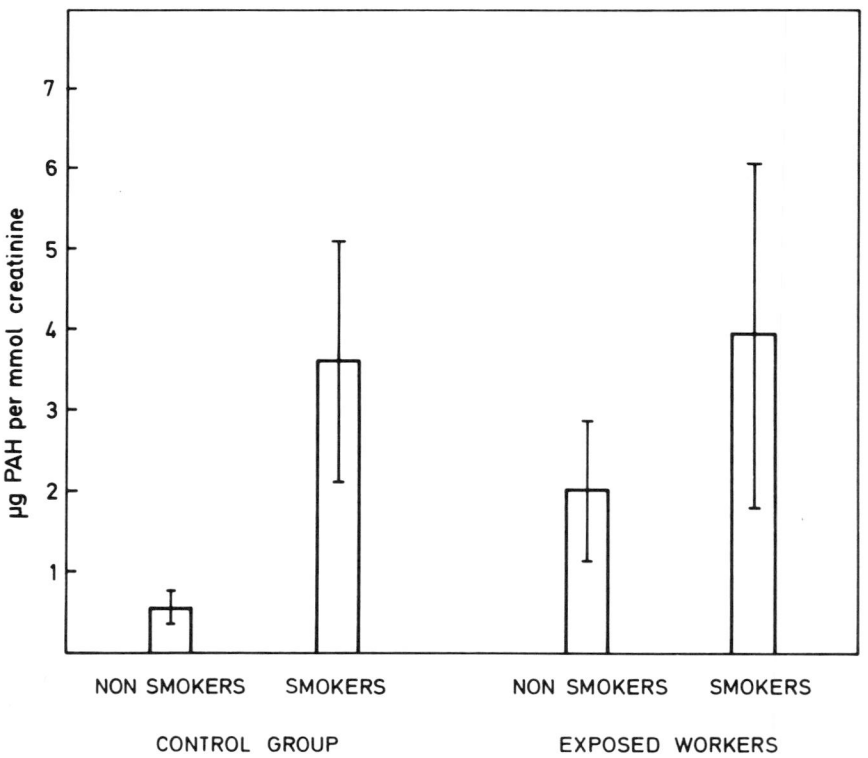

Figure 5
Mean ± SD of PAH levels in urine samples from exposed workers and controls. Reprinted, with permission, from Becher et al. (1984).

of total PAH as 0.21 μg from air, 0.03 μg from water, and 1.6-16 μg from food. In comparison, a smoker of filter cigarettes might inhale 10-40 μg PAH per 20 cigarettes (one pack) (Hoffmann et al. 1978). Thus, cigarette smoking is an important source of PAH exposure. This is reflected in a significant increase in the excretion of PAH and PAH metabolites for smokers in the control group as compared to nonsmokers in this group.

Similar results were obtained by Repetto and Martinez (1974) for benzo[a]-pyrene and by Maly (1971) for dibenzo(a,1)pyrene. On the other hand, Michels and Einbrodt (1979) did not find any significant difference in the content of benz[a]anthracene and benzo[a]pyrene in urine samples from smoking and nonsmoking residents of an industrialized area.

The results from personal sampling of airborne PAH in the potroom of an aluminum plant show that the occupational exposure of workers may be very high. Assuming a breathing volume of 1 m^3/hr, the average exposure for a potroom worker is 1 mg particulate PAH for an 8-hour workshift. This corresponds to smoking 500-2000 cigarettes. However, the analysis of urine samples from potroom workers gives no indication that PAH or PAH metabolites are excreted in high concentrations as a result of the high exposure to airborne PAH. The total amount of PAH in urine from nonsmoking aluminum workers is greater than the value for the respective control group only by a factor of about four.

These results are particularly interesting when the analytical data is compared with epidemiological data on occupational cancer in the aluminum industry. There is no obvious correlation between exposure as measured by air analysis and lung cancer frequency. Recent epidemiological studies indicate that there is no or only a slight excess of lung cancer in aluminum workers, whereas the exposure is up to three orders of magnitude higher than that in urban atmospheres (Doll 1984). On the other hand, analysis of PAH in urine fit well with the epidemiological data, as the excretion of PAH is only slightly increased in exposed workers.

One explanation for these findings might be that PAH are strongly associated with the adsorbing particles found in aluminum smelters and are thus not readily bioavailable. Several experimental studies have shown that the ability of PAH to be desorbed or eluted from particles in the organism may vary greatly depending on the type of carrier particle (Stenbäck et al. 1976). However, very little is known about the bioavailability of PAH adsorbed to airborne particles in workplace environments.

CONCLUSION

The present study shows that the analysis of PAH and PAH metabolites excreted in urine may be used for biological monitoring of PAH exposure. The sensitivity of the method described is high enough to determine PAH in occupationally nonexposed humans. In this group smokers show a significantly higher level of PAH than nonsmokers. However, the high concentration of PAH found in the working atmospheres of an aluminum plant is not reflected to a great extent in the excretion of PAH in urine. These data are in accordance with the very small increase in lung cancer found in epidemiological studies of the aluminum industry. The relevance of PAH air monitoring data may, therefore, be questioned as a measure of the relative safety of the hazard connected with PAH exposure from ambient air.

REFERENCES

Anonymous. 1972. *Biologic effects of atmospheric pollutants. Particulate polycyclic organic matter.* National Academy of Sciences, Washington, D.C.

Becher, G. and A. Bjørseth. 1983. Determination of exposure to polycyclic aromatic hydrocarbons by analysis of human urine. *Cancer Lett.* **17**: 301.

———. 1985. Determination of occupational exposure to PAH by analysis of body fluids. In *Handbook of polycyclic aromatic hydrocarbons* (ed. A. Bjørseth and T. Ramdahl), vol. 2, p. 237. Marcel Dekker, New York.

Becher, G., A. Haugen, and A. Bjørseth. 1984. Multimethod determination of occupational exposure to polycyclic aromatic hydrocarbons in an aluminum plant. *Carcinogenesis* **5**: 647.

Doll, R. 1984. Risk of cancer in the primary aluminium industry: An appraisal. In *PAH-symposium: Polycyclic aromatic hydrocarbons in the primary aluminium industry* (ed. E. Nordheim and T. Guthe). Nordic Aluminium Industry's Secretariat for Health, Environment and Safety, Oslo, Norway.

Doll, R. and R. Peto. 1976. Mortality in relation to smoking: 20 years' observations on male British doctors. *Br. Med. J.* **2**: 1525.

Grimmer, G. 1983. *Environmental carcinogens: Polycyclic aromatic hydrocarbons.* CRC Press, Boca Raton, Florida.

Haugen, A., G. Becher, C. Benestad, K. Vahakangas, G.E. Trivers, M.J. Newan, and C.C. Harris. 1986. Biomonitoring of individuals exposed to high levels of PAH in the work environment. *Cancer Res.* (in press).

Hoffmann, D., I. Schmeltz, S.S. Hecht, and E.L. Wynder. 1978. Tobacco carcinogenesis. In *Polycyclic hydrocarbons and cancer* (ed. H.V. Gelboin and P.O.P. Ts'o), p. 85. Academic Press, New York.

IARC. 1983. *Polynuclear aromatic compounds, part 1, chemical, environmental and experimental data. IARC monographs on the evaluation of the carcinogenic risk of chemicals to humans*, vol. 32. International Agency for Research on Cancer, Lyon, France.

———. *Polynuclear aromatic compounds, part 3, industrial exposures in aluminum production, coal gasification, coke production, and iron and steel founding. IARC monographs on the evaluation of carcinogenic risk of chemicals to humans*, vol. 34. International Agency for Research on Cancer, Lyon, France.

Konieczny, M. and R.G. Harvey. 1979. Efficient reduction of polycyclic quinones, hydroquinones and phenols to polycyclic aromatic hydrocarbons with hydriodic acid. *J. Org. Chem.* **44**: 4813.

Kotin, P., H.L. Falck, and R. Busser. 1959. Distribution, retention, and elimination of C^{14}-3,4-benzpyrene after administration to mice and rats. *J. Natl. Cancer Inst.* **23**: 541.

Maly, E. 1971. A simple test for exposure to polycyclic hydrocarbons. *Bull. Environ. Contam. Toxicol.* **6**: 422.

Michels, S. and H.J. Einbrodt. 1979. Polycyclic aromatic hydrocarbons in human urines collected in a large industrial city–An epidemiological study (in German). *Wiss. Umwelt.* **3**: 107.

Repetto, M. and D. Martinez. 1974. Benzopyrene de cigarette et son excretion urinaire. *Eur. J. Toxicol.* **7**: 234.

Santodonato, J., D. Basu, and P.H. Howard. 1980. Multimedia human exposure and carcinogenic risk assessment for environmental PAH. In *Polynuclear aromatic hydrocarbons: Chemistry and biological effects* (ed. A. Bjørseth and A.J. Dennis), p. 435. Battelle Press, Columbus, Ohio.

Stenbäck, F., J. Rowland, and A. Sellakumar. 1976. Carcinogenicity of benzo(a)pyrene and dusts in the hamster lung (instilled intratracheally with titanium oxide, aluminum oxide, carbon and ferric oxide). *Oncology.* **33**: 29.

Sun, J.D., R.K. Wolff, and G.M. Kanapilli. 1982. Deposition, retention, and biological fate of inhaled benzo(a)pyrene adsorbed onto ultrafine particles and as a pure aerosol. *Toxicol. Appl. Pharmacol.* **65**: 231.

Young, S.K., J. Deutsch, and H.V. Gelboin. 1978. Benzo(a)pyrene metabolism: Activation and detoxification. In *Polycyclic hydrocarbons and cancer* (ed. H.V. Gelboin and P.O.P. Ts'O), vol. 1, p. 205. Academic Press, New York.

COMMENTS

HOFFMANN: The urinary excretion of creatinine is, among others, a function of the physical activity of a person. Have you adjusted your data relative to milligram creatinine or to total daily creatinine excretion? When you took 24-hour urine samples from these workers, did you ever try to see the difference in total creatinine excretion?

BECHER: Unfortunately, 24-hour urine samples could not be obtained in this survey. Instead, spot samples were taken directly after the workshift. The creatinine level was used to correct for varying dilution of the urine samples. Although creatine excretion might vary with factors other than fluid intake, this is a common procedure in biological monitoring of chemical exposure using urine samples.

HOFFMANN: But for the scientist who likes to make up his own mind, were your data adjusted to creatinine?

BECHER: Yes, all data were adjusted to creatinine. However, the data in μg per liter urine are also available.

HOFFMANN: I think that you should consider total creatinine output because, in at least one study, it was shown that a smoker produced less creatinine than a nonsmoker on the same diet. It appears that in general smokers are physically less active. They excrete significantly less creatinine even when diet is standardized, and that in itself is interesting. So one needs to look at the ratio of an excreted compound relative to a unit of creatinine; but, I think, one should also give the data relative to total creatinine output.

BECHER: We had also compared the data in μg PAH per liter urine for the four different categories studied. The results are very similar; however the standard deviation is much greater. The PAH levels in urine samples from smoking workers are about twice as high as for nonsmoking workers. However, this difference is statistically not significant.

WINKELSTEIN: I wonder if the lung cancer rates in smokers and nonsmokers have been examined in the aluminum workers?

BECHER: There are three major epidemiological studies on lung cancer in the aluminum industry from Norway, Canada, and the United States. To the best of my knowledge none of them takes into account the smoking habits and no class differentiation is made between smokers and nonsmokers.

CONNEY: In the rat, most of a dose of benzo[a]pyrene is metabolized and excreted in the bile with only a very small amount in the urine. In addition, polycyclic aromatic hydrocarbons are very lipid-soluble and distribute very extensively in fat. Is it possible that when polycyclic hydrocarbons are absorbed by different routes and with different size particles—cigarette smokers versus aluminum plant workers—that perhaps the distribution of the hydrocarbon is different so that in one type of exposure a higher percent of the dose is excreted in the bile than from the other kind of exposure?

BECHER: Certainly, the route by which PAH are absorbed in the body plays an important role on their biological effect. For the exposure to PAH in both cigarette smoke and aluminum plant inhalation is the principal absorption route. As I pointed out, there is evidence that the physicochemical properties of the particle influence the biological effect and may therefore also alter the distribution in the organism and the excretion of PAH.

HARRIS: Let me ask a question concerning inhalation. You mentioned that the workers were exposed to 1 mg of hydrocarbon a day. What percent of that 1 mg was on respirable size particulates? Because if it is on very large particulates of several microns in size, it would never, in fact, be inhaled and that could be an important factor.

BECHER: The size distribution of PAH containing airborne particles has been studied for aluminum plants. Almost all of the PAH is found on particles in the inhalable size range (up to 7 μm).

HARRIS: So another explanation would be required, such as the one Dr. Conney mentioned.

Modifiers of Endogenous Carcinogen Formation: Studies on In Vivo Nitrosation in Tobacco Users

JAGADEESAN NAIR, HIROSHI OHSHIMA, BRIGITTE PIGNATELLI,
MARLIN FRIESEN, CHRISTIAN MALAVEILLE, SYLVIE CALMELS,
AND HELMUT BARTSCH
International Agency for Research on Cancer
Division of Environmental Carcinogenesis
69872 Lyon cedex 08, France

OVERVIEW

Endogenous formation of N-nitroso compounds (NOC) from ingested precursors appears to be a large source of exposure in the general population; however, quantitation of NOC formed in vivo in humans has not been feasible until recently owing to the lack of noninvasive methods (Bartsch and Montesano 1984). Both nitrosatable amino compounds and nitrosating agents (e.g., nicotine, nitrite, and nitrate) are commonly present in unburned tobacco and in tobacco smoke (Hoffmann et al. 1984). Nitrate is easily reduced to nitrite by bacteria in the oral cavity, hypochloric stomach, or infected urinary bladder. By using a recently developed method for assessing endogenous nitrosation (N-nitrosoproline [NPRO] test, see below) (Ohshima and Bartsch 1981), it has been established unequivocally that NOC are formed in the human body. In addition, inhibitors and catalysts of nitrosation, with which humans come into daily contact, markedly modify exposure to such endogenous NOC (Ohshima et al. 1982a). Increasing attention has thus been paid to the detection of NOC formed in vivo, and in particular in tobacco smokers, chewers of tobacco and of betel quid (which often contains tobacco), and snuff dippers, all of whom are exposed to high levels of precursors and nitrosation modifiers. Results to date indicate that endogenous NOC synthesis occurs at a higher rate in these subjects than in persons without such habits, thus adding to the body burden of carcinogens ingested or inhaled from exogenous intake, as suggested previously (Druckrey and Preussmann 1962). A number of hitherto unknown NOC have been identified recently in human urine and saliva. A fraction of those found in human urine and saliva may be formed through endogenous synthesis and/or may be derived from uptake as preformed compounds.

INTRODUCTION

Preformed N-nitroso compounds (NOC) occur in fermented tobacco products and in tobacco smoke, and this is the most widespread source of human exposure to nitrosamines presently known. Several nitrosamines, in particular tobacco-specific nitrosamines (TSNA), have been detected in high concentrations in tobacco smoke and in even higher concentration in snuff and chewing tobacco; most are potent animal carcinogens (Hoffmann and Hecht 1985). There is a well-established correlation between exposure to tobacco smoke and risk of cancer of the upper respiratory and digestive tracts and of the pancreas, bladder, and renal pelvis (IARC 1985a). This evidence, together with that from experimental studies, strongly suggests that TSNA contribute to the induction of these malignancies. An association has also been confirmed between cancer of the oral cavity and snuff dipping (Winn et al. 1981). Since no chemical carcinogen other than TSNA has been detected in snuff, a direct association between exposure to nitrosamines and induction of cancer in humans must be assumed in this case.

A correlation has been established between oral cancer and chewing of betel quid, which, as used in India and in other southeast Asian countries, often contains tobacco (Bhide et al. 1984; IARC 1985b). It has been shown that nitrosation in vitro of arecoline, an areca nut alkaloid, leads to formation of areca nut-specific nitrosamines (ASNA) and of N-nitroso-N-methylpropionitrile and N-nitroso-N-methylpropionaldehyde, among which the former is a strong carcinogen in experimental animals (Wenke et al. 1984; Brunnemann et al., this volume).

Thus, carcinogens arising from the nitrosation of areca nut and tobacco constituents could play a role in the induction of oral cancer in betel quid and tobacco chewers and contribute to the exposure of smokers to carcinogens. However, the extent to which such endogenous nitrosation reactions take place in the oral cavity, stomach, and urinary bladder of subjects using various tobacco products has not been investigated extensively until recently.

The discovery of a safe substrate, which is readily nitrosatable in vivo in the form of naturally occurring proline, provided the basis for a simple, sensitive, noninvasive test (Ohshima and Bartsch 1981) for the quantitative estimation of endogenous nitrosation in humans. The nitrosated product, NPRO, a noncarcinogen, is excreted almost quantitatively in human urine within 24 hours. To estimate the formation of NOC in human subjects in vivo, they are given vegetable juice containing nitrate and then a solution of L-proline; they fast for 2 hours, and 24-hour urine samples are collected and analyzed for NPRO and other nitrosated amino acids by gas chromatography (GC) using a NOC-specific detector, the thermal energy analyzer (TEA). Alternatively, proline can be added to the diet or ingested three times a day 1 hour after each meal (100 mg each time) and exposure to nitrosating agents and ingested or inhaled nitrosation modifiers (e.g., in tobacco users) can then be assessed by measuring urinary NPRO. Proline can be added to betel quid and/or tobacco samples that are chewed or used by dippers and saliva can subsequently be analyzed for all NPRO content as an index of nitrosation reactions occurring within the oral cavity.

Application of the NPRO test to humans involves no health risk since there is substantial evidence that NPRO is neither carcinogenic nor mutagenic and that > 90% is excreted unmetabolized in humans and animals (Ohshima et al. 1982a).

RESULTS

Increased Excretion of Urinary N-Nitrosamino Acids in Cigarette Smokers: Mechanism of Formation

Endogenous formation of NPRO in human subjects following ingestion of a source of nitrate and of proline was demonstrated unequivocally by Ohshima and Bartsch (1981). It has now been firmly established, using the NPRO test, that inhalation of tobacco smoke containing nitrosating agents results in the formation of nitrosamines in smokers. In a study by Hoffmann and Brunnemann (1983), smoking and nonsmoking subjects were placed on a controlled diet. Excretion of NPRO in 24-hour urine was significantly higher in smokers than in nonsmokers; addition of proline to the diet increased NPRO excretion significantly in smokers but not in nonsmokers; and endogenous NPRO formation in smokers could be inhibited by the daily addition of 1 g ascorbic acid to their diet. Ascorbic acid can also inhibit endogenous nitrosation of proline in nonsmokers (Ohshima and Bartsch 1981; Ohshima et al. 1984).

Ladd et al. (1984) confirmed that the urine of cigarette smokers contains an excess of NPRO following the ingestion of nitrate and proline. The three- to fourfold increase of (mean) urinary NPRO in heavy smokers, as compared to nonsmokers and light smokers, was paralleled by a similar increase in the concentration of salivary thiocyanate (but not that of salivary nitrite), suggesting that the high level of salivary thiocyanate in smokers may be partly responsible for the increased rate of intragastric nitrosation of proline. Thiocyanate catalyzes nitrosation in vitro (Boyland and Walker 1974) and NPRO formation in rats fed proline and nitrite (Ohshima et al. 1982b).

In addition to NPRO, a further indicator of human exposure to exogenously and endogenously formed NOC, their precursors, and nitrosation modifiers is measurement of two new sulfur-containing N-nitrosamino acids (NAA) that have frequently been detected in human urine and identified as N-nitrosothiazolidine 4-carboxylic acid (NTCA), and *trans-* and *cis-*isomers of N-nitroso-2-methylthiazolidine 4-carboxylic acid (NMTCA) (Ohshima et al. 1983a, 1984; Tsuda et al. 1983). NTCA and NMTCA are present in the urine of both smokers and nonsmokers (Ohshima et al. 1984). They can originate from: (1) intake of preformed NOC, (2) intake of the respective parent amino precursor (thiazolidine 4-carboxylic acid and its 2-methyl derivative) and subsequent nitrosation in vivo, or (3) via an endogenous two-step synthesis involving reaction of L-cysteine with an aldehyde (formaldehyde or acetaldehyde) followed by nitrosation (Fig. 1). The latter two

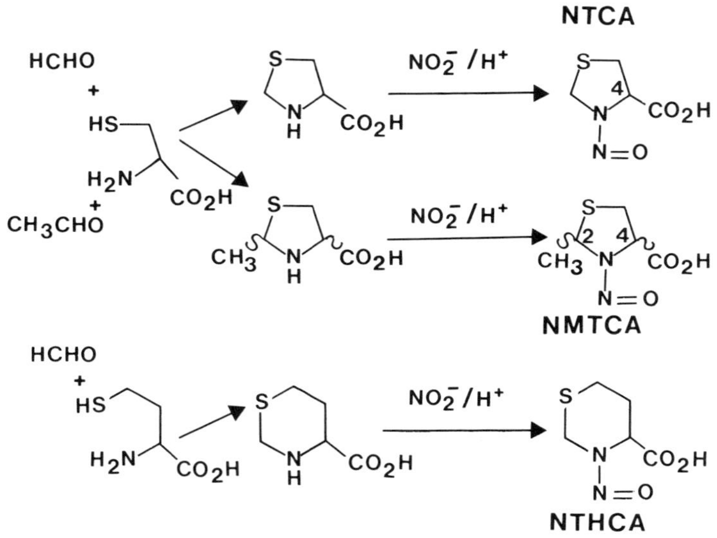

Figure 1
Scheme depicting synthesis of NAA found in human urine from the respective precursors and nitrite

reactions appear to occur to a significant extent in humans, as a diet supplemented with ascorbic acid significantly decreased the levels of NTCA and NMTCA in the urine of one subject (Ohshima et al. 1984). Furthermore, NTCA and NMTCA were found to be formed easily in rats in vivo after ingestion of L-cysteine and nitrite together with formaldehyde and acetaldehyde (Ohshima et al. 1984).

Bartsch et al. (1984) reported that smokers also excrete a higher mean level (twofold) of NAA (sum of NPRO, N-nitrososarcosine, NTCA, and NMTCA) than nonsmokers following ingestion of nitrate and proline. This increase was particularly marked in subjects in whom the pH of fasting gastric juice was 1-2.5.

As shown in a typical GC-TEA chromatogram obtained from the analysis of human urine extract after esterification with diazomethane (Fig. 2), three additional unknown NAA have been observed occasionally at relatively low concentrations. They were recently identified as 3-(N-nitroso-N-methyl-amino) propionic acid (NMPA), N-nitrosoazetidine-2-carboxylic acid (NAZCA), and N-nitrosotetrahydro-4H-1,3-thiazine 4-carboxylic acid (NTHTCA) (H. Ohshima et al. in prep.). The latter compound may be formed in a manner similar to NTCA, by reaction of formaldehyde with homocysteine (instead of cysteine) and subsequent nitrosation (Fig. 1).

The urinary levels of these and other NAA in smokers and nonsmokers are summarized in Table 1. Whether or not smokers excrete more of these three NAA remains to be determined and requires monitoring of nonsmokers for passive ex-

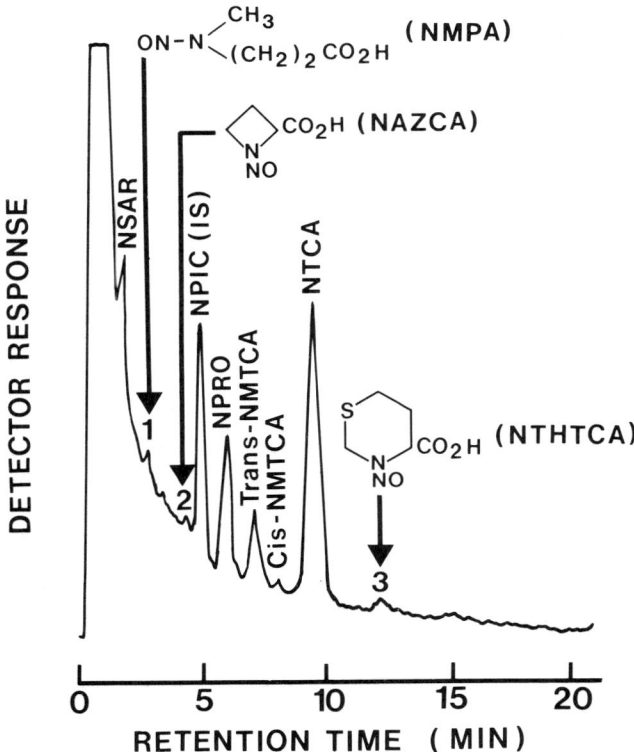

Figure 2
Typical GC-TEA chromatogram of human urine extract after esterification with diazomethane. A 2 m X 3 mm id glass column packed with 5% FFAP on Chromosorb W-HP (80-100 mesh) was employed at a column oven temperature of 180°C. Peaks *1, 2,* and *3* were identified as NMPA, NAZCA, and NTHTCA, respectively.

posure to smoke. Consistent with previous findings, the sum of urinary NAA (μg/24-hour urine) was higher in active smokers (mean, 33.4 μg) than in nonsmokers (mean, 16.8 μg).

NMPA and 4-(N-nitroso-N-methylamino)butyric acid (NMBA) were detected at ng per ml levels in saliva samples collected from subjects from Bombay, India, who were cigarette smokers, tobacco chewers, or chewers of betel quid with tobacco (Nair et al. 1985). Subjects with no such habit had no detectable levels of these NOC in their saliva. The origin of these two NOC was traced to the tobacco added to betel quid (Ohshima et al. 1985).

Excretion of NPRO and NTCA has been measured in the 24-hour urine of a small number of male subjects from Bombay, India, who were smokers of western-

Table 1
Levels of NAA Detected in Urine Samples from Nonsmoking and Cigarette Smoking Volunteers[a]

Subject	NMPA	NAZCA	NTHTCA	NSAR	NPRO	NMTCA	NTCA	Total NAA[b]
				(μg/24-hr urine)				
Nonsmoker								
A	0.5	0.4	ND	0.9	10.5	0.6	11.4	24.3
	0.6	ND	1.1	0.5	4.5	10.5	8.0	25.2
B	ND	ND	ND	0.2	0.9	0.8	3.0	4.9
	ND	ND	ND	0.3	1.7	1.0	2.8	5.8
C	0.5	0.5	ND	ND	10.3	2.2	21.4	34.9
	ND	ND	ND	ND	1.1	1.1	1.7	3.9
D	0.8	2.0	0.8	ND	2.4	0.8	11.6	18.4
Smoker								
E	0.8	ND	2.0	0.6	12.4	5.0	35.0	55.8
	ND	ND	ND	1.1	2.2	1.0	11.4	15.7
F	0.4	0.6	12.0	3.0	7.6	3.9	16.0	43.5
	ND	0.5	ND	ND	6.1	5.2	3.1	14.9
G	0.6	ND	ND	ND	6.7	9.3	34.0	50.6
	ND	ND	ND	ND	1.6	2.5	3.1	7.2
H	0.5	1.1	1.5	0.4	4.5	19.8	18.4	46.2

[a]NAA were determined in urine extracted and analyzed as previously described (Ohshima et al. 1984); duplicate samples were collected from several subjects.
[b]Sum of all seven NAA
ND = not detected

type cigarettes and of bidis (native cigarette) or chewers of betel quid containing Indian tobacco (Table 2) (J. Nair, in prep.). The mean levels tended to be increased in groups with either habit, being most pronounced in cigarette and bidi smokers, as compared to subjects without such habits. However, large interindividual variations were observed. It was interesting to note that the absolute levels of urinary NPRO excreted after proline ingestion in this study were much lower than those found in subjects living on a western diet (Ohshima and Bartsch 1981; Hoffmann and Brunnemann 1983).

In a larger study, Lu et al. (1984) collected about 250 samples of 24-hour urine from inhabitants of high- and low-risk areas for esophageal cancer in Northern China, according to three protocols: from undosed subjects, subjects who had ingested 100 mg proline three times a day 1 hour after each meal, and subjects who had ingested 100 mg ascorbic acid together with 100 mg proline three times a day 1 hour after each meal. Inhabitants of the high-risk area excreted more NAA than those in the low-risk area; smokers (mostly males) excreted greater amounts of NPRO, NTCA, and NMTCA in the urine than did nonsmokers ($P < 0.01$).

Table 2
Urinary Excretion of NAA (ng/24 hr) in Indian Tobacco Users and in Controls with No Tobacco Habit

Study group	NPRO		NTCA	
	Without proline	With proline	Without proline	With proline
No habit (control)	324 ± 141[a]	545 ± 120	651 ± 173	731 ± 416
	(4/4)[b]	(4/4)	(3/4)	(3/4)
Cigarette smokers	808 ± 509	2844 ± 1272	3321 ± 2702	2196 ± 1098
	(6/6)	(5/6)	(6/6)	(4/6)
Bidi smokers	422 ± 60	634 ± 284	2305 ± 1124	2322 ± 1120
	(5/5)	(5/5)	(5/5)	(4/5)
Chewers of betel quid with tobacco	280 ± 70	1856 ± 1113	1767 ± 817	935 ± 303
	(5/5)	(5/5)	(4/5)	(5/5)

[a]Mean ± SE from 4–6 subjects
[b]Number of samples with detectable NOC/total number of samples analyzed

Urinary excretion of NAA in groups of subjects from Bombay, India, who had or had not ingested 100 mg proline 1 hour after each meal three times a day, and who had smoked one or more cigarettes of one or more bidis or who had chewed one or more betel quids after each meal. Controls (no habit group) did or did not receive proline. Urine was collected for 24 hours and analyzed for NPRO, NTCA, NMTCA, and NSAR as previously described (Ohshima et al. 1984). As the latter two NAA were either not found or were at negligible concentrations, they are not listed.

In Vivo Formation of NOC in the Oral Cavity of Chewers of Betel Quid with or without Tobacco: Studies with Vitamin C as a Nitrosation Inhibitor

It has been reported that TSNA and ASNA are present in the saliva of chewers of betel quid with tobacco (BQT) and without tobacco (BQ) (Nair et al. 1985; Brunnemann et al., this volume). In particular, the higher levels of N-nitrosoanatabine (NAT), N-nitrosoguvacoline (NGCO), and N-nitrosoguvacine (NGCI) found in the saliva of BQT and BQ chewers than in controls and the observation that these NOC are present only in traces or not at all in BQT or BQ samples suggest that they could be formed during the chewing process, i.e., from arecoline or tobacco alkaloids in the presence of salivary nitrite and thiocyanate and possibly through catalysis of phenolic compounds present in betel quid (IARC 1985b; Nair et al. 1985). Evidence to support this theory was obtained from in vitro nitrosation experiments under conditions simulating those prevailing in the saliva (pH 7.4) or in the stomach (pH 2.1) (Table 3). In three BQT samples (obtained from local shops in Bombay), a marked increase in the concentration of NAT, NGCI, and NGCO, (and of NNN only at pH 2.1) was observed with nitrosation, which was more pronounced at acidic pH. NGCI and NGCO levels in BQ samples were increased to a similar degree after nitrosation (Table 3).

Further evidence that synthesis of NOC occurs during the chewing of BQT or BQ was obtained in the following study in ten healthy male subjects who were asked to chew sequentially: (A) an unmodified BQT (or BQ) sample; (B) one to which 100 mg of proline had been added; and (C) one to which 100 mg proline and 100 mg ascorbic acid had been added. Saliva was collected from each subject for over 20 minutes, and analyzed for nicotine, arecoline, NPRO, TSNA, and ASNA (J. Nair, et al. in prep.; data not shown). When the results were expressed as a ratio of NPRO (ng/ml) to nicotine (μg/ml) in saliva (Fig. 3), all ten BQT chewers had an increased NPRO content after chewing BQT with proline (A versus B). In the case

Table 3
Levels of Nitrosamines before and after In Vitro Nitrosation of Betel quid Samples with (BQT) or without (Indian) Tobacco (BQ)

Incubation	BQT sample				BQ sample	
	NNN	NAT	NGCO	NGCI	NGCO	NGCI
			(ng per g wet weight)			
None	56	tr	0	5	0	2
pH 7.4, 1 hr	68	35	52	111	169	18
pH 2.1, 1 hr	1239	6859	81	330	115	194

Values are means from experiments each with three BQT or BQ samples. Nitrosation was carried out at 20°C at the pH indicated in presence of NO_2^- (50 ppm) and SCN^- (100 ppm) (from Nair et al. 1985).
tr = trace

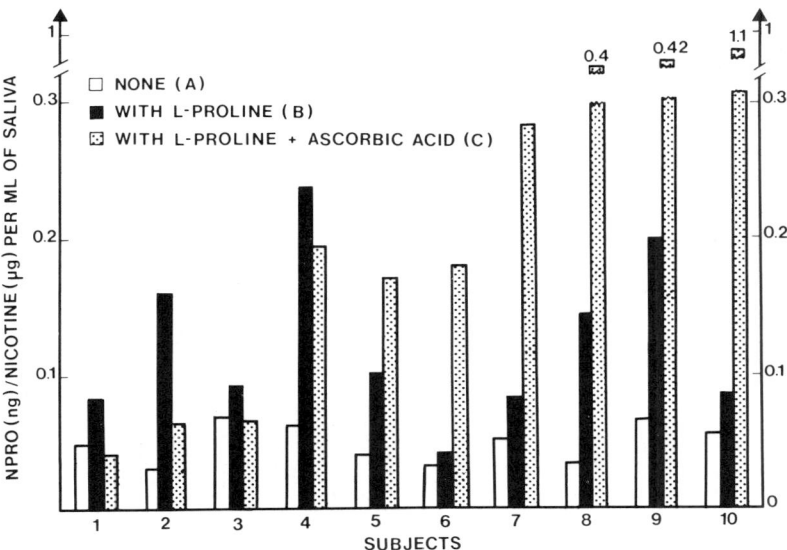

Figure 3
Nitrosation in the saliva of chewers of betel quid containing Indian tobacco (BQT). Ten subjects chewed for 20 minutes sequentially: (*A*; □) A BQT sample, (*B*; ■) a quid to which 100 mg proline had been added, and (*C*; ▨) a quid to which 100 mg proline plus 100 mg ascorbic acid had been added. Saliva was collected from each subject during a 20-min period and analyzed for presence of nicotine, arecoline, and NPRO (also for NO_2, SCN^-, TSNA, and BSNA, not shown) as described previously (Nair et al. 1985).

of BQ chewers, when the results were expressed as a ratio of NPRO (ng/ml) to arecoline (μg/ml), a similar increase in NPRO content was also observed (*A* versus *B*, Fig. 4). However, in only four out of ten BQT chewers and five out of ten BQ chewers was there inhibition of the increased nitrosation by ascorbic acid (*B* versus *C* in Figs. 3 and 4), and the remainder showed increased levels of NPRO in saliva when ascorbate was present. The mechanism of this accelerating effect of ascorbic acid on NPRO formation under these experimental conditions remains to be elucidated, although ascorbate has been reported to catalyze nitrosation in vitro under certain conditions (Chang et al. 1979). However, a number of simple phenolic and polyphenolic compounds are known to be strong nitrosation modifiers (Pignatelli et al. 1982), and tobacco and betel quid constituents (areca nut and catechu) contain tannins and a large variety of (poly)phenols (e.g., catechol, catechin, chlorogenic acid). Studies have shown that certain of these polyphenols, such as catechin and betel nut extracts, can both catalyze and inhibit *N*-nitrosation reactions in vitro, in experimental animals, and in humans (Pignatelli et al. 1982; Stich et al.

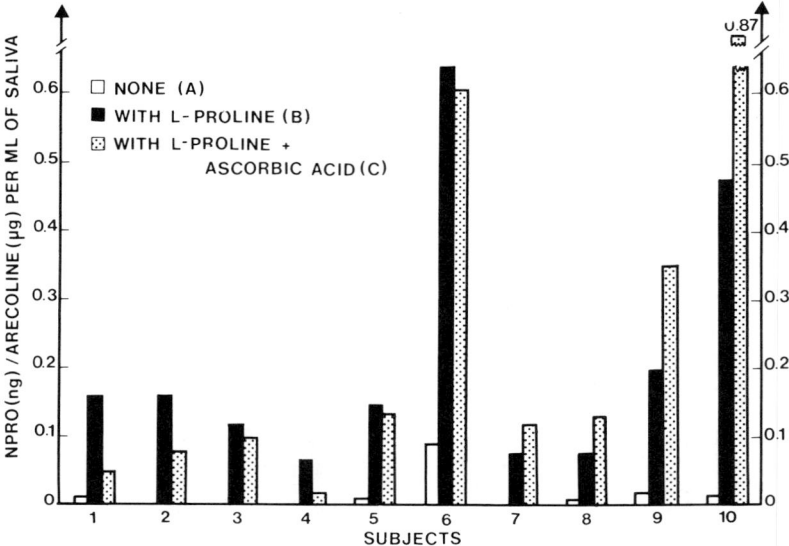

Figure 4
Nitrosation in the saliva of chewers of betel quid without tobacco (BQ). (*A*; □) Unmodified quid; (*B*; ■) sample supplemented with 100 mg proline; (*C*; ▨) sample with 100 mg proline and 100 mg ascorbic acid. Saliva was collected and analyzed for arecoline and NPRO (also for NO_2, SCN^-, and BSNA, not shown) as described previously (Nair et al. 1985).

1983, 1984). The effect depends strongly on pH, the nature of the phenolic compound involved and the ratio of the concentrations of nitrite to polyphenols present in the reaction mixture.

DISCUSSION

Use of tobacco products results in heavy exposures to preformed nitrosamines, in particular TSNA, which are present both in tobacco smoke and in various tobacco products. Further exposure to NOC is due to their endogenous synthesis, which has been demonstrated unequivocally to occur in smokers as well as in users of noncombusted tobacco and betel quid, which often contains tobacco. Several studies involving smokers from several countries, using different tobacco products, indicated increased excretion of NAA (mainly NPRO and NTCA) in urine. In one study in cigarette smokers, the addition of the nitrosation inhibitor, ascorbic acid, to the diet diminished NPRO formation. As urinary NPRO has been shown to be a reliable index of endogenous nitrosation of other amines yielding carcinogenic NOC (Ohshima et al. 1983b; Ohshima and Bartsch 1984), the present findings infer increased formation in tobacco users as a result of increased exposure to nitrosamine precursors and nitrosation modifiers (Hoffmann et al. 1984; Hoffmann and Hecht 1985; IARC 1985a,b). Smokers of > 20 cigarettes may be exposed to up to 12 mg of nitrogen oxides, which act as nitrosating agents, and 30 mg of nicotine and other nitrosatable amines. Heavy smokers have salivary levels of thiocyanate, a potent nitrosation catalyst, that are increased to mmolar levels. Since thiocyanate has a plasma half-life of about 2 weeks, its presence in saliva, plasma, and urine may lead to increased endogenous synthesis of nitrosamines from nontobacco-related precursors, even after cessation of smoking. Tobacco smoke contains a number of simple and polyphenolic compounds ($\sim$ 600 μg per cigarette), of which resorcinol-type compounds could act as nitrosation catalysts; this remains to be verified. Exposure to smoke results in increased uptake of precursors for certain NAA (NTCA, NMTCA), i.e., formaldehyde and acetaldehyde (about 1 mg/cigarette), possibly leading to an increased two-step synthesis in vivo (Fig. 1).

In addition to smokers, consumers of unburned tobacco have increased exposure to nitrosamines, and ng/ml of TSNA in saliva have been detected in snuff users, tobacco chewers, and betel quid chewers. Nitrosation appears to occur in the oral cavity of betel quid chewers, as shown by increased NPRO formation during a 20-minute period of chewing betel quid to which proline had been added. Chewers of tobacco or of betel quid containing tobacco also appeared to excrete more NAA in their urine than did no habit controls.

Tobacco users have heavier exposure than nonusers to nitrosamines, their precursors, and nitrosation modifiers in a number of ways. Snuff dippers and chewers of tobacco ingest milligram levels of nitrite and 100-mg levels of both nitrate and nicotine (Hoffmann et al. 1984). Nitrate is reduced to nitrite in the oral cavity by the bacterial flora; and thiocyanate has been found in the saliva of users of noncombusted tobacco products. Furthermore, tobacco and other betel quid ingredients (areca nut and catechu) contain high concentrations of tannins and polyphenols, some of which could act as nitrosation catalysts at neutral pH. In vitro nitrosation of betel quid with and without tobacco under conditions simulating those prevailing in the oral cavity or stomach led to large increases in the levels of certain TSNA, i.e., NAT, and of the ASNA, i.e., NGCO and NGCI (Table 3). The much greater increase in the levels of these NOC formed at gastric pH suggests that chewers of tobacco and betel quid may produce higher concentrations of endogenous NOC than nonusers when tobacco- and areca nut-related amines, catalysts, and nitrite reach their stomachs. This possibility is likely in chewers who swallow the saliva in which these ingredients occur. This hypothesis is being tested in an ongoing long-term carcinogenicity study in hamsters fed betel nut powder (2% in the diet) and nitrite (0.2% in drinking water) for 1 year (U. Mohr et al., unpubl.).

An additional site of nitrosation is the urinary bladder. An increased risk of bladder cancer has been reported among individuals with a history of urinary infections and especially among cigarette smokers (Kantor et al. 1984). Nitrate and thiocyanate, together with the tobacco-derived alkaloids (nicotine) and cotinine, are present in the urine of smokers, and nitrosation could take place at acidic pH when nitrate-reducing bacteria are present. Recently, several microorganisms isolated from humans with urinary infections have been shown to catalyze nitrosation of secondary amines at neutral pH, possibly through the action of a bacterial enzyme (Calmels et al. 1985). Similarly, smokers of cigarettes of black tobacco have about a twofold higher risk for bladder cancer than those using bright tobacco (Vineis et al. 1984). Black tobacco generally contains more TSNA and their precursors than bright tobacco (Hoffmann et al. 1984). In a study in progress (in collaboration with B. Terracini and P. Vineis, Turin, Italy and J. Estéve, IARC), we are comparing urinary mutagenicity and excretion of NAA, thioethers, nicotine, and cotinine in smokers of black and of bright tobacco.

The identification of a number of hitherto unknown NAA in the urine and saliva of human subjects deserves special attention and further investigation. It is not yet clear whether NMPA, NAZCA, and NTHTCA, which have been detected in the urine of smokers and nonsmokers, are produced via in vivo synthesis and/or are ingested as preformed compounds from tobacco products or dietary components. Since they may be metabolic products of other NOC, and thus indicators of hitherto unknown exposures to NOC, their sources, pathways of endogenous synthesis, and toxicological properties remain to be investigated.

CONCLUSIONS

TSNA are major carcinogenic agents, alone and in combination with other tobacco constituents, in tobacco-associated cancers in both smokers and, to an even greater degree, in users of noncombusted tobacco products (Hoffmann and Hecht 1985). A substantial fraction (as yet undetermined) of TSNA and other NOC appear to be synthesized in vivo, in the oral cavity, in the acidic gastric environment, and possibly in the (infected) urinary bladder. Ascorbic acid, shown to be an effective inhibitor of nitrosation in humans (Ohshima et al. 1984), also inhibits endogenous NOC synthesis in smokers (Hoffmann and Brunnemann 1983). Epidemiological studies have shown that tobacco smoking and alcohol drinking are risk factors for cancer of the upper digestive tract (Tuyns et al. 1977; IARC 1985a); it has been hypothesized that ethanol facilitates metabolic activation of TSNA (Swann 1984), notably in the target organs of nitrosamine carcinogenicity. Regular consumption of vegetables and fresh fruits, a potential source of ascorbic acid, has some protective effect against these malignancies (Tuyns 1983), and it can be assumed that this protective effect is attributable mainly to an inhibitory action of ascorbate on nitrosamine formation, although various other modifiers of carcinogenesis are present in these food items. The absence of an effect of ascorbate on nitrosation during betel quid chewing found in most subjects in our study, however, should encourage further research for more effective nitrosation inhibitors. A lowering of the effect of nitrosation catalysts may be a promising avenue for further investigations.

Given the limited possibilities available today for reliably lowering exposure of tobacco users to tobacco-derived nitrosamines and other carcinogens (e.g., by reducing the levels of precursors [nitrate and nicotine] in tobacco products and by using nitrosation inhibitors, dietary anticarcinogens, and other chemopreventive agents), avoidance or cessation of tobacco use appears to be the only certain way of eliminating the cancer risk associated with exposure to tobacco and tobacco smoke.

ACKNOWLEDGMENTS

Part of the work reported in this paper was undertaken during the tenure of a Research Training Fellowship awarded to J.N. by the International Agency for Research on Cancer. We wish to thank Dr. S.V. Bhide, Bombay, India and coworkers for collaborative efforts on betel quid studies, and Miss M.C. Bourgade and Mrs. L. Garren for technical assistance. One of the TEA detectors was provided on loan by the National Cancer Institute of the United States under contract NO1 CP-55715. The authors are grateful to Mrs. E. Heseltine for editorial assistance and to Miss Y. Granjard for secretarial help.

REFERENCES

Bartsch, H. and R. Montesano. 1984. Commentary: Relevance of nitrosamines to human cancer. *Carcinogenesis* **108**: 1381.

Bartsch, H., H. Ohshima, N. Muñoz, M. Crespi, V. Cassale, V. Ramazotti, R. Lambert, Y. Minaire, J. Forichon, and C.L. Walters. 1984. In-vivo nitrosation, precancerous lesions and cancers of the gastrointestinal tract. On-going studies and preliminary results. In *N-Nitroso compounds: Occurrence, biological effects and relevance to human cancer* (ed. I.K. O'Neill, R.C. von Borstel, C.T. Miller, J. Lone, and H. Bartsch), publ. 57, p. 957. International Agency for Research on Cancer, Lyon, France.

Bhide, S.V., A. Shah, J. Nair, and D. Nagarajrao. 1984. Epidemiological and experimental studies on tobacco-related oral cancer in India. In *N-Nitroso compounds: Occurrence, biological effects and relevance to human cancer* (ed. I.K. O'Neill, R.C. von Borstel, C.T. Miller, J. Lone, and H. Bartsch), publ. 57, p. 851. International Agency for Research on Cancer, Lyon, France.

Boyland, E. and S.E. Walker. 1974. Effect of thiocyanate on nitrosation of amines. *Nature* **248**: 601.

Calmels, S., H. Ohshima, P. Vincent, A.-M. Gounot, and H. Bartsch. 1985. Screening of microorganisms for nitrosation catalysis at pH 7 and kinetic studies on nitrosamine formation from secondary amines by *E. coli* strains. *Carcinogenesis* **6**: 911.

Chang, S.K., G.W. Harrington, M. Rothstein, W.A. Shergalis, D. Swern, and S.K. Vohra. 1979. Accelerating effect of ascorbic acid on N-nitrosamine formation and nitrosation by oxyhyponitrite. *Cancer Res.* **39**: 3871.

Druckrey, H. and R. Preussmann. 1962. Die Bildung carcinogener Nitrosamine am Beispiel des Tabakrauchs. *Naturwissenschaften* **49**: 498.

Hoffmann, D. and K.D. Brunnemann. 1983. Endogenous formation of N-nitrosoproline in cigarette smokers. *Cancer Res.* **43**: 5570.

Hoffmann, D. and S.S. Hecht. 1985. Nicotine-derived N-nitrosamines and tobacco-related cancer: Current status and future directions. *Cancer Res.* **45**: 935.

Hoffmann, D., K.D. Brunnemann, J.D. Adams, and S.S. Hecht. 1984. Formation and analysis of N-nitrosamines in tobacco products and their endogenous formation in tobacco consumers. In *N-Nitroso compounds: Occurrence, biological effects and relevance to human cancer* (ed. I.K. O'Neill, R.C. von Borstel, C.T. Miller, J. Lone, and H. Bartsch), publ. 57, p. 743. International Agency for Research on Cancer, Lyon, France.

International Agency for Research on Cancer (IARC). 1985a. *IARC monographs on the evaluation of the carcinogenic risk of chemicals to humans: Tobacco habits other than smoking; betel-quid and areca-nut chewing; and some related nitrosamines*, vol. 37. International Agency for Research on Cancer, Lyon, France.

―――. 1985b. *IARC monographs on the evaluation of the carcinogenic risk of chemicals to humans: Tobacco smoking,* vol. 38. International Agency for Research on Cancer, Lyon, France.

Kantor, A.F., P. Hartige, R.N. Hoover, A. Narayama, J.W. Sullivan, and J.F. Fraumeni, Jr. 1984. Urinary tract infection and risk of bladder cancer. *Am. J. Epidemiol.* **119**: 510.

Ladd, K.F., H.L. Newmark, and M.C. Archer. 1984. N-Nitrosation of proline in smokers and non-smokers. *J. Natl. Cancer Inst.* **73**: 83.

Lu, S.H., H. Ohshima, and H. Bartsch. 1984. Recent studies on N-nitroso compounds as possible etiological factors in oesophageal cancer. In *N-Nitroso compounds: Occurrence, biological effects and relevance to human cancer* (ed. I.K. O'Neill, R.C. von Borstel, C.T. Miller, J. Lone, and H. Bartsch), publ. 57, p. 947. International Agency for Research on Cancer, Lyon, France.

Nair, J., H. Ohshima, M. Friesen, A. Croisy, S.V. Bhide, and H. Bartsch. 1985. Tobacco-specific and betel-nut-specific N-nitroso compounds: Occurrence in saliva and urine of betel quid chewers and formation in vitro by nitrosation of betel quid. *Carcinogenesis* **6**: 295.

Ohshima, H. and H. Bartsch. 1981. Quantitative estimation of endogenous nitrosation in humans by monitoring N-nitrosoproline excreted in the urine. *Cancer Res.* **41**: 3658.

Ohshima, H. and H. Bartsch. 1984. Monitoring endogenous nitrosamine formation in man. In *Monitoring human exposure to carcinogenic and mutagenic agents* (ed. A. Berlin, M. Draper, K. Hemminki, and H. Vainio), publ. 59, IPCS Joint Symposia no. 7, p. 233. International Agency for Research on Cancer, Lyon, France.

Ohshima, H., B. Pignatelli, and H. Bartsch. 1982a. Monitoring of excreted N-nitrosamino acids as a new method to quantitate endogenous nitrosation in humans. In *Banbury Report 12: Nitrosamines and human cancer* (ed. P.N. Magee), p. 297. Cold Spring Harbor Laboratory, Cold Spring Harbor, New York.

Ohshima, H., J.-C. Bereziat, and H. Bartsch. 1982b. Monitoring N-nitrosamino acids excreted in the urine and feces of rats as an index for endogenous nitrosation. *Carcinogenesis* **3**: 115.

Ohshima, H., M. Friesen, I. O'Neill, and H. Bartsch. 1983a. Presence in human urine of a new N-nitroso compound, N-nitrosothiazolidine 4-carboxylic acid. *Cancer Lett.* **20**: 183.

Ohshima, H., G.A.T. Mahon, J. Wahrendorf, and H. Bartsch. 1983b. Dose-response study of N-nitrosoproline formation in rats and a deduced kinetic model for predicting carcinogenic effects caused by endogenous nitrosation. *Cancer Res.* **43**: 5072.

Ohshima, H., I.K. O'Neill, M. Friesen, J.-C. Bereziat, and H. Bartsch. 1984. Occurrence in human urine of new sulphur-containing N-nitrosamino acids, N-nitrosothiazolidine 4-carboxylic acid and its 2-methyl derivative, and their formation. *J. Cancer Res. Clin. Oncol.* **108**: 121.

Ohshima, H., J. Nair, M.-C. Bourgade, M. Friesen, L. Garren, and H. Bartsch. 1985. Identification and occurrence of two N-nitrosamino acids in tobacco products: 3-(N-nitroso-N-(methyl-amino)propionic) acid and 4-(N-nitroso-N-(methylamino)butyric) acid. *Cancer Lett.* **26**: 153.

Pignatelli, B., J.C. Bereziat, G. Descotes, and H. Bartsch. 1982. Catalysis of nitrosation *in vitro* and *in vivo* in rats by catechin and resorcinol and inhibition by chlorogenic acid. *Carcinogenesis* **3**: 1045.

Stich, H.F., B.P. Dunn, B. Pignatelli, H. Ohshima, and H. Bartsch. 1984. Dietary phenolics and betel nut extracts as modifiers on N-nitrosation in rat and man. In *N-Nitroso compounds: Occurrence, biological effects and relevance to human cancer* (ed. I.K. O'Neill, R.C. von Borstel, C.T. Miller, J. Lone, and H. Bartsch), pub. 57, p. 213. International Agency for Research on Cancer, Lyon, France.

Stich, H.F., H. Ohshima, B. Pignatelli, J. Michelon, and H. Bartsch. 1983. Inhibitory effect of betel nut extracts on endogenous nitrosation in humans. *J. Natl. Cancer Inst.* **70**: 1047.

Swann, P.F. 1984. Effect of ethanol on nitrosamine metabolism and distribution. Implications for the role of nitrosamines in human cancer and for the influence of alcohol consumption on cancer incidence. In *N-Nitroso compounds: Occurrence, biological effects and relevance to human cancer* (ed. I.K. O'Neill, R.C. von Borstel, C.T. Miller, J. Lone, and H. Bartsch), pub. 57, p. 501. International Agency for Research on Cancer, Lyon, France.

Tsuda, M., T. Hirayama, and T. Sugimura. 1983. Presence of N-nitroso-L-thioproline and N-nitroso-L-methylthioprolines in human urine as major N-nitroso compounds. *Gann* **74**: 331.

Tuyns, A.J. 1983. Protective effect of citrus fruit on esophageal cancer. *Nutr. Cancer* **5**: 195.

Tuyns, A.J., G. Pequignot, and O.M. Jensen. 1977. Le cancer de l'oesophage en Ille et Vilaine en fonction des niveaux de consommation d'alcool et de tabac. *Bull. Cancer* **64**: 45.

Vineis, P., J. Esteve, and B. Terracini. 1984. Bladder cancer and smoking in males: Types of cigarettes, age of start, effect of stopping and interaction with occupation. *Int. J. Cancer* **34**: 165.

Wenke, G., K.D. Brunnemann, and D. Hoffmann. 1984. A study of betel quid carcinogenesis IV. Analysis of the saliva of chewers. A preliminary report. *J. Cancer Res. Clin. Oncol.* **108**: 110.

Winn, D.M., W.J. Blott, C.M. Shy, L.W. Pickle, A. Toledo, and J.F. Fraumeni, Jr. 1981. Snuff-dipping and oral cancer among women in the Southern United States. *New Engl. J. Med.* **304**: 745.

COMMENTS

HOFFMANN: Has nitrosoproline been tested for carcinogenic activity in experimental animals other than rats?

MAGEE: Not to my knowledge.

BARTSCH: I haven't heard of any study.

HOFFMANN: Now that's one thing to be concerned about. We find this compound in such significant concentrations and just because nitrosoproline is not carcinogenic in rats, we cannot assume that this is so in all species.

BARTSCH: We have studied the nitrosation rates of various amino acids and we could demonstrate that this reaction occurs rapidly.

HOFFMANN: Where? In the stomach?

BARTSCH: In vitro, as well as in rats, likely in the stomach.

MAGEE: What is the possible biological implication of finding nitrosarcosine? Isn't it a carcinogen?

BARTSCH: Yes, but this compound is found in rather small amounts, and not every time in human urine samples; but it is there. We don't know where it comes from because we haven't checked for the intake of preformed nitrososarcosine or precursors, but it could be derived from other sources, e.g., metabolic pathways, as well.

HECHT: I'm curious about nitrosohydroxyproline. I was rereading one of your papers, Dr. Bartsch, and you said that 50% of it is excreted in the feces of rats. Do you have any ideas why that might be?

BARTSCH: No, but noticing this different excretion profile as compared to nitrosoproline, we had another idea. We thought we could use hydroxyproline for monitoring nitrosation in the colon. But we haven't done it yet.

HECHT: Are any of your other compounds excreted in the feces? You haven't looked at the other compounds to determine distribution between urine and feces?

BARTSCH: For the nitrosothioprolines (NTCA and NMTCA) and for nitrosarcosine, we have published papers showing that in rats they are mostly excreted in the urine, like nitrosoproline.

Hemoglobin Adducts of Tobacco-related Aromatic Amines: Application to Molecular Epidemiology

STEVEN R. TANNENBAUM,* MATTHEW S. BRYANT,* PAUL L. SKIPPER,*
AND MALCOLM MACLURE†
*Department of Applied Biological Sciences
Massachusetts Institute of Technology
Cambridge, Massachusetts 02139
†Department of Epidemiology
Harvard School of Public Health
Boston, Massachusetts 02115

INTRODUCTION/OVERVIEW

Molecular epidemiology is a rapidly growing field of research devoted to the study of environmental chemicals that pose a hazard to human health. It differs from conventional epidemiology in the manner of exposure quantification. Instead of environmental sampling to determine ambient concentrations for estimating exposure, one measures the reaction products with cellular targets such as DNA or protein. The concentrations of these products may ultimately be related to risk, or may, with appropriate animal models for interpretation, be used to quantify intake.

This approach is designed to circumvent several shortcomings of the environmental sampling approach. Foremost of these is the extrapolation from ambient toxin levels to actual tissue burden. Ambient levels are commonly determined by spot sampling. The individual's burden may be incorrectly estimated if his environment is significantly different from that at the point of sampling. In the case of tobacco carcinogenesis, individual exposure is particularly difficult to assess because of such additional variables as the carcinogen yield from different products and individual smoking habits.

Even if the actual intake of a toxin can reasonably be estimated from environmental sampling, other postconsumption variables are also important, primarily metabolic processing. Many carcinogens and genotoxins must be metabolically activated before they exert their toxic effects. Simultaneously, other enzymes are engaged in detoxification. The relation between these competing pathways is both constitutive and, in many cases, inducible. Thus, the true tissue burden will vary from one individual to another.

As a means of circumventing these various sources of uncertainty about the true tissue burden, it has been proposed to measure the end product of carcinogen exposure—the adducts formed between cellular nucleophiles and the ultimate metabolite responsible for initiation of tumorogenesis. The measurements ideally would be made in the target tissue. This will rarely be possible, however, so a substitute matrix needs to be used. The most readily available specimens, which also contain sufficient adduct levels, are generally blood or urine. In this paper, we will discuss the use of one type of dosimetry, that based upon adducts formed with blood proteins, to monitor exposure to carcinogens of tobacco origin.

ALBUMIN AND HEMOGLOBIN AS DOSIMETERS

In the blood, two proteins, albumin and hemoglobin, dominate carcinogen binding. Each has advantages for the purpose of dosimetry, and may provide information complementary to that obtained from the other. Hemoglobin has a lifetime of about 120 days in humans; thus, circulating levels of carcinogen-modified hemoglobin will reflect the level of exposure during a period of nearly 4 months. It also possesses some metabolic competence, particularly, the ability to oxidize aromatic hydroxylamines to nitroso compounds which react quite efficiently with sulfhydryl groups. Albumin also has a relatively slow turnover which leads to a half-life of 20-25 days in humans. This protein does not possess metabolic capacity other than, perhaps, some esterase activity. In contrast to hemoglobin, though, it is not segregated by the erythrocyte membrane and might be the target for a greater number of carcinogens. It is present and is synthesized in the same cells in which the reactive metabolic intermediates of carcinogens are primarily formed, the hepatocytes. Also, albumin has a number of high affinity binding sites for a broad spectrum of xenobiotics, which may enhance its ability to attract and react with electrophiles.

A detailed review of the background and history of the use of hemoglobin as a biological dosimeter is beyond the scope of this paper. Ehrenberg and his colleagues pioneered this area of research for small alkylating agents such as ethylene oxide and have derived and tested the equations that describe the properties of the hemoglobin dosimeter (Osterman-Golkar et al. 1976). Whenever the covalently bound adduct has the lifetime of an erythrocyte, the adduct level formed following an acute dose will decrease linearly with time. As stated earlier, for humans, this period is approximately 120 days. During chronic dosing the adduct level would accumulate for 120 days to a level 60 times higher than that given by an acute dose, and then remain at that level.

4-AMINOBIPHENYL

This paper will focus on 4-aminobiphenyl (4-ABP), which is one of a large number of amines found in tobacco smoke (Patrianakos and Hoffmann 1979), some of which are listed in Table 1. All of these are found in much greater amounts in sidestream smoke than in mainstream smoke, suggesting the possibility that significant aromatic amine exposure might also result from passive smoking. Our interest in 4-ABP in particular was stimulated by its known tumorigenicity in humans (Melick

Table 1
Aromatic Amines in Sidestream Smoke and Mainstream Smoke[a]

Compound	Sidestream	Mainstream
Aniline	10,800	364
2-Toluidine	3,030	162
3-Toluidine	2,080	30.4
4-Toluidine	1,730	33.8
2-Ethylaniline + 2,6-dimethylaniline	1,240	54.2
2,5-Dimethylaniline	2,370	87.2
3-Ethylaniline + 2,4-dimethylaniline	1,200	56.7
4-Ethylaniline + 2,3-dimethylaniline	494	27.3
1-Naphthylamine	103	2.5
2-Naphthylamine	67	1.7
2-Aminobiphenyl	110	3.0
3-Aminobiphenyl	132	5.0
4-Aminobiphenyl	143	4.6
2-Methyl-1-naphthylamine	117	3.6

[a]ng/cigarette (commercial, 70-mm, nonfilter French cigarette)
Reprinted, with permission, from Patrianakos and Hoffmann (1979).

et al. 1971), as well as by its very favorable yield of hemoglobin reaction products in experimental animals relative to many of the other amines.

In some species, 4-ABP is a potent hepato- or mammary gland carcinogen (Poupko et al. 1983; Garner et al. 1984). The metabolic steps believed to be important in these activities are reviewed elsewhere (Garner et al. 1984). In general, in animal species that more readily acetylate the amine or its hydroxylamine, the major site of action is the liver, mammary gland, or intestine. In species such as the dog, which does not N-acetylate amines, bladder cancer is the resulting lesion. Humans exhibit genetic polymorphism with respect to acetylator phenotype (Glowinski et al. 1978), so the target organ may differ from one individual to another.

The N-hydroxylation of 4-ABP and other aromatic amines is a critical step in the activation of these compounds. The acute toxicity of 4-ABP in humans and dogs is due to the ability to induce methemoglobinemia. The mechanism of methemoglobin formation by aromatic amines has been studied extensively by Kiese (1974) and others and has been shown to be related to hydroxylamine formation. One consequence of methemoglobin formation is the production of nitroso intermediates which are predominantly the species that react further with hemoglobin to form stable adducts.

The feasibility of monitoring exposure to 4-ABP via quantification of the hemoglobin binding has now been established. Studies with the rat have shown that greater than 90% of ABP bound to hemoglobin is in the form of a cysteine sulfinic acid amide, a product formed by the intermediate, nitrosobiphenyl. The bound ABP can be released by mild hydrolysis and detected as the parent amine. The structure of the principal hemoglobin adduct as a sulfinamide of cysteine β-93 has now been confirmed by x-ray crystallography (D. Ringe et al., in prep.). Between 5 and 11% of a single dose becomes bound to the total hemoglobin. During chronic administration of 4-ABP, the level bound to hemoglobin increases to a plateau value of about 30 times greater than that resulting from a single dose. Bound ABP persists in circulation until a full erythrocyte lifetime has elapsed. The dose-response relationship for a single dose is linear between 500 ng/kg to 5 mg/kg (Green et al. 1984).

A method has been developed to quantify 4-ABP adducted to hemoglobin (4-ABP-Hb). It utilizes basic hydrolysis of the isolated hemoglobin, followed by extraction of the regenerated amine into hexane. After clean-up, the amine is derivatized with pentafluoropropionic anhydride and analyzed on a capillary gas chromatograph (GC) coupled to a mass spectrometer (MS). An ABP analog, 4'-F-ABP, is added at the beginning to serve as an internal standard. The method is sensitive to levels below 10 pg (50 fmole) per 10 ml blood.

PRELIMINARY STUDIES OF 4-ABP-HEMOGLOBIN ADDUCT LEVELS IN HUMAN SMOKERS/NONSMOKERS

Two studies have been undertaken using blood samples from human subjects classified as smokers or nonsmokers. Information about the two studies is listed below.

Study 1

Blood samples of 1-3 ml were obtained from another study done at a melanoma clinic. The smoking histories of the subjects had been obtained in the questionnaire for that study. Since it was expected that about 10 ml of blood (5 ml red cells) would be necessary for the adduct measurement, samples from 2-5 individuals of like smoking status were combined to form suitably sized samples. Fourteen combined samples were assembled from a total of 48 individual samples.

Study 2

Samples were obtained from F. Perera, R.M. Santella, and D. Brenner of the Columbia University School of Public Health in a coded, blind fashion (the samples were numbered from 1000-1 to 1021-1, and the smoking status was not known to us at the time of analysis). Each sample consisted of the washed red blood cells and the serum, in separate tubes, from 10 ml blood samples. The red cells were analyzed for 4-ABP-Hb adduct levels by the GC-MS methodology.

Histograms of the adduct levels in the samples versus the number of samples of the same adduct level (frequency) were plotted for the smoker and nonsmoker samples in the two studies (Fig. 1). It can be seen from these figures that the

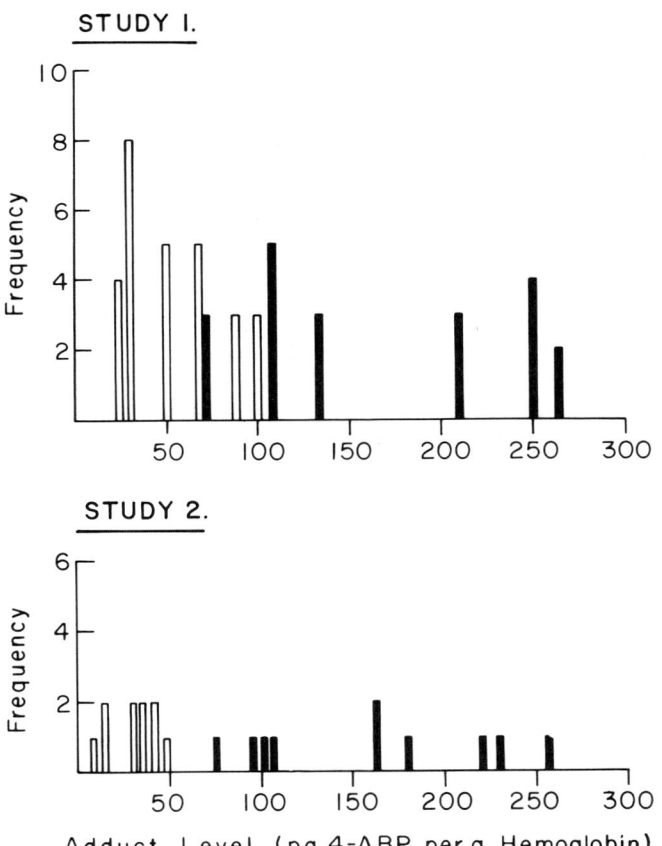

Figure 1
Distribution of observed adduct levels of 4-ABP-Hb among individuals who have either never smoked or who are currently cigarette smokers. *Study 1* (□) nonsmokers, $\bar{x}$ = 53, (■) smokers, $\bar{x}$ = 166; *study 2* (□) nonsmokers, $\bar{x}$ = 1, SE = 13, (■) smokers, $\bar{x}$ = 158, SE = 63.

smoker samples consistently had a higher level of 4-ABP-Hb adducts than the nonsmoker samples. The mean values and ranges for each category are shown below:

Study 1
Nonsmokers (n = 28); mean 53 ± 26 pg 4-ABP/g Hb
; range = 28 to 99 pg/g Hb
Smokers (n = 20); mean = 166 ± 76 pg 4-ABP/g Hb
; range = 65 to 265 pg/g Hb

Study 2
Nonsmokers (n = 10); mean = 31 ± 13 pg 4-ABP/g Hb
; range = 7 to 99 pg/g Hb
Smokers (n = 10); mean = 158 ± 63 pg 4-ABP/g Hb
; range = 75 to 256 pg/g Hb

Combined (Studies 1 and 2)
Nonsmokers (n = 38); mean = 47 ± 25 pg 4-ABP Hb
; range = 7 to 99 pg/g Hb
Smokers (n = 30); mean = 163 ± 71 pg 4-ABP/g Hb
; range = 65 to 265 pg/g Hb

Although the smokers have a mean adduct level about 3.3 times higher than the nonsmokers, there is still a significant adduct level in the nonsmokers. None of the human samples tested thus far have shown an adduct level below 7 pg 4-ABP/g Hb. This suggests that there may be human exposure to 4-ABP other than through direct smoking, such as passive smoking, dietary contamination, or air pollution.

ESTIMATION OF AVERAGE DAILY EXPOSURE TO 4-ABP

Using the human adduct levels and the chronic dosing model confirmed experimentally in the rat, one can estimate the average daily exposure values for the human subjects tested. The following assumptions are operative in extending this model to the human situation:

1. The exposure values are normalized to those for a 70-kg individual for ease of calculation. A 70-kg individual is further assumed to have 150 mg of hemoglobin per ml of blood and a total blood volume of 5 liters. Thus, a 70-kg individual would have 750 g of hemoglobin.
2. The measured adduct levels are steady-state values which result from chronic exposure (i.e., daily), and are thus related to the daily adduction level by a factor of $1/2 \times T_{er}$, where T_{er} is the average lifetime of a human erythrocyte.
3. The dose-response relationship between 4-ABP intake and the amount adducted to hemoglobin is estimated to be 5-11% based on experiments with the rat (5-11%) and the dog (5%).

Calculating an estimate of the average daily intake of 4-ABP is done as follows (using the combined nonsmoker mean values of the two studies as an example):

Measured steady-state adduct level = 0.047 ng 4-ABP/g Hb
4-ABP in a 70-kg individual = (0.047 ng/gm Hb) x (750 g Hb)
= 35.3 ng

$$\text{Daily adduction level} = \frac{\text{steady state adduction level}}{1/2 \times \text{Ter}}$$
$$= \frac{35.3 \text{ ng 4-ABP}}{64 \text{ days}}$$
$$= 0.55 \text{ ng 4-ABP/day}$$

$$\text{Average daily intake} = \frac{\text{daily adduction level}}{\% \text{ of dose adducted}}$$
$$= \frac{0.55 \text{ ng 4-ABP/day}}{0.05\text{-}0.11}$$
$$= 5\text{-}11 \text{ ng 4-ABP/day}$$

The same calculation for the mean of the smoker samples from studies 1 and 2 results in an average daily intake of 17-38 ng 4-ABP. Table 2 shows how the estimated exposure values for the low, high, and mean value for the two categories vary according to the one value which we will not be able to confirm experimentally, the percent of dose which becomes adducted to hemoglobin in the human. We will thus have to rely on the values determined in the various animal models to provide us with estimated exposure values for the human subjects.

Table 2
Human Exposure Values as Function of Dose-response Estimate

Adduct levels (pg 4-ABP/g Hb)	Exposure (ng 4-ABP/day)		
	5%	8%	11%
Smokers			
65 (low)	15	10	7
163 (mean)	38	24	17
265 (high)	62	39	28
Nonsmokers			
7 (low)	1.6	1	0.7
47 (mean)	11	7	5
99 (high)	23	14	11

HOW ACCURATE IS THE HEMOGLOBIN DOSIMETER FOR 4-ABP?

This is clearly a crucial question if this method is going to be useful for epidemiological studies. The range of estimated intake for smokers calculated from the Hb adduct data is 15-35 ng per day. The range of 4-ABP in cigarettes (Patrianakos and Hoffmann 1979) is 1-5 ng per cigarette or 20-100 ng per day for a one pack per day smoker. Thus our estimate based upon analysis of the smoker's blood is of the same order of magnitude as that expected from an average smoker's cigarette consumption. Given all of the assumptions described above, as well as the difficulties of extrapolating from rat to human, we conclude that this approach has great potential for 4-ABP and similar compounds.

ACKNOWLEDGMENTS

This work was supported by grant No. 5-P0-ES00597-13 from the National Institute of Environmental Health Sciences, the Toxicology Training Grant, No. 2-T32-ES07020 from NIH, and a grant from the American Cancer Society, No. SI6-10-I.

REFERENCES

Garner, R.C., C.N. Martin, and D.B. Clayson. 1984. Carcinogenic aromatic amines and related compounds. In *Chemical carcinogens*, 2nd ed. (ed. C.E. Searle), ACS Monograph 182, chp. 4. American Chemical Society, Washington, D.C.

Glowinski, I.B., H.E. Radtke, and W.W. Weber. 1978. Genetic variation in N-acetylation of carcinogenic arylamines by human and rabbit liver. *Mol. Pharmacol.* **14**: 940.

Green, L.C., P.L. Skipper, R.J. Turesky, M.S. Bryant, and S.R. Tannenbaum. 1984. *In vivo* dosimetry of 4-aminobiphenyl in rats via a cysteine adduct in hemoglobin. *Cancer Res.* **44**: 4254.

Kiese, M. 1974. *Methemoglobinemia: A comprehensive treatise*, CRC Press, Cleveland, Ohio.

Melick, W.F., J.J. Naryka, and R.E. Kelly. 1971. Bladder cancer due to exposure to para-aminobiphenyl: A 17-year follow-up. *J. Urol.* **106**: 220.

Osterman-Golkar, S., L. Ehrenberg, D. Segerback, and I. Hallstrom. 1976. Evaluation of genetic risks of alkylating agents. II. Haemoglobin as a dose monitor. *Mutat. Res.* **34**: 1.

Patrianakos, C. and D. Hoffmann. 1979. Chemical studies on tobacco smoke. LXIV. On the analysis of aromatic amines in cigarette smoke. *J. Anal. Toxicol.* **3**: 150.

Poupko, J.M., T. Radomski, R.M. Santella, and R.M. Radomski. 1983. Organ, species and compound specificity in the metabolic activation of primary aromatic amines. *J. Natl. Cancer Inst.* **70**: 1077.

COMMENTS

HOFFMANN: Curt Harris and I felt that this conference should bring us in the tobacco sciences closer to the biochemists and molecular biologists studying chemical carcinogenesis. In respect to the significance of aromatic amines in tobacco smoke and bladder carcinogenesis, I personally had rather ambiguous feelings. This is in part due to an influence by our epidemiologists who do not believe that the low concentrations in tobacco smoke of β-naphthylamine and other carcinogenic amines are significant in respect to the increased risk of cigarette smokers for bladder cancer. However, Doll has published a paper in which he compared the exposure to aromatic amines and the bladder cancer rates of British gas oven workers with those of cigarette smokers. He concluded that the aromatic amines in cigarette smoke may very well explain the increased risk of cigarette smokers for bladder cancer. Another exciting observation was made in a study by Terracini and his coworkers in Torino, Italy in collaboration with Bartsch's group. This study finds that long-term smokers of black cigarettes, rich in nitrate, have a significantly higher bladder cancer risk than those men who are long-term smokers of blond cigarettes, low in nitrate. We have clearly shown that the nitrate content of cigarette tobacco is the primary determinant for the smoke yields of aromatic amines. The higher the nitrate concentration of cigarette smoke, the higher the yield of aromatic amines in mainstream and sidestream smoke. Thus, it would be most desirable to study, with Tannenbaum's method, the yields of 4-aminobiphenyl adducts in the blood of smokers of black and of blond cigarettes.

BARTSCH: May I give some details? In this study, done in collaboration with Vineis, Terracini (Turin), and Malaveille, Estève (IARC), we were interested to see if smokers of black tobacco excrete more mutagens in the urine than those smoking blonde tobacco. Some preliminary results are available and this study is progressing well. So, if you need blood samples from these smokers, we could try to get them, after consultation with our colleagues.

TANNENBAUM: We should talk about this because I think that would be very interesting.

BRUNNEMANN: Steve [Tannenbaum], did you ever consider using this elegant method to verify or estimate cigarette smoke uptake in passive smokers also?

TANNENBAUM: The question is, where does the aminobiphenyl come from in nonsmokers. We are definitely going to do a passive smoking study, but there are other possible sources of aminobiphenyl in the environment. I should point out that our methodology cannot distinguish between exposure to amino aromatics and nitro aromatics. Nitrobiphenyl gives exactly the same adducts as aminobiphenyl. It goes through the same intermediate. Another question is whether nitrobiphenyl is present in cigarette smoke.

HOFFMANN: No, it is not. The burning zone of a cigarette is a reducing atmosphere. Thus, possibly formed nitroaromatic hydrocarbons would be reduced to the corresponding aromatic amines. Karam El-Bayoumy in our laboratory studied this in depth, and we failed to detect nitroaromatics in cigarette smoke (< 10 ng/cigarette).

CONNEY: It would be of great interest to see if the level and duration of adducts in a population of dogs given aminobiphenyl or in carefully matched cigarette smokers would be predictive of bladder cancer risk. Would the individuals with the largest amount of adduct be the ones that later develop bladder cancer?

TANNENBAUM: We and Fred Kalubar have been proposing to do that precise study in the dog, i.e., to try to characterize why some animals get tumors and other animals don't. With regard to your other comment, I think that would also be very interesting because we don't have enough data to really make a statement about the population. It's clear that some people have very high levels and others do not. At this point it does not appear to be related simply to the smoking behavior.

BELAND: In your animal experiment was the plateau dependent upon the concentration of the compound being administered?

TANNENBAUM: That plateau level is characteristic of the daily dose. There is an amplifying factor. If you vary the daily dose, then what you would get would be an amplification of the average daily dose over that period of time.

MAGEE: Is aminobiphenyl carcinogenic in the rat?

TANNENBAUM: Yes. Unfortunately there isn't enough dose-response information. There is a study in which dogs were dosed with 1 mg/kg per day, 5 days a week. That's the lowest dose I know. In 3 years they had a yield of 50% bladder tumors. It is a very potent bladder carcinogen in the dog.

HOFFMANN: Although studies with dogs were the first bioassays that induced bladder cancer with aromatic amines, such as β-naphthylamine, we are now in a position to induce bladder cancer with aromatic amines in Syrian golden hamsters within 2 years. Therefore, the less expensive hamster model should be preferred to the costly and time-consuming assay in dogs for examining the potential of chemicals to induce bladder cancer.

TANNENBAUM: We haven't done any carcinogenicity studies with hamsters.

BELAND: Fred Kadlubar and I have considered this. We are aware that the hamsters are good models and that they develop bladder tumors. We feel, however, that we will be able to measure more biological parameters using a larger experimental animal and we will be able to get bladder tumors in about 2-3 years.

CORREA: The association between bladder cancer and black tobacco is very interesting because the risk in smokers of light tobacco is two times greater than in nonsmokers, while in smokers of black tobacco it is about four times greater. Larynx cancer is also associated with black tobacco; so, it may be interesting to look at this in patients with larynx cancer because, for some reason, black tobacco plays a role in both bladder and larynx cancer.

PEGG: This may not be very important and may actually already be known, but is it not possible that in heavy smokers the half-life of the erythrocytes is actually somewhat different, which would affect your calculations?

TANNENBAUM: I don't know if it's known. If so, we've underestimated the results.

HALEY: In a study of several thousand smokers in Israel, it was noted that there were alterations in the numbers of erythrocytes and the median size of red cells in the circulation of heavy smokers.

BARTSCH: How does that fast and slow acetylator phenotype differ in your study?

TANNENBAUM: What we proposed to do, but which has become very difficult, is to look at the phenotype by looking at both albumin and hemoglobin. But nature is full of surprises, and we have a paper in press in which the albumin adduct has been characterized as a tryptophan adduct. Aminobiphenyl reacts with very exclusive sites on proteins. The only amino acid residue that it reacts with in albumin is the sole tryptophan in human albumin. The problem is that it reacts to give a compound in which there is a new ring system formed, so you no longer have either a tryptophan ring system or an aminobiphenyl ring system. We had set out to make antibodies to aminobiphenyl, which would be able to characterize this adduct.

ENZELL: With the technique you are using in detecting the aminobiphenyl adduct, it would be quite easy to detect other amines, too, wouldn't it?

TANNENBAUM: Yes.

ENZELL: If these are also bound to hemoglobin, can't you correlate them with the ones in smoke and see if there is a consistent pattern?

TANNENBAUM: Let me mention the ones that we have found in human hemoglobin, which we have shown are definitely not artifacts. Incidentally, that's a very important part of this work. A tremendous amount of the effort goes into showing that what you're measuring is characteristic of the blood sample and not of the analytical procedure.

ENZELL: Did you do this by the same monitoring technique?

TANNENBAUM: Yes.

BELAND: How did the level of Trp-P-1 compare to the level of 4-aminobiphenyl?

HOFFMANN: The smoke of a cigarette contains about 1-4 ng of 4-aminobiphenyl and, according to a Japanese study, 30-300 ng of the two 2-amino-α-carbolines.

PEGG: I think if you're going to be looking for some of these compounds in the urine of cases versus noncases, you would want to look at both cases of bladder cancer in smokers and nonsmokers, and probably also at other cancers, such as lung cancer or cervical cancer. It seems to be very hard to conceive that it's all going to be chemical-specific, or is it? I mean, are the sites going to be specific to particular agents?

HARRIS: Not necessarily, because there could be cofactors and cocarcinogens that can alter sites and in which under one condition you would have, perhaps, liver cancer and in another condition you'd have colon cancer. Data in experimental animals indicates that you can shift the site by altering the host. Another point is that the aromatic amines can be effectively metabolized by a variety of different types of human tissues, not only bladder epithelium. They could play some contribution to cancer at other sites in addition to bladder.

HOFFMANN: Yes, there are slow and fast acetylators among cigarette smokers. Despite the relatively low incidence rates of bladder cancer among cigarette smokers (10-30 per 100,000 per year), the difference between slow and fast acetylators in respect to the risk for bladder cancer is of great interest and importance. However, it will take many years of research before we will fully comprehend this aspect.

BELAND: If you look at the difference between slow and fast acetylators in relation to the incidence of bladder cancer, the difference is not all that great. In low-risk populations, 65% of the bladder cancer patients are slow acetylators, as opposed to 59% in the control population. When you talk about an acetylator phenotype, it is an operational definition. You are considering the ability of an individual to acetylate a particular type of amine. There may be considerable variation between various aromatic amines which may contribute to the observation that there is a relatively small difference between acetylator phenotype and bladder tumor induction in low-risk populations. However, when individuals are exposed to a very specific class of aromatic amines, significant differences may be found. This could explain why 23 out of 24 individuals who developed bladder cancer and worked in a dye manufacturing plant were slow acetylators.

HARRIS: We have a "mind set" that bladder cancer is caused only by aromatic amines. N-Nitrosamines and other compounds also cause bladder cancer in experimental animals. So it's very difficult to sort out the causative agents, especially when you have a complex mixture, such as tobacco smoke.

HOFFMANN: We have searched intensely in cigarette smoke for di-n-butylnitrosamine, which is a known bladder carcinogen in rats. So far, we have not detected this compound in tobacco smoke. The five tobacco-specific nitrosamines bioassayed to date were not carcinogenic to the bladder. However, at least two other compounds still need to be tested.

Analysis of Aniline and o-Toluidine in Human Urine

KARAM EL-BAYOUMY, JEAN DONAHUE, STEPHEN S. HECHT AND
DIETRICH HOFFMANN
Naylor Dana Institute for Disease Prevention
American Health Foundation
Valhalla, New York 10595

OVERVIEW

Cigarette smoking is associated with an increased risk for bladder cancer. Aromatic amines, which are known to be bladder carcinogens in experimental animals and humans, have been detected in cigarette smoke. The objective of this study was to quantify the levels of two aromatic amines, aniline and o-toluidine, in the urine of smokers. Using gas chromatography with electron capture detection and combined gas chromatography-mass spectrometry, aniline and o-toluidine were positively identified in the urine of smokers, in concentrations ranging from 0.8 to 11.2 μg/24 hr. They were also detected in nonsmokers' urine, up to 3.2 μg/24 hr. The results of this study provide new evidence on human exposure to aromatic amines.

INTRODUCTION

Epidemiologic studies of exposed workers in the dye, chemical, and rubber industries have established that aromatic amines, such as 2-naphthylamine and 4-aminobiphenyl, are known to cause bladder cancer in humans (Parkes and Evans 1984). Cigarette mainstream smoke and sidestream smoke contain aromatic amines (Schmeltz and Hoffmann 1977; Patrianakos and Hoffmann 1979). Concentrations of these compounds in mainstream smoke range from 1-2 ng/cigarette for 2-naphthylamine and 4-aminobiphenyl to 30-400 ng/cigarette for aniline and o-toluidine. Their levels in sidestream smoke are 20-40 times higher than in mainstream smoke (Patrianakos and Hoffmann 1979). According to the 1982 Report of the Surgeon General, between 30 and 40% of all bladder cancers in the United States are related to smoking (U.S. Department of Health and Human Services 1982). It is therefore plausible that the aromatic amines of cigarette smoke are important factors in the increased risk of smokers to develop bladder cancer. Nevertheless, little information is available on the concentrations of aromatic amines or their metabolites in the urine of smokers. We are aware of only one report: Connor et al. (1983) tentatively identified unspecified amounts of 2-naphthylamine and 2-amino-7-naphthol in a smoker's urine.

Since aniline and o-toluidine are present in cigarette smoke in higher concentrations than any of the other aromatic amines, we have focused on quantifying their levels in smokers' urine. They may be good indicators of aromatic amine exposure. o-Toluidine is carcinogenic in rats. When it is administered in the diet, it causes bladder tumors and fibroma of the skin and spleen, as well as mammary and peritoneal tumors (Weisburger et al. 1978; NIH 1979; Hecht et al. 1982). High levels of dietary aniline have been shown to cause spleen tumors in rats (NIH 1978). According to the International Agency for Research on Cancer, there is sufficient evidence for the carcinogenicity of o-toluidine in experimental animals, but limited evidence for aniline (IARC 1982).

The scheme for analysis of aniline and o-toluidine in human urine is summarized in Figure 1. In preliminary studies, we found that recoveries of parts per million amounts of underivatized o-toluidine from human urine were low. Therefore, a derivatizing agent, diethyl pyrocarbonate, was added to the urine collection bottles along with ethanol to inhibit bacterial growth and to increase solubility of the diethyl pyrocarbonate. Diethyl pyrocarbonate reacts with aromatic amines to give the corresponding carbamates. Urine was collected for 24 hours and [methyl-^{14}C]-o-toluidine (1.9×10^4 dpm, 180 ng) was added as an internal standard. After a brief incubation period to derivatize the internal standard, the urine was lyophil-

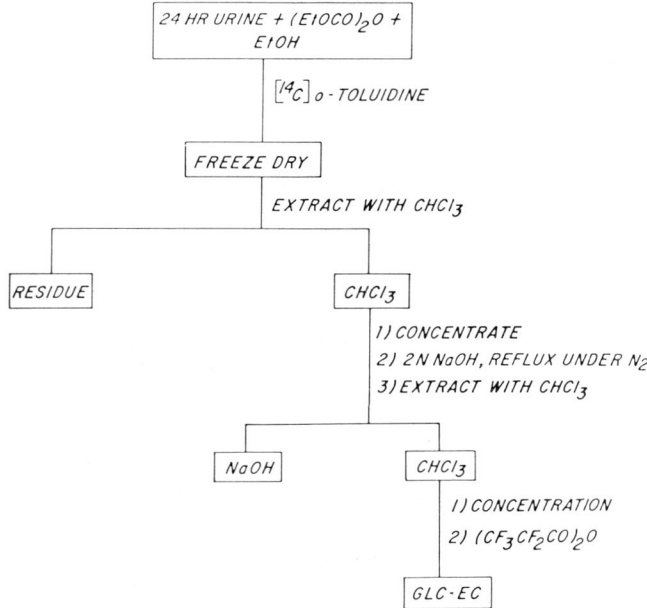

Figure 1
Analysis of aromatic amines in human urine

ized and the residue was extracted with $CHCl_3$. The $CHCl_3$ extracts were concentrated and the resulting material was heated under reflux, in an atmosphere of N_2, with aqueous NaOH. This procedure converted the carbamates back to the aromatic amines. The resulting mixture was extracted with $CHCl_3$. The extracts were concentrated and derivatized with pentafluoropropionic acid anhydride. This procedure is used to convert the aromatic amines to the corresponding pentafluoropropionamides, which are amenable to detection by capillary gas chromatography with an electron capture detector.

RESULTS

Figure 2 is a typical gas chromatogram of the derivatized aromatic amine fraction from a smoker's urine. Peaks corresponding in retention time to the pentafluoropropionamide derivatives of aniline and o-toluidine were observed as indicated. Electron capture detection of these compounds was extremely sensitive; 0.5 pg was readily detected. The aromatic amine fraction was then analyzed by combined gas chromatography-mass spectrometry with selected ion monitoring. The three major

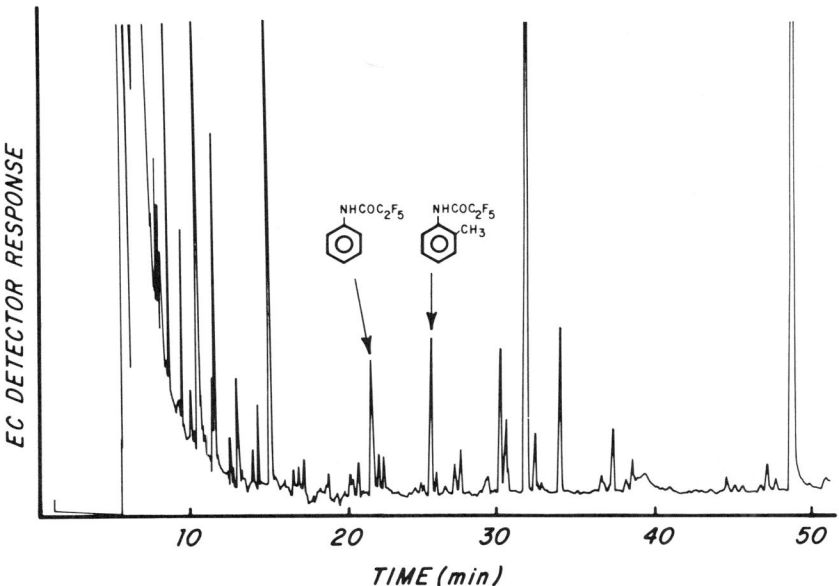

Figure 2
Gas chromatogram of aromatic amine fraction of a smoker's urine

peaks in the mass spectra of the pentafluoropropionamide derivatives of aniline and o-toluidine are the molecular ions, and the peaks due to loss of C_2F_5 and loss of $NHCOC_2F_5$. These are m/e 239, 120, and 77 for aniline and 253, 134, and 91 for o-toluidine. Selected ion monitoring demonstrated that these three ions were present only at the correct gas chromatographic retention times of aniline and o-toluidine. Further confirmation of the identities of aniline and o-toluidine was obtained from their chemical ionization mass spectra (Figs. 3 and 4).

Analyses of 24-hr urine samples from nonsmokers were also performed. Peaks corresponding in retention time to aniline and o-toluidine were observed. These peaks were not detected in an H_2O blank.

Table 1 summarizes the results of the analyses carried out on smokers. Levels of aniline and o-toluidine ranged from 0.8 to 11.2 µg/24 hr urine sample from smokers. Levels varied widely on different days for the same subject, smoking the same number of cigarettes. Amounts of aniline and o-toluidine in the urine of nonsmokers are summarized in Table 2. Recoveries of internal standard in these analyses were generally in the range of 30-50%.

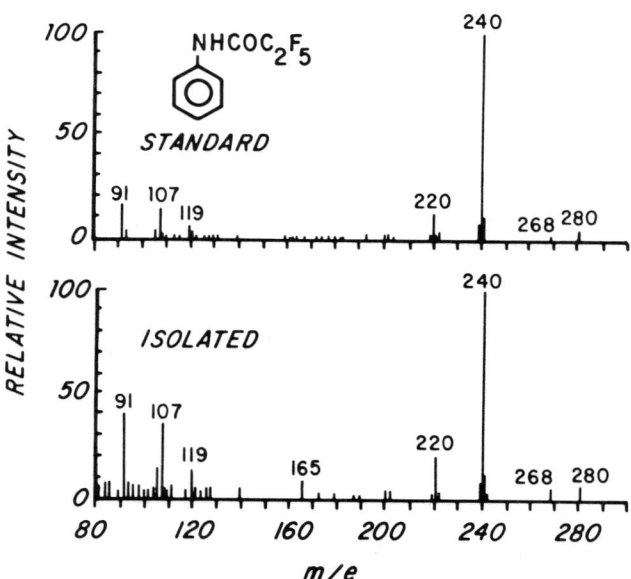

Figure 3
Mass spectra of pentafluoropropionamide derivative of aniline. (*Top panel*) Standard; (*bottom panel*) isolated from a smoker's urine.

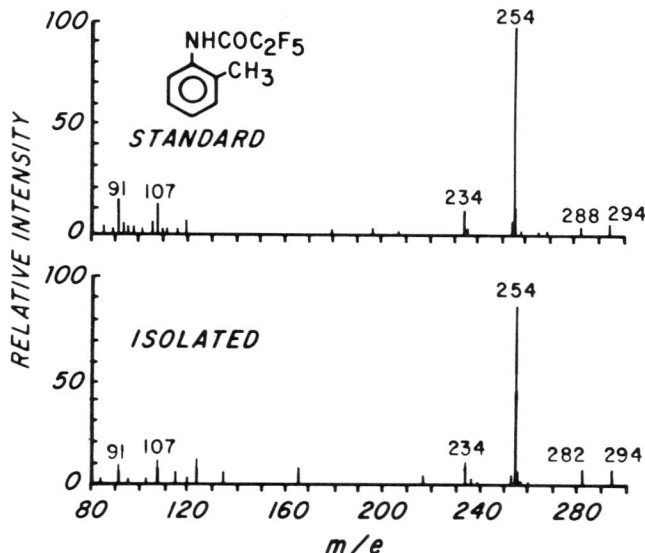

Figure 4
Mass spectra of pentafluoropropionamide derivative of o-toluidine. (*Top panel*) Standard; (*bottom panel*) isolated from a smoker's urine.

Table 1
Aniline and o-Toluidine in Smokers' Urine

Smoker	Day	Number of cigarettes	μg/24 hr Aniline	o-Toluidine
1	1	40	4.0	5.7
	2	40	4.8	11.2
	3	40	2.6	6.2
			3.7 ± 1.1	7.7 ± 3.1
2	1	20	1.1	6.1
	2	20	0.8	11.2
	3	20	8.8	8.4
			3.6 ± 4.5	8.6 ± 2.5
3	1	20	2.2	2.6
	2	20	0.8	3.5
	3	20	1.4	1.4
			1.5 ± 0.7	2.5 ± 1.1

Table 2
Aniline and o-Toluidine in Nonsmokers' Urine

Nonsmoker	Day	μg/24 hr	
		Aniline	o-Toluidine
1	1	0.02	—
	2	0.3	0.3
2	1	3.4	3.1
	2	2.7	2.0
3	1	7.8	3.1
4	1	4.9	5.1

DISCUSSION

These results demonstrate that aniline and o-toluidine are present in the urine of smokers as well as nonsmokers. Their levels in smokers' urine were higher than we expected. Assuming that the mainstream smoke of a cigarette contains 100 ng of either aniline or o-toluidine, their intake from 20 cigarettes should be about 2 μg each. Metabolism studies have shown that in mammalian systems, aniline and o-toluidine are extensively converted to conjugates of their ring-hydroxylated derivatives (Parke 1960; Son et al. 1980). If 10% were excreted unchanged, we would expect levels of approximately 0.2 μg in the 24-hr urine of smokers. Instead, concentrations of aniline and o-toluidine ranged from 0.8 to 11.2 μg/24 hr, 4–56 times higher than expected. One possible explanation for the differences between observed and expected levels is that machine smoking does not accurately reflect human smoking behavior. Differences between machine smoking estimates of uptake and actual uptake are well known for nicotine and related smoke components (N.J. Haley et al., this volume). However, these differences alone are unlikely to account for our results. It is more likely that there are additional sources of exposure to aniline and o-toluidine. One possible source is sidestream smoke. Reported amounts of aniline and o-toluidine in sidestream smoke are 10 μg and 3 μg per cigarette, respectively (Patrianakos and Hoffmann 1979).

However, the relatively high levels of aniline and o-toluidine in nonsmokers' urine indicate that there are other important sources of exposure to aniline and o-toluidine or their precursors. Aniline and o-toluidine are major industrial chemicals, and they have been detected in surface water samples from rivers. The presence of aniline in drinking water has been reported. Limited information on their presence in air pollution seems to be available, but o-toluidine was present in the air of an o-toluidine manufacturing plant (Hoffmann and Wynder 1977; IARC 1982). Aniline has been detected in ppm quantities in a variety of vegetables, including cauliflower, carrots, and celery, as well as in maize, rhubarb, and apples (Neurath et al. 1977). Aniline and o-toluidine have been identified in the volatile aroma compounds of black tea (Vitzthum et al. 1975). Limited information seems to be available on levels of aromatic amines in cooked foods (Committee on Diet, Nutrition, and Cancer 1982; Grasso 1984), but aniline is a common constituent observed in pyrolysis studies of amino acids and proteins (Chortyk and Schlotzhauer 1973; Mabrouk 1976) and its presence in broiled foods would be expected.

Endogenous formation of aniline or o-toluidine could occur from anthranilic acid or related metabolites of tryptophan. Other potential metabolic precursors to aniline and o-toluidine include azo-dyes used in food coloring or related products, and nitrobenzenes, which are known constituents of cigarette smoke and may also be present in the general environment (Hoffmann and Rathkamp 1970; Schuetzle 1983). Further studies using subjects on controlled diets are necessary to assess the role of these various factors in contributing to urinary aromatic amines.

SUMMARY

Aniline and o-toluidine were positively identified in the urine of smokers. Their levels ranged from 0.8 to 11.2 μg/24 hr. They were also detected in the urine of nonsmokers. The levels of aniline and o-toluidine in smokers' urine were higher than expected based on machine smoking measurements, and their presence in nonsmokers' urine indicates that exposures other than tobacco smoke contribute to urinary aromatic amines. The method developed for this study should be widely applicable for analysis of aromatic amines in urine.

REFERENCES

Chortyk, O.T. and W.S. Schlotzhauer. 1973. Studies on the pyrogenesis of tobacco smoke constituents (a review). *Beitr. Tabakforsch.* **7**: 165.

Committee on Diet, Nutrition, and Cancer. 1982. *Diet, nutrition, and cancer*, chapt. 13. National Academy Press, Washington, D.C.

Connor, T.H., V.M. Sadagopa Ramanujan, J.B. Ward, Jr., and M.S. Legator. 1983. The identification and characterization of a urinary mutagen resulting from cigarette smoke. *Mutation Res.* **133**: 161.

Grasso, P. 1984. Carcinogens in food. In *Chemical carcinogens, second edition* (ed. C.E. Searle) p. 1205. American Chemical Society, Washington, D.C.

Hecht, S.S., K. El-Bayoumy, A. Rivenson, and E. Fiala. 1982. Comparative carcinogenicity of o-toluidine hydrochloride and o-nitrosotoluene in F344 rats. *Cancer Lett.* **16**: 103.

Hoffmann, D. and G. Rathkamp. 1970. Quantitative determination of nitrobenzenes in cigarette smoke. *Anal. Chem.* **42**: 1643.

Hoffmann, D. and E.L. Wynder. 1977. Organic particulate pollutants—Chemical analysis and bioassays for carcinogenicity. In *Air pollution*, third edition (ed. A. Stern), p. 361. Academic Press, New York.

International Agency for Research on Cancer. 1982. *IARC Monographs on the evaluation of the carcinogenic risk of chemicals to humans. Some aromatic amines, anthraquinones and nitroso compounds, and inorganic fluorides used in drinking-water and dental preparations*, vol. 27, p. 39. IARC, Lyon, France.

Mabrouk, A.F. 1976. Non-volatile nitrogen and sulfur compounds in red meats and their relation to flavor and taste. In *Phenolic, sulfur, and nitrogen compounds in food flavors* (ed. G. Charalambus and I. Katz), p. 146. American Chemical Society, Washington, D.C.

National Cancer Institute Carcinogenesis Technical Report Series No. 130, (NIH). 1978. *Bioassay of aniline hydrochloride for possible carcinogenicity*. DHEW Publication No. (NIH) 78-1385. Washington, D.C.

National Cancer Institute Carcinogenesis Technical Report Series No. 153, (NIH). 1979. *Bioassay of o-toluidine hydrochloride for possible carcinogenicity*. DHEW Publication No. (NIH) 79-1709. Washington, D.C.

Neurath, G.B., M. Dünger, F.G. Pein, D. Ambrosius, and O. Schreiber. 1977. Primary and secondary amines in the human environment. *Food Cosmet. Toxicol.* **15**: 275.

Parke, D.V. 1960. Studies in detoxication: 84. The metabolism of [^{14}C] aniline in the rabbit and other animals. *Biochem. J.* **77**: 493.

Parkes, H.G. and A.E.J. Evans. 1984. Epidemiology of aromatic amine cancers. In *Chemical carcinogens*, second edition (ed. C.E. Searle), p. 277. American Chemical Society, Washington, D.C.

Patrianakos, C. and D. Hoffmann. 1979. On the analysis of aromatic amines in cigarette smoke. *J. Anal. Toxicol.* **3**: 150.

Schmeltz, I. and D. Hoffmann. 1977. Nitrogen-containing compounds in tobacco and tobacco smoke. *Chem. Rev.* **77**: 295.

Schuetzle, D. 1983. Sampling of vehicle emissions for chemical analysis and biological testing. *Environ. Health Perspect.* **47**: 65.

Son, O.S., D.W. Everett, and E.S. Fiala. 1980. Metabolism of o-[methyl-^{14}C]-toluidine in the F344 rat. *Xenobiotica* **10**: 457.

U.S. Department of Health and Human Services. 1982. *The health consequences of smoking: Cancer. A report of the surgeon general*, p. vii. U.S. Government Printing Office, Washington, D.C.

Vitzthum, O.G., P. Werkhoff, and P. Hubert. 1975. New volatile constituents of black tea aroma. *J. Agric. Food Chem.* **23**: 999.

Weisburger, E.K., A.B. Russfield, F. Homburger, J.H. Weisburger, E. Boger, C.G. Van Dongen, and K.C. Chu. 1978. Testing of twenty-one environmental aromatic amines or derivatives for long-term toxicity or carcinogenicity. *J. Environ. Pathol. Toxicol.* **2**: 325.

^{32}P-Postlabeling Test for Smoking-related DNA Adducts in Animal and Human Tissues

KURT RANDERATH,* M. VIJAYARAJ REDDY,* TOMMIE A. AVITTS,*
ROBERT H. MILLER,† RICHARD B. EVERSON,** AND ERIKA
RANDERATH*
*Department of Pharmacology
†Department of Otorhinolaryngology
Baylor College of Medicine
Houston, Texas 77030
**Epidemiology Branch, Biometry and Risk Assessment Program
National Institute of Environmental Health Sciences
Research Triangle Park, North Carolina 27709

OVERVIEW

Environmental exposure to DNA-reactive (mutagenic/carcinogenic) chemicals can be measured by a newly developed ^{32}P-postlabeling assay (Randerath et al. 1981; Gupta et al. 1982; Reddy et al. 1984). Radiolabel (^{32}P) is incorporated into mononucleotides in enzymatic digests of adducted DNA by enzymatic [^{32}P]-phosphate transfer from (γ-^{32}P]ATP; then the ^{32}P-labeled adducts are separated by thin-layer chromatography and detected by autoradiography. The assay responds to low levels of DNA damage (one adduct in 10^8–10^{10} DNA nucleotides) and has been applied to a total of ~100 chemical carcinogens. As reported here, the test enables one to fingerprint altered DNA nucleotides in tissues of experimental animals and humans exposed to crude environmental mixtures containing DNA-reactive chemicals, such as components of tobacco smoke. The ^{32}P-postlabeling test holds promise as a tool for the detection and identification of chemical agents that most severely damage human DNA.

INTRODUCTION

A large number of (but not all) chemical carcinogens can be categorized as electrophilic, DNA-reactive agents, i.e., such chemicals or their metabolites are capable of forming covalent bonds with nucleophilic centers in DNA (O-, N-, and C-atoms) (Miller and Miller 1981; Hemminki 1983; Reddy et al. 1984). The formation of such DNA adducts in vivo is generally regarded to be a key element in the initiation of chemical carcinogenesis. Unless the adducted DNA nucleotides are promptly repaired, miscoding may ensue upon DNA replication, leading to point mutations, activation of oncogenes, and chromosomal alterations (Farber 1984). The human environment contains a great (and increasing) number of genotoxic chemicals, only a fraction of which have been identified to date. Since genotoxic chemicals may be of natural or man-made origin and may be present in air, water, or food, exposure to them cannot be completely eliminated. It appears prudent, however, to minimize human contact with chemicals that may alter DNA readouts in somatic and reproductive tissues. A number of powerful short-term in vitro tests have been developed recently to detect genotoxic activity of chemicals (Ames 1979; De Serres and Ashby 1981; Stich and San 1981). However, since the fate of a chemical in the intact mammalian organism in vivo is the result of a delicate balance of pharmacokinetic and metabolic effects, such assays do not accurately reflect the potential genotoxic activity of chemicals in intact animals or humans. Therefore, tests are needed that allow one to measure this property directly in vivo.

The determination of DNA adduct levels in humans may potentially serve three purposes:

1. The estimation of exposure of target tissue DNA to potentially carcinogenic and mutagenic agents, i.e., for environmental monitoring. Data may relate to exposure patterns and can be used to reduce exposure. Adduct levels may also reflect interindividual differences, which may underlie susceptibility to cancer or other adverse effects.
2. The design of cancer chemotherapy. It appears possible to define interindividual differences in DNA adduction by alkylating agents. This may be important for designing more efficacious and less toxic cancer treatment regimens.
3. The identification of potentially mutagenic and carcinogenic components in complex mixtures. Work in progress to detect and identify the products of tobacco smoke leading to DNA adducts will be presented in this paper.

RESULTS

^{32}P-Postlabeling Assay for DNA Adducts

The basic features of the ^{32}P-postlabeling assay (Randerath et al. 1981; Gupta et al. 1982; Reddy et al. 1984) are illustrated in Figure 1. The DNA to be tested for the presence of covalent carcinogen/mutagen adducts is first digested enzymatically to deoxyribonucleoside 3′-monophosphates of normal and (if present) adducted nucleotides. The digestion products are subsequently converted to 5′-^{32}P-labeled deoxyribonucleoside 3′,5′-bisphosphates via incubation with [γ-^{32}P]ATP and T4 polynucleotide kinase. The radiolabeled reaction products are resolved by thin-layer chromatography into individual normal and adducted nucleotides and detected by autoradiography utilizing high-speed x-ray film (e.g., Kodak XAR) and efficient intensifying screens (e.g., du Pont Lightning Plus). For quantitation, spots of ^{32}P-labeled normal and adducted nucleotides are excised from the chromatograms and evaluated by scintillation (Cerenkov) assay. The ratio of count rates of adduct(s) to count rates of normal nucleotides (with appropriate correction for the

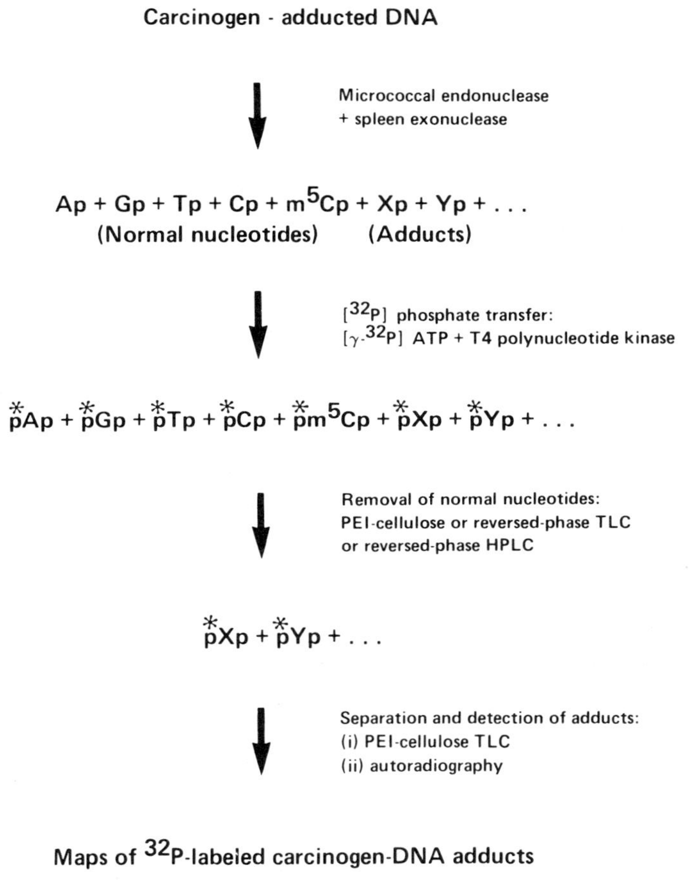

Carcinogen - adducted DNA

↓ Micrococcal endonuclease + spleen exonuclease

Ap + Gp + Tp + Cp + m^{5}Cp + Xp + Yp + ...
(Normal nucleotides)   (Adducts)

↓ [^{32}P] phosphate transfer:
[γ-^{32}P] ATP + T4 polynucleotide kinase

$\overset{*}{p}$Ap + $\overset{*}{p}$Gp + $\overset{*}{p}$Tp + $\overset{*}{p}$Cp + $\overset{*}{p}$m^{5}Cp + $\overset{*}{p}$Xp + $\overset{*}{p}$Yp + ...

↓ Removal of normal nucleotides:
PEI-cellulose or reversed-phase TLC
or reversed-phase HPLC

$\overset{*}{p}$Xp + $\overset{*}{p}$Yp + ...

↓ Separation and detection of adducts:
(i) PEI-cellulose TLC
(ii) autoradiography

Maps of ^{32}P-labeled carcinogen-DNA adducts

Figure 1
^{32}P-Postlabeling assay for carcinogen-adducted DNA involves four steps: Digestion of DNA, ^{32}P-labeling of the digestion products, removal of ^{32}P-labeled nonadduct components, and TLC mapping of the [^{32}P] adducts.

dilution of the normal nucleotides for chromatographic analysis) is calculated and defined as a relative adduct labeling (= RAL) value. The data are given in RAL x 10^7 units: These represent the number of adducts in 10^7 DNA nucleotides and may be converted to pmole adduct/mg DNA values by multiplication with 0.3. In the standard version of the procedure (Randerath et al. 1981; Gupta et al. 1982), an excess of [γ-^{32}P] ATP over the substrate nucleotides to be labeled is employed, while in a modified (adduct intensification) version (Randerath et al. 1985a), [γ-^{32}P] ATP is deficient relative to substrate. This results in the preferential labeling of many adducts and affords a considerably greater sensitivity of the overall procedure, especially if carrier-free [γ-^{32}P] ATP (9120 Ci/mmole) is used as donor of the label.

For the ^{32}P-postlabeling scheme to serve as a test for the capacity of chemicals to bind covalently to DNA, it must be applicable to many genotoxic chemicals. Thus, a major question to be answered during the development of the method was whether it could be applied to a large number of DNA adducts of diverse structure (Reddy et al. 1984; Randerath et al. 1985b). A total of ~100 test compounds comprising arylamines and derivatives, azo compounds, nitroaromatics, polycyclic aromatic hydrocarbons, methylating agents (Reddy et al. 1984), heterocyclic polycyclic aromatics (Schurdak and Randerath 1985), estrogens (Liehr et al. 1985, 1986), and mycotoxins (Reddy et al. 1985) were studied. In every case, ^{32}P-labeling of carcinogen-DNA derivatives was readily detected.

An important part of the analytical procedure is the separation of adducts from the (usually large) excess of normal DNA nucleotides. This is conveniently done by anion-exchange TLC on PEI-cellulose (Gupta et al. 1982; Reddy et al. 1984) and is particularly successful with carcinogens having 2-6 aromatic rings. In the case of less aromatic carcinogens (such as alkenylbenzenes, sterigmatocystin, aflatoxin B_1, and mitomycin C), removal of normal nucleotides is preferably accomplished by C18 reversed-phase TLC (Randerath et al. 1984).

Although the ^{32}P-postlabeling assay has been applied to date mainly in studies of the formation (Gupta et al. 1982; Randerath et al. 1983, 1984; Reddy et al. 1984; Schurdak and Randerath 1985) and persistence (Randerath et al. 1983, 1985a; Phillips et al. 1984; Reddy et al. 1985) of DNA adducts formed in tissues of experimental animals exposed to authentic genotoxic chemicals (for examples, see Figs. 2 and 3), its utility in the detection of DNA damage from unknown DNA-reactive substances has now become clear. For example, use of the assay has demonstrated that various carcinogenic estrogens, during renal carcinogenesis in the Syrian hamster (Kirkman 1959), do not give rise to adducts containing estrogen moieties in kidney DNA, but rather induce the organ-specific formation of an unknown endogenous DNA-reactive compound (or compounds) in target tissue (Liehr et al. 1985, 1986).

^{32}P-Postlabeling Assay of Cigarette Smoke Condensate-induced DNA Adducts in Mouse Skin

Tobacco smoke contains several thousand chemicals, including many identified genotoxic, mutagenic, or carcinogenic compounds (U.S. Department of Health and Human Services 1982; Hoffmann and Hecht 1985; Loeb et al. 1984). It is not clear which of these compounds are primarily responsible for human carcinogenesis, thus it is important to identify compounds in this complex mixture that are capable of binding to the DNA of experimental animals and humans in vivo. It was of interest,

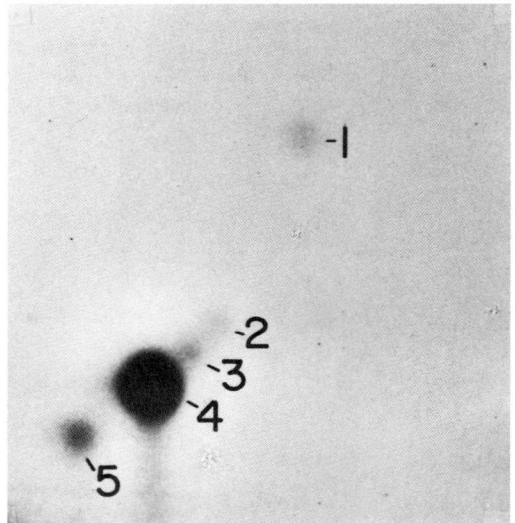

Figure 2
PEI-cellulose map of benzo[a]pyrene-induced DNA adducts in mouse skin. Skin DNA was isolated 24 hr after the last of four topical applications of benzo[a]pyrene (1.2 μmole/200 μl acetone each, given at 0, 6, 30, and 54 hr). Labeled digest of DNA (0.17 μg) was prepared according to the scheme shown in Figure 1 under standard labeling conditions (Reddy et al. 1984). Labeled adducts were separated on a PEI-cellulose thin layer in two directions in 3.5 M Li formate, 7 M urea, pH 3.5 (from bottom to top), and in 0.8 M LiCl, 0.5 M Tris HCl, 8.5 M urea, pH 8.0 (from left to right), and located by screen-enhanced autoradiography for 1.5 days at $-80°C$. Adduct spots are numbered 1–5. The major adduct (4) is the reaction product of (+)antiBPDE with N^2 of guanine.

therefore, to apply the ^{32}P-postlabeling assay to DNA of experimental animals exposed to cigarette smoke condensate (CSC).

^{32}P-Fingerprints of DNA adducts induced in mouse skin by topical treatment with CSC are shown in Figure 4. The condensate, which was prepared by collecting smoke from burning cigarettes in vacuo at $-80°C$, followed by acetone/ether extraction, was applied to the shaved backs of female ICR mice. One hundred μl of condensate, diluted with acetone and corresponding to 0.75 cigarette, was given each on day 1 and day 2 and 200 μl each of condensate was given on days 3–7. Mice were sacrificed on days 4 and 8 after having received condensate equivalent to a total of three and nine cigarettes, respectively (Fig. 4b and c). Control mice (Fig. 4a) were treated with acetone. DNA (4 μg) extracted from skin was analyzed by ^{32}P-postlabeling assay under adduct intensification conditions (Randerath et al. 1985a).

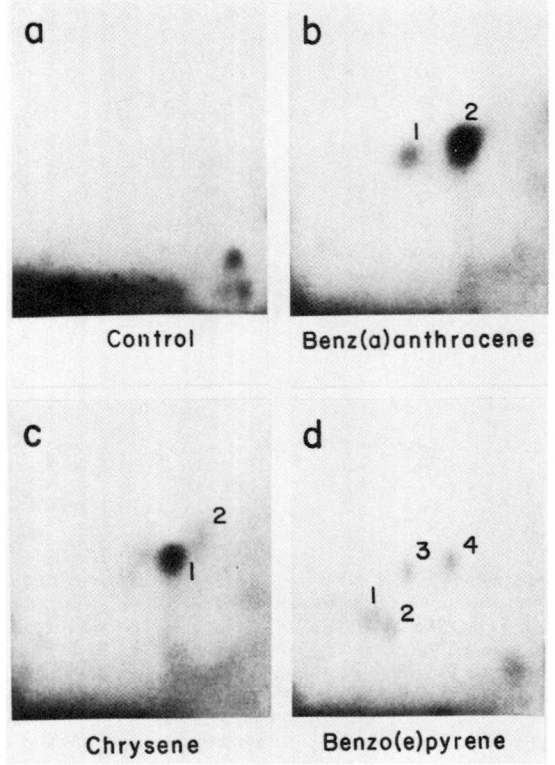

Figure 3
PEI-cellulose maps of DNA adducts induced in mouse skin by benz[a]anthracene, chrysene, and benzo(e)pyrene, respectively. Treatment with the polycyclic aromatic hydrocarbons was as described in the legend to Figure 2. Control mice (a) received acetone. Labeled digest of DNA (3 μg) was prepared by an adduct enrichment procedure (K. Randerath et al., in prep.) involving the removal before labeling of nonadduct components from the DNA digests by reversed-phase (C18) chromatography and the use of carrier-free $[\gamma-^{32}P]$ATP. Labeled adducts were separated as described in the legend for Figure 2, except that 8.5 M urea was used in the acidic solvent. Screen-enhanced autoradiography was performed for 3 hr at $-80°C$. Adduct spots are indicated by numbering.

A comparison of the fingerprints derived from CSC-exposed DNA (b and c) with a map of labeled digest from unexposed control DNA (a) showed several adducts that accumulated during treatment. While exposure to condensate from three cigarettes for 4 days induced one major adduct (1) and several minor adducts (2-5), DNA from skin exposed to nine cigarettes for 8 days had three additional major adducts (7-9) and one additional minor adduct (6). A diagonal radioactive

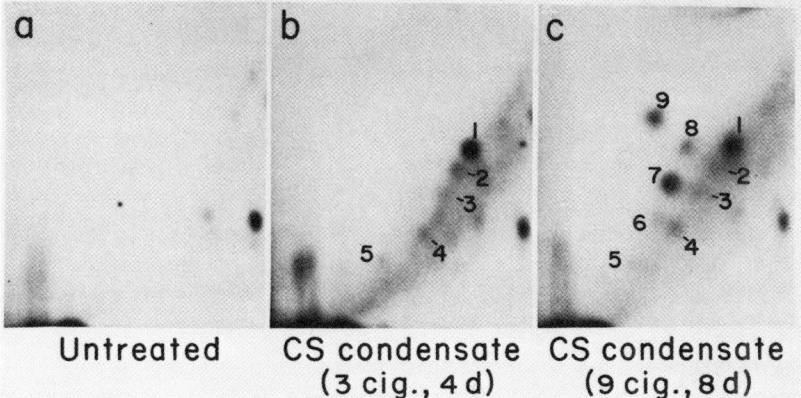

Figure 4
PEI-cellulose maps of CSC-induced DNA adducts in mouse skin. (*a*) Labeled digest of mouse skin DNA exposed to acetone only; (*b* and *c*) labeled DNA digests derived from CSC-treated skin. Labeled digests of DNA (4 μg) were prepared according to the scheme shown in Figure 1 under adduct intensification conditions (Randerath et al. 1985a). Labeled adducts were separated in two directions on PEI-cellulose thin layers in 4.2 M Li formate, 7.5 M urea, pH 3.5 (from bottom to top), and in 0.8 M LiCl, 0.5 M Tris HCl, 8.5 M urea, pH 8.0 (from left to right), and located by screen-enhanced autoradiography for 4.5 days at −80°C. The control sample exhibited several background spots that were also present on the other autoradiograms. Adduct spots are indicated by numbering.

zone, which was not seen for control DNA and increased with the duration of exposure, appeared to be derived, also, from damaged DNA. In view of the presence of numerous compounds in tobacco smoke known to cause cancer in animal bioassays, at least part of this radioactive material probably represented low levels of additional adducts.

All the adducts noted on the fingerprints were presumably derivatives of aromatic or bulky unsaturated compounds due to the selectivity of the chromatographic procedure used. In an attempt to identify adduct 1, CSC-exposed DNA was mixed with test DNA preparations containing known aromatic carcinogen-DNA adducts and then subjected to ^{32}P-postlabeling assay. The test DNAs were isolated from the skin or livers of mice treated with the compound of interest. In these experiments, adduct 1 did not appear to be related to several aromatic genotoxic chemicals known to occur in cigarette smoke: benzo[*a*]pyrene, benz[*a*]anthracene, dibenz[*ah*]anthracene, pyrene, chrysene, fluoranthene, benzo[*ghi*]perylene, 4-aminobiphenyl, β-naphthylamine, or certain nicotine-derived tobacco-specific *N*-nitrosamines. However, one of the benz[*a*]anthracene- and one of the chrysene-DNA adducts cochromatographed with spot 7 (Fig. 4c). None of the radioactive adducts shown in Figure 4c comigrated with the major benzo[a]pyrene DNA adduct (Fig.2), i.e., the reaction product of (+) antiBPDE with N^2 of guanine.

^{32}P-Postlabeling Assay of DNA Adducts in Tissues of Smokers

^{32}P-Fingerprints of labeled DNA digests from placentas (Everson et al. 1985) and bronchi (K. Randerath et al., unpubl.) of smokers and nonsmokers are shown in Figure 5. Placentas were obtained at delivery and bronchi were autopsy specimens.

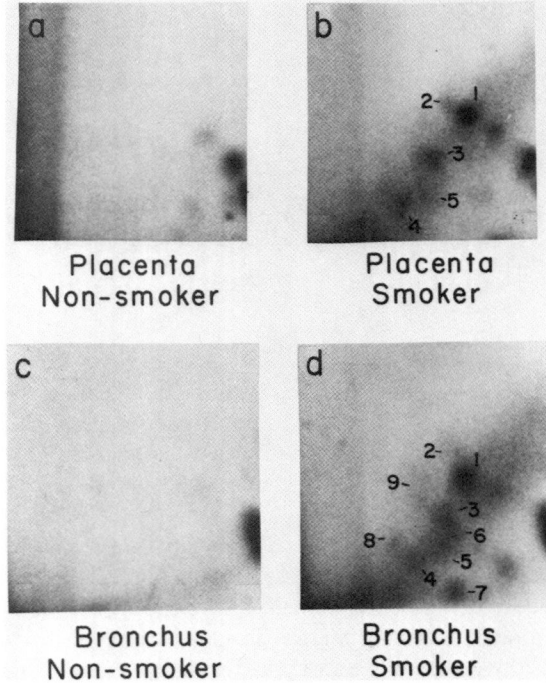

Figure 5
PEI-cellulose maps of labeled DNA digests derived from placental and bronchial tissue of smokers and nonsmokers. For details of the procedure, see legend to Figure 4. Labeled adducts were separated in 3.6 M Li formate, 6.4 M urea, pH 3.5 (from bottom to top), and 0.6 M LiCl, 0.37 M Tris HCl, 6.4 M urea, pH 8.0 (from left to right). The control sample exhibited several background spots that were also present on the adduct maps. Adduct spots are numbered *1-5* (*b*) and *1-9* (*d*). The spot to the lower right of adduct *1* (*b* and *d*) may contain an adduct cochromatographing with a background spot (Everson et al. 1985).

Tissues were kept at −80°C until DNA extraction. DNA was assayed by the same procedure as CSC-exposed DNA.

Comparison of *a* and *b* in Figure 5 revealed several labeled DNA adducts (1-5) in a smoker's placenta that were not seen in placental DNA from a nonsmoker. Similarly, adducts (*d*, adducts 1-9) were only present in bronchial DNA from a smoker, but not from a nonsmoker (*c*). Interestingly, a diagonal radioactive zone was again seen in DNA samples from exposed tissues (*b* and *d*), but not from unexposed tissues (*a* and *c*), indicating that this diffuse radioactivity might reflect DNA damage. Smokers' placental and bronchial DNAs had adducts 1-5 in common. The additional adducts present in bronchial DNA may be due to the direct exposure to cigarette smoke. Adduct 1 was found to be strongly related to maternal smoking during pregnancy: It was present in placental DNA from 29 of 30 smokers and was not found in placental DNA from 21 of 24 nonsmokers (Everson et al. 1985 and unpubl.). Of the three nonsmokers, who exhibited a very weak adduct 1 spot, two were passive smokers. Furthermore, adduct 1 was also found in the DNA of a number of other tissues from smokers, such as lung parenchyma, aryepiglottic fold, and tonsils, but was not detectable in DNA of corresponding tissues from nonsmokers (K. Randerath et al., unpubl.). Its level in the placental sample (b) was estimated to be one adduct in $> 10^8$ nucleotides. Cochromatography experiments revealed adduct 1 from smokers' tissues to be identical with adduct 1 from DNA of CSC-exposed mouse skin (K. Randerath et al., unpubl.). Experiments are now under way to identify adduct 1 by using CSC fractions for DNA adduction in mouse skin and analyzing the resultant adducts by ^{32}P-post-labeling assay.

DISCUSSION

Evidence was presented that the ^{32}P-postlabeling assay, originally developed for the analysis of DNA adducts of pure carcinogens (Randerath et al. 1981), is suitable, also, for the detection of genotoxic activity of components of crude environmental mixtures, such as cigarette smoke or its condensate. The assay was found to be applicable to DNA from exposed experimental animals and humans. In the case of tissue DNA from smokers, the assay yielded an unexpected result, i.e., the detection of a single major adduct (adduct 1) in these samples. The chromatographic behavior of this compound suggested an aromatic adduct which, however, did not seem derived from several known polycyclic aromatic hydrocarbons or aromatic amines. More specifically, adduct 1 did not correspond to the DNA adducts obtained from the administration of these carcinogens to mouse skin. Further experiments are necessary to determine which component (or components) of cigarette smoke is responsible for this DNA lesion. Our observation that adduct 1 seemed to be formed also as a major adduct in mouse skin DNA treated in vivo with CSC is currently exploited in attempts to purify and characterize the responsible parent compound. The ^{32}P-postlabeling assay will be a principal tool in these experiments.

Additional experiments (Everson et al. 1985) indicated that, among smokers, placental adduct 1 was related only weakly to the intensity of smoking exposure, as measured by questionnaire and biochemical data. This may have been due to modulation of adduct levels by individual susceptibility factors (Omenn and Gelboin 1984). These observations suggest that the ^{32}P-postlabeling assay may be suitable for monitoring of human exposure to tobacco smoke (and possibly other environmental agents) at the level of the individual and thus contribute to the assessment of risk in relation to individual differences in susceptibility to environmental chemicals.

SUMMARY

A recently developed highly sensitive ^{32}P-postlabeling assay enables the detection and quantitation of DNA adducts in experimental animals and humans exposed to pure genotoxic chemicals or mixtures of such compounds. When this assay was applied to DNA of tissues of smokers and to mouse skin DNA after topical treatment with cigarette smoke condensate, several adducts were detected. One of these (adduct 1) was one major smoking-associated aromatic adduct in human tissues. Mouse skin DNA exposed in vivo to cigarette smoke condensate also gave adduct 1 as a predominant modified nucleotide. Preliminary experiments have thus far excluded several polycyclic aromatic hydrocarbons and aromatic amines known to occur in tobacco smoke as the source of adduct 1.

ACKNOWLEDGMENTS

This work was made possible by grants from USPHS, National Cancer Institute (CA 13591, CA 32157, CA 10893 (P6)), and an Occupational and Environmental Health Grant from du Pont Chemical Company.

REFERENCES

Ames, B.N. 1979. Identifying environmental chemicals causing mutations and cancer. *Science* **204**: 587.

De Serres, F.J. and J. Ashby. 1981. *Evaluation of short-term tests for carcinogens: Report of the international collaborative program.* Elsevier, New York.

Everson, R.B., E. Randerath, R.M. Santella, R.C. Cefalo, T.A. Avitts, and K. Randerath. 1986. Detection of smoking-related covalent DNA adducts in human placenta. *Science* **231**: 54.

Farber, E. 1984. The multistep nature of cancer development. *Cancer Res.* **44**: 4217.

Gupta, R.C., M.V. Reddy, and K. Randerath. 1982. ^{32}P-Postlabeling analysis of non-radioactive aromatic carcinogen-DNA adducts. *Carcinogenesis* **3**: 1081.

Hemminki, K. 1983. Nucleic acid adducts of chemical carcinogens and mutagens. *Arch. Toxicol.* **52**: 249.

Hoffmann, D. and S.S. Hecht. 1985. Nicotine-derived N-nitrosamines and tobacco-related cancer: Current status and future directions. *Cancer Res.* **45**: 935.

Kirkman, H. 1959. *Estrogen-induced tumors of the kidney in the Syrian hamster. Natl. Cancer Inst. Monogr.* **1**.

Liehr, J.G., K. Randerath, and E. Randerath. 1985. Target organ-specific covalent DNA damage preceding diethylstilbestrol-induced carcinogenesis. *Carcinogenesis* **6**: 1067.

Liehr, J.G., T.A. Avitts, E. Randerath, and K. Randerath. 1986. Estrogen-induced endogenous DNA adduction: A novel possible mechanism of hormonal cancer. *Proc. Natl. Acad. Sci. U.S.A.* (in press).

Loeb, L.A., V.L. Ernster, K.E. Warner, J. Abbotts, and J. Laszlo. 1984. Smoking and lung cancer: An overview. *Cancer Res.* **44**: 5940.

Miller, E.C. and J.A. Miller. 1981. Searches for ultimate chemical carcinogens and their reactions with cellular macromolecules. *Cancer* **47**: 2327.

Omenn, G.S. and H.V. Gelboin (eds.). 1984. *Banbury report 16: Genetic variability in responses to chemical exposure.* Cold Spring Harbor Laboratory, Cold Spring Harbor, New York.

Phillips, D.H., M.V. Reddy, and K. Randerath. 1984. ^{32}P-Postlabelling analysis of DNA adducts formed in the livers of animals treated with safrole, estragole and other naturally-occurring alkenylbenzenes. II. Newborn male B6C3F$_1$ mice. *Carcinogenesis* **5**: 1623.

Randerath, K., M.V. Reddy, and R.C. Gupta. 1981. ^{32}P-Labeling test for DNA damage. *Proc. Natl. Acad. Sci. U.S.A.* **78**: 6126.

Randerath, E., H.P. Agrawal, M.V. Reddy, and K. Randerath. 1983. Highly persistent polycyclic aromatic hydrocarbon-DNA adducts in mouse skin: Detection by ^{32}P-postlabeling analysis. *Cancer Lett.* **20**: 109.

Randerath, K., R.E. Haglund, D.H. Phillips, and M.V. Reddy. 1984. ^{32}P-Postlabelling analysis of DNA adducts formed in the livers of animals treated with safrole, estragole and other naturally-occurring alkenylbenzenes. I. Adult female CD-1 mice. *Carcinogenesis* **5**: 1613.

Randerath, E., H.P. Agrawal, J.A. Weaver, C.B. Bordelon, and K. Randerath. 1985a. ^{32}P-Postlabeling analysis of DNA adducts persisting for up to 42 weeks in the skin, epidermis, and dermis of mice treated topically with 7,12-dimethylbenz(a)-anthracene. *Carcinogenesis* **6**: 1117.

Randerath, K., E. Randerath, H.P. Agrawal, R.C. Gupta, M.E. Schurdak, and M.V. Reddy. 1985b. Postlabeling methods for carcinogen-DNA adduct analysis. *Environ. Health Perspect.* **62**: 57.

Reddy, M.V., T.R. Irvin, and K. Randerath. 1985. Formation and persistence of sterigmatocystin-DNA adducts in rat liver determined via ^{32}P-postlabeling analysis. *Mutat. Res.* **152**: 85.

Reddy, M.V., R.C. Gupta, E. Randerath, and K. Randerath. 1984. ^{32}P-Postlabeling test for covalent DNA binding of chemicals in vivo: Application to a variety of aromatic carcinogens and methylating agents. *Carcinogenesis* **5**: 231.

Schurdak, M.E. and K. Randerath. 1985. Tissue-specific DNA adduct formation in mice treated with the environmental carcinogen 7H-dibenzo(c,g)carbazole. *Carcinogenesis* **6**: 1271.

Stich, H.F. and R.H.C. San. 1981. *Short-term tests for chemical carcinogens.* Springer Verlag, New York.

U.S. Department of Health and Human Services. 1982. *The health consequences of smoking, a report of the Surgeon General.* U.S. Government Printing Office, Washington, D.C.

COMMENTS

CONNEY: I'm not convinced that the ^{32}P profiles that you find after treatment with cigarette smoke or estrogen really represent adducts. I think that there could be other explanations of your data.

RANDERATH: It is important to realize that the enzyme we use for ^{32}P-incorporation, T4 polynucleotide kinase, exhibits absolute specificity for labeling of 5'-hydroxyls of ribo- or deoxyribopolynucleotides and ribo- or deoxyribonucleoside 3'-monophosphates. An intact nucleic acid base is required: No labeling occurs with depurinated or depyrimidinated nucleotides. However, as we have found, the enzyme readily accepts base-substituted deoxyribonucleoside 3'-monophosphates (mononucleotide adducts) as substrates; in many cases, it labels these at a greater rate than it does the normal, unsubstituted nucleotides. During the development of the method, we have studied a number of model adducts of known structure and have shown that adducts obtained from in vivo experiments with procarcinogens cochromatographed with the corresponding reference adducts. This work has been published in detail. Therefore, if you treat one group of animals or cells with a test chemical and another group with vehicle only, and you detect extra spots on the TLCs in the first group only, you can be confident, I believe, that the extra spots represent ^{32}P-labeled derivatives of DNA adducts.

TANNENBAUM: I couldn't understand how you got adducts with cholesterol.

RANDERATH: There were no adducts with cholesterol in hamster kidney DNA.

TANNENBAUM: But you got some spots?

RANDERATH: A small amount of label is incorporated into background material. This can be easily identified in most cases by running a vehicle-treated control.

TANNENBAUM: I see. It seems to me, carrying this one step further, that you're relying on your knowledge of the TLC behavior to say that these are hydrophobic adducts. I mean, in other words, it's a combination of the way they behave in chromatography, plus the fact that they get ^{32}P-labeled.

RANDERATH: Plus you don't see them at all in your control.

MAGEE: Have studies ever been done in the more conventional way for example with highly radioactive estrogens?

RANDERATH: Yes. There are studies by Lutz and coworkers in Switzerland. He found that 8 hours after administration of radioactive estrogen, very low levels of label were associated with DNA, but no adducts were detected upon DNA digestion and chromatography. All attempts to isolate radioactive estrogen-DNA adducts from animal tissue have failed thus far.

BARTSCH: Could it be possible that the DNA adducts arising from estrogens are coming from lipid proxidation breakdown products?

E. RANDERATH: Yes, we are considering that.

RANDERATH: The major point I was making is this: Normally, if you look at adducts formed with different carcinogens, they give different "fingerprints." The only exception we have seen to date are the estrogens. They give chromatographically identical adducts in seven systems on PEI-cellulose TLC and in two systems on C18 (reversed-phase) TLC. We take this as evidence that the structurally diverse estrogens do not by themselves bind to DNA in hamster kidney; instead they induce the DNA binding of some unknown metabolite. We have no idea about the nature of this metabolite and the resulting adduct structures, except that our chromatographic evidence suggests that the adducts contain bulky unsaturated or aromatic moieties. This is a novel mechanism of DNA adduction (and possibly of cancer initiation).

PEGG: I have two related questions. I don't have any doubt at all that you are measuring adducts; I mean, if you use a loose definition of adducts. But one thing that bothers me a little bit is that it seems to me that the quantitation depends on your knowing that the enzyme which you're using to digest the DNA to nucleotides will actually split all of the bonds. You know, if it works very slowly at the sites at which certain adducts are located, then you wouldn't get a complete digestion, although you'd still get a pattern. I wonder how you know about that.

RANDERATH: M.V. Reddy, E. Randerath, and I have done extensive digestion studies with DNAs containing model adducts (such as benzo[a] pyrene, 7,12-dimethylbenz[a] anthracene, safrole, 2-acetylaminofluorene, and 2-aminofluorene), and the conditions have been optimized so that complete digestion to mononucleotides is obtained in most cases. With unknown adducts, for which no model compounds are available, one can also do preliminary experiments to make sure that a plateau of digestion is attained. In addition, one studies whether the adduct spots, after isolation from TLC, can be further digested by other nucleases, for example, nuclease P_1 or DNase I. This would indicate whether the adduct is a mono- or oligonucleotide. Digestion to oligonucleotides was observed by us only for aflatoxin B_1- and sterigmatocystin-DNA adducts.

PEGG: For the second part of my question, I was going to ask the actual level of adducts that you were getting in the smokers. But what you are really saying is that unless you can tell what the adduct is, you can't really do the quantitation, isn't that right? I mean, unless you know what it is, you don't know what the optimal digestion conditions for it will be; so you couldn't put a number on it with as much precision as you would like.

RANDERATH: That is correct to some extent. Absolute quantitation by our "intensification procedure" depends on the determination of intensification factors, which requires running the assay under conditions of excess ATP and needs adduct levels of one adduct in $3-5 \times 10^7$ normal nucleotides. If the adduct levels are lower than this, the "intensification procedure" still allows you to do comparative quantitations of samples containing the same adducts, and this is essentially what we have done with the human smokers' adducts.

HALEY: With regard to the background you note and to genetic damage, do you find any such markers in placentas of women passively exposed to sidestream smoke?

E. RANDERATH: We would have to look at it again because we looked at these samples early on, and only lately have we observed that we consistently get a hazy background. We had too few specimens from passive smokers to answer this.

BELAND: I would like to consider quantitation for a minute. Randerath is working with adducts from known carcinogens, including aromatic hydrocarbons and aromatic amines, and yet he did not detect any of these adducts in the placental samples. I believe this is important.

PEGG: Yes, that's quite right. You can say there is less than a certain number.

BELAND: Perhaps Randerath's data means that we have been working with the wrong carcinogens. I have a second question: In your mouse skin experiment, the major spot, adduct number 1, is the fastest to form and the slowest to be repaired. This suggests that it should increase in intensity upon repeated administration, but it does not. Does this mean that saturation in DNA binding is occurring?

E. RANDERATH: One does not really know the details of what is going on with such a complex mixture in vivo. The mixture contains initiators (DNA-damaging), metabolic inhibitors, perhaps chemicals affecting DNA repair and adduct persistence, and tumor promoters. So I do not expect that these adducts will show kinetics that we are familiar with from pure carcinogens.

The Use of Micronuclei in Tracing the Genotoxic Damage in the Oral Mucosa of Tobacco Users

HANS F. STICH*
Environmental Carcinogenesis Unit
British Columbia Cancer Research Centre
Vancouver, B.C. V5Z 1L3, Canada

OVERVIEW

Millions of people use smokeless tobacco, such as snuff, chewing tobacco, nass or nasswar (tobacco, slaked lime, ash and oil mixture), Khaini tobacco (tobacco and slaked lime), or as part of a simple betel quid (areca nut, tobacco, lime, betel leaf), or a complex "pan" (betel quid with catechin seeds, perfumes, and silver foils). These habits are involved in the etiology of oral cancer, which should be amenable to primary prevention when applied in the early stages of carcinogenesis.

To accomplish this goal, markers are needed that can quantitate carcinogen-induced damage in a tissue during the preneoplastic stage and that indicate the level of relative risk for cancer. The micronucleus test, as applied to exfoliated cells from the oral mucosa, appears to be a suitable tool with which to quantitate tobacco-induced damage in the target tissue, to uncover enhancing (e.g., smoking and alcohol drinking) factors, to predict a risk for developing oral carcinomas (comparing the effect of various chewing patterns), and to follow the response of a carcinogen-exposed tissue towards the administration of chemopreventive agents, as exemplified by the reduced frequency of micronuclei in exfoliated human cells (MEC) in snuff dippers following a beta-carotene regime (180 mg/week for 10 weeks).

INTRODUCTION

Mankind's fascination with tobacco has led to a great variety of customs (Volger 1981), including the smoking of cigarettes, cigars, pipes, and waterpipes, smoking cigars in a reverse manner (chutta: burning end within the mouth), the chewing of tobacco and various tobacco-containing mixtures (betel quid), placing tobacco into the lower or upper groove (snuff) or tobacco/lime mixtures (nass, nasswar), brushing the teeth and gums with tobacco paste, blowing tobacco dust into the

---

*This paper was presented at the Banbury Conference by Dr. Miriam P. Rosin.

nostrils, and introducing tobacco in an enema (de Smet 1983). In addition, there is a wide array of tobacco types. Sun-dried tobacco (Khaini), which frequently contains several species of molds (Stich et al. 1983a), is used as plugs (Bihar, India) and by betel quid chewers among the hill tribes of Luzon (Philippines), female Khasis of Meghalaya (India), and by Nepalese. Fermented tobacco pieces and tobacco pastes containing a great variety of perfumes and spices are commonly used in the preparation of a typical Indian "pan." By comparing the various chewing patterns with the incidence of preneoplastic lesions and carcinomas within the oral cavity, it should be possible to pinpoint the causative agents. One of the difficulties with this approach has been a lack of cellular or biochemical markers that would reveal and quantitate cell or tissue damage caused by exposures to carcinogenic chewing mixtures. To resolve this problem, an active search for markers suitable for quantitating events in the early stages of carcinogenesis was initiated. Sperm (morphological anomalies), erythrocytes (hemoglobin changes), and lymphocytes (chromosome aberrations or sister chromatid exchange) are among the cells used to monitor carcinogen-induced damage in humans. However, there appears to be one drawback to this approach. Sperm, erythrocytes, and lymphocytes are not the actual targets for most carcinogens, nor do they give rise to carcinomas, the most frequent type of human cancers. Since every human tissue has its own way of handling compounds, a relevant marker should be applicable to tissues which are the targets of carcinogens and from which preneoplastic lesions and carcinomas will later develop. The micronucleus test on exfoliated human cells is directly applicable to human tissues (Stich and Rosin 1983a, 1984, 1985) that contain a host of defense mechanisms. Since this test can be used in in vivo and in vitro systems, it should be ideally suited to trace the source of carcinogens and help in the identification of compounds responsible for the genotoxic damage in human tissues.

RESULTS

Micronuclei in Exfoliated Human Cells as Markers

An increase of micronuclei which result from chromosome and chromatid fragments should be found in the early stages of carcinogenesis. First, most chemical carcinogens are active clastogens and should induce a variety of chromosome aberrations in human tissues exposed to carcinogenic mixtures. Second, many, if not all, carcinomas seem to have altered chromosome numbers and chromosomal rearrangements, some of which involve particular regions (Rowley 1983; Mitelman 1985). These abnormal karyotypes in transformed cells must evolve from chromosome aberrations during the preneoplastic stage. The third argument is based on a more theoretical consideration. Amplification and transposition of oncogenes seem to be mechanisms involved in neoplastic transformation and progression of a malignant phenotype. These oncogene changes result from chromatid breaks and exchanges that can be indirectly detected by the appearance of micronucleated cells in preinvasive stages. With this working hypothesis in mind, we applied the micronucleus test to exfoliated cells of individuals at elevated risk for cancer in the oral cavity (Stich et al. 1982a,b; Stich and Rosin 1983b), esophagus (Zaridze et al. 1985), urinary bladder (Raafat et al. 1984) and cervix (H. Stich, unpubl.). A significant increase in the frequency of micronuclei in exfoliated human cells (MEC) was found in virtually all examined individuals at elevated risk for cancer. Moreover, an elevated frequency of MEC was also observed in various tissues of individuals who are afflicted with a cancer-predisposing syndrome such as Bloom's syndrome or ataxia telangiectasia (Rosin and German 1985; M. Rosin and H. Ochs, in prep.).

There are considerable advantages of applying the micronucleus test directly to tissues of carcinogen-exposed individuals: (1) The frequency of MEC can be readily estimated in smear preparations of exfoliated cells or in cell suspensions obtained from biopsies following treatment with pronase and/or collagenase. Thus genotoxic damage can actually be measured in tissues which are the targets for carcinogens. (2) Exfoliated cells and biopsies can also be used to estimate the levels of retinol, beta-carotene, or a number of other chemopreventive agents. Thus a localized deficiency in protective agents which could increase the sensitivity towards the action of carcinogens can be estimated in the tissue in which carcinogen-induced genotoxic damage can also be quantitated. (3) Since exfoliated cells can be sampled from small areas, the distribution of MEC within a tissue can be mapped. Thus it should be possible to link foci with high frequencies of MEC with regions in which preneoplastic lesions, carcinoma in situ, or carcinomas preferentially develop. (4) The scoring of MEC, which is currently a time- and manpower-consuming task, lends itself to automation so that thousands of cells can be screened within minutes for the presence of micronuclei.

However, we would be remiss if we did not point to some of the restrictions of using the frequency of MEC as markers for carcinogen-exposed tissues: (1) Only two groups of carcinogens (or conceivably promoters) will lead to the formation of micronucleated cells: (a) Carcinogens which induce chromosome and/or chromatid aberrations, and (b) carcinogens which can induce aberrant chromosomes. Since most, if not all, chemical and physical carcinogens are also clastogenic and/or mutagenic, this issue may not prove to be of great concern. Nevertheless, it may be prudent to ascertain in sensitive in vitro bioassays whether or not a carcinogen, mixture of carcinogens, or promoters under investigation can actually induce chromosome and chromatid aberrations or mitotic aneuploidy. (2) Of greater concern is the sampling time following exposure to carcinogens. The micronucleus test on exfoliated cells seems to provide reliable information when applied to tissues which are chronically or repeatedly exposed to carcinogens. However, a wave of MEC resulting from a single short-term exposure to a carcinogen could be missed. Similarly, past exposures that occurred 2 or more months prior to the sampling period may not be readily detectable. The frequency of MEC is greatly reduced within approximately 1 month following the cessation of a micronucleus-causing insult (e.g., cessation of radiotherapy to the head/neck region for oral mucosa cells or to the pelvic region for urinary bladder cells) (Stich et al. 1983b; Stich and Rosin 1985). If the time interval between sampling of exfoliated cells and the original exposure to a carcinogen exceeds 1 month, one may not find an elevated frequency of MEC. (3) Micronuclei can only be formed during a cell division. Thus, apart from the concentration of the carcinogen, the proliferation rate of the carcinogen-exposed tissue also has an effect on the frequency of MEC. No elevation of MEC may be seen in a nonproliferating tissue even if the carcinogen should cause chromatid or chromosome breaks and fragments in the interphase nucleus.

Elevated Frequency of Micronucleated Cells in the Oral Cavity of Tobacco Users

Smokeless tobacco is used in many different ways and in many different combinations with other chewing ingredients. By comparing the effect of the various habits on the frequency of MEC, the incidence of preinvasive lesions and the incidence of carcinomas, it should be possible to assess the contribution of various components to the genotoxic effect, and, by implication, the carcinogenic activity of particular ingredients in tobacco-containing chewing mixtures (Table 1). The results show that the frequency of MEC in the oral mucosa of individuals who chew complex mixtures is considerably greater than that found in persons who use tobacco only. The risk for developing oral cancer seems to follow a comparable pattern: A relatively high risk among individuals who chew betel quid (pan) consisting mainly of tobacco, areca nut, betel leaf, and slaked lime (IARC 1985), and among persons who place nass, a mixture of tobacco, slaked lime, ash, and oil, under the tongue (Paches and Milievskaya 1980; Napalkov et al. 1983); and a lower risk among snuff users (Winn et al. 1981, 1984) and tobacco chewers (Wynder et al. 1957). In contrast to the relatively high genotoxic damage caused by placing smokeless tobacco

Table 1
Frequency of MEC in the Oral Cavity of Individuals with Various Tobacco Habits

Tobacco type	Population group	Area of exposure	Number of individuals	Frequency of MEC (%)
Snuff	Inuits	Gingiva	20	2.1 (0.6-3.8)
Khaini tobacco	India	Gingiva	27	2.1 (0.8-4.9)
Nass	Uzbekis	Floor of mouth	15	4.1 (2.7-5.7)
Betel quid + tobacco:				
+ fermented tobacco	India	Buccal mucosa	20	7.2 (3.3-13.1)
+ dried tobacco	Philippines	Buccal mucosa	132	3.1 (1.3-6.5)

into the mouth, the inhalation of cigarette smoke has a virtually undetectable effect on the MEC frequency of the oral mucosa. Even the smoking of cigarettes or cigars by holding the burning end within the mouth does not seem to increase the frequency of MEC in all individuals with this unique habit.

Factors Modulating the Frequency of MEC and the Risk for Oral Cancer

Epidemiological evidence points to a synergistic effect between cigarette smoking and alcohol consumption in the induction of oral cancers (Wynder et al. 1957; Rothman 1975; Schottenfeld 1979). The question has been raised whether a synergistic action of these two habits can be detected by the frequency of micronucleated cells in the buccal mucosa (Stich and Rosin 1983b). The results clearly demonstrated an elevated frequency of MEC in individuals with both smoking and drinking habits compared to nonsmokers and nondrinkers of alcoholic beverages (Fig. 1). Of particular interest is the fact that a synergistic effect can be uncovered many years prior to the appearance of preinvasive oral lesions or carcinomas.

The usefulness of the frequency of MEC as predictors for carcinogenicity was further tested on snuff dippers following the administration of beta-carotene which seems to be an efficient chemopreventive compound (Peto et al. 1981; Peto 1983). The twice weekly administration of beta-carotene (180 mg/week) for 10 weeks resulted in a significant reduction of MEC in the oral mucosa of snuff dippers (Stich et al. 1985) (Fig. 2). Whether a lower genotoxic damage in the mucosa will be reflected by a decrease in preinvasive and invasive oral lesions can only be revealed by a long-term chemoprevention trial.

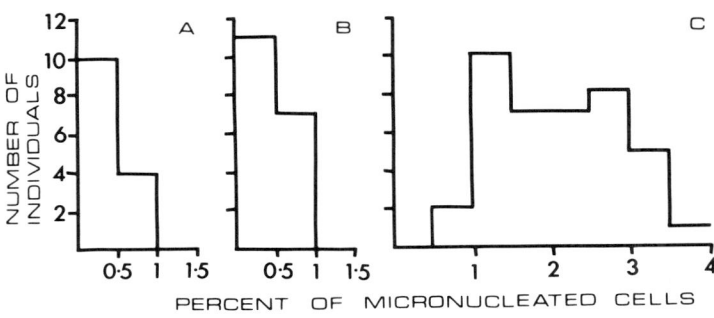

Figure 1
Number of individuals with indicated frequency of MEC in the oral mucosa. (*A*) Smokers (40-75 cigarettes/day); (*B*) alcohol drinkers; (*C*) smokers (40-75 cigarettes/day) and alcohol drinkers.

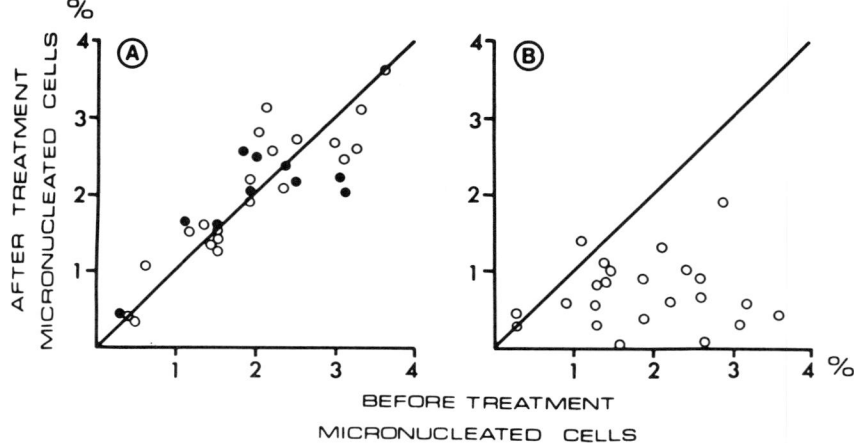

Figure 2
Frequency of MEC in the lower gingival groove of snuff users. (A) Frequency of MEC at the oral site where the tobacco is located; (●) before and after a 10-week ingestion of placebo capsules; (○) before and after the 10-week trial period (no treatment); (B) changes in the frequency of MEC before and after a 10-week administration of beta-carotene (180 mg/week).

Genotoxicity of Saliva of Tobacco Chewers

In the past little attention has been given to the mutagenic or clastogenic activity of various body fluids of humans exposed to carcinogenic mixtures (Stich and Stich 1982). Such an approach should have a high relevance value since it can provide quantitative information on the distribution kinetics and metabolism of carcinogens in man. One can assume that in the case of snuff dippers and tobacco chewers, carcinogenic and/or genotoxic agents will be released into the saliva from whence they can be absorbed by the oral mucosa or, on swallowing, pass into the digestive system and later into the blood. The appearance of chromosome-damaging activity in the saliva of users of various brands of tobacco is shown in Table 2.

The In Vitro Induction of Micronuclei by Various Tobacco Brands and Mixtures

The formation of MEC, which was used to detect genotoxic damage in the oral mucosa of chewers, was also employed to test aqueous extracts of various tobacco brands or tobacco-containing mixtures (Table 3). All the examined tobacco samples elevated the frequency of micronuclei in Chinese hamster ovary (CHO) cells following a 3-hour exposure. All the examined tobacco extracts also induced, as would be expected, chromatid breaks and exchanges. This observation is in agreement with

Table 2
Induction of Micronuclei in CHO Cells Exposed for 3 Hours to the Saliva of Chewers of Different Brands of Tobacco (4-Minute Chewing)

Tobacco type	Dilution of saliva[a] (%)	Cells with micronuclei (%)	Metaphases with chromatid aberrations (%)
Snuff L	50	5.9	4.5
Snuff K	50	3.1	2.0
Chewing RM	50	4.8	4.7
Zarda (India)	20	20.8	14.1
Khaini (Bihar)	50	16.2	9.8

[a] 2 g of each type of tobacco was held in the mouth for 10 min and the saliva (10 ml total) collected over this period
CHO = Chinese hamster ovary

the assumption that micronuclei seen in exfoliated cells of chewers originated from chromatid and chromosome aberrations that occurred in the proliferating basal cell layer of the oral mucosa.

DISCUSSION

The many in vitro tests for mutagenicity, clastogenicity, and recombinogenicity of chemicals or complex mixtures are ill-suited to reveal their actual carcinogenic

Table 3
Induction of Micronuclei in CHO Cells Exposed for 3 Hours to Aqueous Extracts of Various Brands of Tobacco

Tobacco type	Country	Dose[a] (mg/ml)	Cells with micronuclei (%)	Metaphases with chromatid aberrations (%)
Snuff L	Canada	70	11.6	21.4
Snuff K	Canada	70	12.5	27.3
Chewing RM	United States	60	9.2	16.7
Chewing BN	Canada	80	11.5	20.0
Zarda	India	4	8.6	29.4
Khaini	Bihar	6	12.3	24.3
Gorathin	Orissa	12	15.2	22.9
Toothpaste	Orissa	25	8.6	20.0
Nass A	Uzbekistan	250	18.2	28.8
Nass D	Uzbekistan	250	8.6	35.1

[a] The amount of tobacco used to prepare an aqueous extraction

and/or genotoxic actions in man. The defense mechanisms of an entire organism are difficult, if not impossible, to simulate in the short-term assays using microorganisms or cultured mammalian cells. The application of the micronucleus test to exfoliated human cells could conceivably bridge the existing gap between results obtained in in vitro assays and those gained by examining the human target tissues directly, since the frequency of micronuclei can be estimated in human tissues (Stich and Rosin 1983a, 1984, 1985), in tissues of experimental animals (Heddle et al. 1982; Goldberg et al. 1983; Wargovich et al. 1985), and in cultured cells exposed to aqueous extracts of the same carcinogenic mixtures or isolated carcinogens. Since the same endpoint can be used in all of these different carcinogen-exposed cell systems, it should be possible to assess the potential genotoxic capacity of carcinogens and the actual genotoxic damage induced in tissues of humans exposed to complex carcinogenic mixtures.

The application of the micronucleus test to the oral mucosa of individuals engaged in placing tobacco plugs into the mouth, chewing tobacco or tobacco-containing quids, smoking cigarettes, or using tobacco as toothpaste has revealed the usefulness of this approach. A relatively good correlation was observed between the frequency of MEC and the risk of developing oral cancer. A highly elevated frequency of MEC in one location of the mucosa within the oral cavity even seems to be indicative for the site at elevated risk for carcinomas (Stich et al. 1982a,b; Stich and Rosin 1984). Another advantage of this method can be found in its capacity to uncover factors that can modulate the genotoxic damage and, by implication, the carcinogenic hazard caused by the use of tobacco. The enhancing effect of alcohol consumption on the carcinogenicity of cigarette smoking is reflected by an increase in MEC of the oral mucosa. On the other hand, the administration of beta-carotene led to a reduction of MEC in the mucosa of snuff dippers. The latter observation is in agreement with the epidemiological results pointing to a protective effect of ingesting beta-carotene-containing vegetables on the oral cancer incidence among snuff dippers (Winn et al. 1984).

The question must be raised as to the significance of the micronucleated cells in neoplastic transformation. Obviously, the micronucleated exfoliated cells from the oral cavity are moribund. However, the micronuclei indicate the occurrence of chromatid breaks and exchanges in the dividing cell population of the basal layer, as well as the loss of a chromosome, which do not become included in the daughter nuclei following a cell division. Such anomalies will lead to the formation of cells with reshuffled gene sequences, chromosomes with multiple gene copies, and/or aneuploid chromosome complements which can be characterized by monosomy or polysomy of particular chromosomes. Some of these chromosomal anomalies may be involved in oncogene amplification (Schwab et al. 1983; Alitalo 1985) or their activation (Rowley 1983; Klein and Klein 1984; Yunis and Soreng 1984). In order to gain a particular transposition, duplication of gene sequences, or double minutes, a relatively large number of chromatid aberrations must occur. The appearance of micronuclei in the early stages of carcinogenesis and their elevated frequency over prolonged preneoplastic periods seems to indicate the period of genome reshuffling. An elevation in the frequency of micronucleated cells should reflect an increased probability of obtaining one of the changes in DNA sequences which involve the changed function of oncogenes. If this assumption is correct, then any increase in chromosome aberrations, as seen in an elevated frequency of micronucleated cells, should enhance the probability of neoplastic transformation.

CONCLUSION

The frequency of MEC provides a simple, reliable indicator for genotoxic damage in human tissues which are exposed to carcinogens and from which carcinomas will develop. The level of MEC seems to reflect the integrated effect of enhancing (e.g., smoking plus alcohol ingestion), inhibiting (e.g., beta-carotene administration), genetic (e.g., Bloom's Syndrome) (Rosin and German 1985), and physical (e.g., pH of saliva) factors. Studies on the MEC frequencies in human tissues can be supplemented by estimating in vitro the capacity of body fluids (e.g., saliva of chewers) and of aqueous extracts of the carcinogen mixtures (e.g., nass or betel quids) to induce micronucleated cells.

In the future, emphasis should be placed on studies to yield insight into the link between MEC and DNA adduct formation in the oral mucosa of tobacco users, as well as the link between MEC and the incidence of preinvasive lesions or carcinomas. Only additional evidence on these issues will prove the reliability of the frequency of MEC as a predictor of cancer incidence.

REFERENCES

Alitalo, K. 1985. Amplification of cellular oncogenes in cancer cells. *Trends Biochem. Sci.* **10**: 194.

de Smet, P.A.G.M. 1983. A multidisciplinary overview of intoxicating enema rituals in the Western hemisphere. *J. Ethnopharmacol.* **9**: 129.

Goldberg, M.T., D.H. Blakey, and W.R. Bruce. 1983. Comparison of the effects of 1,2-dimethylhydrazine and cyclophosphamide on micronucleus incidence in bone marrow and colon. *Mutat. Res.* **109**: 91.

Heddle, J.A., D.H. Blakey, A.M.V. Duncan, M.T. Goldberg, H. Newmark, M.J. Wargovich, and W.R. Bruce. 1982. Micronuclei and related nuclear anomalies as a short-term assay for colon carcinogens. In *Banbury report 13: Indicators of genotoxic exposure* (ed. B. Bridges, B.E. Butterworth, and I.B. Weinstein), p. 367. Cold Spring Harbor Laboratory, Cold Spring Harbor, New York.

IARC. 1985. *Monographs on the evaluation of the carcinogenic risk of chemicals to humans: Tobacco habits other than smoking; betel-quid and areca-nut chewing; and some related nitrosamines,* vol. 37. International Agency for Research on Cancer, Lyon, France.

Klein, G. and E. Klein. 1984. Oncogene activation and tumor progression. *Carcinogenesis* **5**: 429.

Mitelman, F. 1985. *Catalog of chromosome aberrations in cancer*, 2nd edition. *Progress and topics in cytogenetics*, vol. 5. Alan R. Liss, New York.

Napalkov, N.P., G.F. Tserkovny, V.M. Merabishvili, D.M. Parkin, M. Smans, and C.S. Muir, eds. 1983. *Cancer incidence in the USSR*, IARC Sci. Publ. no. 48. International Agency for Research on Cancer, Lyon, France.

Paches, A.I. and I.L. Milievskaya. 1980. An epidemiologic study of carcinoma of the mucous membrane of the oral cavity in the USSR. In *Cancer epidemiology in the USA and USSR* (ed. D.L. Levin), NIH Publ. no. 80-2044, p. 177. Bethesda, Maryland.

Peto, R. 1983. The marked differences between carotenoids and retinoids: Methodological implications for biochemical epidemiology. *Cancer Surv.* **2**: 327.

Peto, R., R. Doll, J.D. Buckley, and M.B. Sporn. 1981. Can dietary beta-carotene materially reduce human cancer rates? *Nature (Lond.)* **290**: 201.

Raafat, M., S. El-Gerzawi, and H.F. Stich. 1984. Detection of mutagenicity in urothelial cells of bilharzial patients by "the micronucleus test." *J. Egypt. Natl. Cancer Inst.* **1**: 63.

Rosin, M.P. and J. German. 1985. Evidence for chromosome instability in vivo in Bloom syndrome: Increased numbers of micronuclei in exfoliated cells. *Hum. Genet.* **71**: 187.

Rothman, K.J. 1975. Alcohol. In *Persons at high risk of cancer* (ed. J.F. Fraumeni), p. 139. Academic Press, New York.

Rowley, J.D. 1983. Human oncogene locations and chromosome aberrations. *Nature (Lond.)* **301**: 290.

Schottenfeld, D. 1979. Alcohol as a co-factor in the etiology of cancer. *Cancer* **43**: 1962.

Schwab, M., K. Alitalo, H.E. Varmus, J.M. Bishop, and D. George. 1983. A cellular oncogene (c-Ki-*ras*) is amplified, overexpressed, and located within karyotypic abnormalities in mouse adrenocortical tumour cells. *Nature (Lond.)* **303**: 497.

Stich, H.F. and M.P. Rosin. 1983a. Micronuclei in exfoliated human cells as an internal dosimeter for exposures to carcinogens. In *Carcinogens and mutagens in the environment: Naturally occurring compounds: Endogenous formation and modulation* (ed. H.F. Stich), vol. II, p. 17. CRC Press, Boca Raton, Florida.

———. 1983b. Quantitating the synergistic effect of smoking and alcohol consumption with the micronucleus test on human buccal mucosa cells. *Int. J. Cancer* **31**: 305.

———. 1984. Micronuclei in exfoliated human cells as a tool for studies in cancer risk and cancer intervention. *Cancer Lett.* **22**: 241.

———. 1985. Towards a more comprehensive evaluation of a genotoxic hazard in man. *Mutat. Res.* **150**: 43.

Stich, H.F. and W. Stich. 1982. Chromosome-damaging activity of saliva of betel nut and tobacco chewers. *Cancer Lett.* **15**: 193.

Stich, H.F., W. Stich, and B.B. Parida. 1982a. Elevated frequency of micronucleated cells in the buccal mucosa of individuals at high risk for oral cancer: Betel quid chewers. *Cancer Lett.* **17**: 125.

Stich, H.F., J.R. Curtis, and B.B. Parida. 1982b. Application of the micronucleus test to exfoliated cells of high cancer risk groups: Tobacco chewers. *Int. J. Cancer* **30**: 553.

Stich, H.F., B. Bohm, K. Chatterjee, and J. Sailo. 1983a. The role of saliva-borne mutagens and carcinogens in the etiology of oral and esophageal carcinomas of betel nut and tobacco chewers. In *Carcinogens and mutagens in the environment: Naturally occurring compounds: Epidemiology and distribution* (ed. H.F. Stich), vol. III. p. 43. CRC Press, Boca Raton, Florida.

Stich, H.F., R.H.C. San, and M.P. Rosin. 1983b. Adaptation of the DNA repair and micronucleus tests to human cell suspensions and exfoliated cells. *Ann. N.Y. Acad. Sci.* **407**: 93.

Stich, H.F., A.P. Hornby, and B.P. Dunn. 1985. A pilot beta-carotene intervention trial with Inuits using smokeless tobacco. *Int. J. Cancer* **36**: 321.

Volger, G. 1981. Rausch und Realität. Drogen im Kultur-Vergleich. *Ethnologia* **9**: 25.

Wargovich, M.J., V.W.S. Eng, and H.L. Newmark. 1985. Inhibition by plant phenols of benzo(a)pyrene-induced nuclear aberrations in mammalian intestinal cells: A rapid in vivo assessment method. *Food Chem. Toxicol.* **23**: 47.

Winn, D.M., W.J. Blot, C.M. Shy, L.W. Pickle, M.A. Toledo, and J.F. Fraumeni, Jr. 1981. Snuff dipping and oral cancer among women in the southern United States. *New Engl. J. Med.* **304**: 745.

Winn, D.M., R.G. Ziegler, L.W. Pickle, G. Gridley, W.J. Blot, and R.N. Hoover. 1984. Diet in the etiology of oral and pharyngeal cancer among women from the southern United States. *Cancer Res.* **44**: 1216.

Wynder, E.L., I.J. Bross, and R.M. Feldman. 1957. A study of the etiological factors in cancer of the mouth. *Cancer* **10**: 1300.

Yunis, J.J. and A.L. Soreng. 1984. Constitutive fragile sites and cancer. *Science* **226**: 1199.

Zaridze, D.G., M. Blettner, N.N. Trapeznikov, J.P. Kuvshinov, E.G. Matiakin, B.P. Poljakov, B.K. Poddubni, S.M. Parshikova, V.I. Rottenberg, F.S. Chamrakulov, M.C. Chodjaeva, H.F. Stich, M.P. Rosin, D.I. Thurnham, D. Hoffmann, and K.D. Brunnemann. 1985. Survey of a population with a high incidence of oral and oesophageal cancer. *Int. J. Cancer* **36**: 153.

COMMENTS

TANNENBAUM: Have you measured beta-carotene in these exfoliated cells?

ROSIN: We collect these cells by brushing the buccal mucosa vigorously with a moistened toothbrush and then rinsing the mouth with water. The cells are centrifuged down and frozen in liquid nitrogen. The extraction procedures involve a pronase digestion treatment with KOH/methanol and, finally, preparation of a hexane extract.

TANNENBAUM: You're talking about very low levels. You are measuring nanograms—less than nanograms.

ROSIN: Yes. Determination of beta-carotene content involves HPLC analysis.

TANNENBAUM: You can measure nanograms of beta-carotene that way?

ROSIN: Yes. We can actually measure subnanogram quantities.

HOFFMANN: Please let me pose a question which may only reflect my lack of knowledge in regard to the micronucleus test. I see this assay as an indicator for cell damage, though presently, I do not see the results of the test as an early indicator for a precancerous lesion. Can you explain this point to us?

ROSIN: Actually I see two questions in your comments. The first involves the mechanism by which micronucleus frequencies are reduced in individuals receiving beta-carotene. The second question concerns the relationship between micronucleus formation and cancer. As to the first question, it is possible that the beta-carotene protection involves an increased mucous secretion or an acceleration in repair. We can't eliminate these possibilities. However, what we think is occurring is that the damage just isn't happening. We think what we're doing is trapping the free radicals so they don't damage the DNA. That's our theory. Micronucleus frequencies decreased because there was a reduction in chromosomal breakage in the dividing basal cells. The individual was using the same amount of tobacco but less carcinogen damage was occurring in these cells. We're using the micronucleus test to measure quantitatively genotoxic damage by carcinogens to a target tissue. This would mean that we're looking at early initiation events in carcinogenesis since genotoxicity is felt to be involved at this stage. We are not specifically measuring the production of a premalignant cell. The current feeling is that genotoxic damage occurs over a wide time frame in carcinogen-exposed individuals and that the specific genetic alteration involved in early neoplasia occurs randomly sometime during this exposure. We are using the micronucleus test to study this ongoing genetic change. If I could speculate, chromosomal rearrangement is currently postulated to be involved in oncogene expression. Well, if that's true, then that means that any process which stimulates micronucleus formation, which measures chromosomal breakage and rearrangement, is going to enhance your chance of obtaining the specific genetic change required for oncogene expression.

TANNENBAUM: Has the basic biology been done on these kinds of cells?

ROSIN: The majority of our knowledge on the basic biology of micronucleus formation in exfoliated cells is derived from a series of studies done on cancer patients receiving radiotherapy. Individuals receiving radiation to the buccal mucosa were sampled by swabbing this area and collecting exfoliated cells prior to and then throughout the course of the radiotherapy. Micronucleus frequencies did not change for 7-9 days after treatment began. This is the time required for 1-2 divisions of the basal epithelial cells where the micronuclei are formed, plus the time required for the daughter cells containing the micronuclei to migrate to the surface of the epithelium where they could be collected. After this time period, we observed a dose-dependent increase in the frequency of micronucleated exfoliated cells. When radiation treatment stopped, it required 7-10 days before the micronucleus frequencies began to fall; then a gradual decrease in the frequencies was observed until background levels were attained 2-3 weeks after radiation therapy ended. These data provide us with a time frame for interpretation of studies on carcinogens in exposed populations. The remainder of our knowledge on the basic biology of micronucleus formation in exfoliated cells stems from three sources. First, numerous studies on control populations have established "spontaneous" limits for this event in individuals not receiving carcinogen exposure of 0.2-0.8%. Second, these levels are significantly elevated in all high-risk populations comprised of individuals exposed to oral carcinogens, primarily tobacco chewers. The increase appears to be quantitatively linked to carcinogen exposure. Third, we have recently studied two genetic groups known to have spontaneous chromosomal instability and to be at elevated risk for cancer. These groups were patients with Bloom's syndrome or ataxia telangiectasia. The elevated chromosomal fragmentation characteristic of such individuals was reflected in a five- to tenfold elevation in micronucleus frequencies in exfoliated cells from the oral cavity and urinary bladder.

Validation of Smoking History with the Micronuclei Test

ELIZABETH FONTHAM, PELAYO CORREA, ELSIE RODRIGUEZ, AND
YOUPING LIN
Department of Pathology
Louisiana State University Medical Center
New Orleans, Louisiana 70112

OVERVIEW

The micronucleus test was applied to exfoliated cells of the oral cavity, bladder, uterine cervix, and bronchus from four patient groups to detect smoking-induced nuclear damage. Significantly elevated frequencies of micronuclei were observed in epithelial cells of smokers compared to nonsmokers for each of the four sites. The findings demonstrate tobacco-associated genotoxicity in both epithelial cells from tissue in direct contact with tobacco carcinogens as well as cells from distant sites, presumably exposed via the circulation.

INTRODUCTION

Epidemiologic studies often point to exposure of human populations to environmental carcinogens, but frequently lack means of validating such exposure. The micronucleus test was proposed as an in vivo assay to detect environmental carcinogens by Schmid in 1973. Experimental studies (Wargovich and Bruce 1983a; Wargovich et al. 1983b) have established that the test has the same site-specificity as several chemical carcinogens. Stich and Rosin (1984) have extensively used exfoliated cells as indicators of environmental carcinogens.

Our study was designed to investigate whether tobacco smoke, which has been epidemiologically associated with increased risk of cancers of the bronchus, oral cavity, bladder, and uterine cervix, is associated with an increase in micronuclei in epithelial cells from these tissues.

RESULTS

A group of 486 persons, who were patients at Charity Hospital in New Orleans, were participants in this study. Each study subject was asked to submit one type of specimen and was administered a brief questionnaire to determine tobacco and alcohol history as well as other variables of interest. Two hundred women undergoing routine gynecologic examination as outpatients submitted a duplicate cervical smear made at the time of Papanicolaou screening. Buccal mucosal cells were obtained from 51 study subjects by swabbing the mucosa of both cheeks. Samples of sputum were collected from 98 patients and urine samples from 137. The age-sex-race distribution is shown in Table 1 and reflects the population at Charity Hospital.

Cells from buccal smears, cervical smears, and sputum were transferred directly onto precleaned microscopic slides. Urine samples were filtered and cells transferred to dry-coated slides. Slides were fixed in 95% methanol and stained with the Feulgen method. No counterstain was used. A total of 500 intact epithelial cells for each sample were screened for the presence of micronuclei according to criteria previously described (Stich and Rosin 1983a).

The coded slides were read by a pathologist trained in micronuclei techniques. All readings were made without knowledge of demographic or exposure data. Intra-observer precision was assessed by "blinded" duplicate readings. Exact agreement in first and second readings was found for 94% of the slides read. For the remaining 6%, the difference between the first and second reading was 1 micronucleus per 500 cells in each case.

A group of persons (n = 19) receiving therapeutic radiation to the site from which the specimen was obtained was studied with the same methods. Radiation exposure, a known genotoxic event, was examined as a measure of the validity of the test to detect genotoxic agents. Results showed a significantly elevated mean proportion of micronucleated cells among persons receiving irradiation compared to nonirradiated subjects: 0.63 (SE 0.09) versus 0.20 (SE 0.01), $P < 0.001$. These 19 study subjects and an additional three persons receiving both radiation and chemotherapy were excluded from the remainder of the analyses.

Table 2 contrasts the proportion of micronucleated cells for current cigarette smokers and nonsmokers. A 2½-fold elevation ($P < 0.005$) in the percent of micronucleated cells from the bronchus was found for smokers; a 3½-fold elevation ($P < 0.05$) in buccal mucosal cells among smokers; and a five-fold ($P < 0.001$) and sixfold ($P < 0.001$) excess for smokers in percent micronucleated cells from the uterine cervix and urinary bladder, respectively.

Alcohol consumption and cigarette smoking were examined simultaneously. There was no evidence of a significant genotoxic effect of alcohol alone nor a synergistic effect of smoking and alcohol for any of the four organ sites. Table 3

Table 1
Age-Sex-Race Distribution of Population by Specimen Type

| | White | | Nonwhite | | | Mean |
	Male	Female	Male	Female	Total	age (yrs)
Buccal mucosa	9	6	18	18	51	42
Bronchus	16	5	58	19	98	54
Urinary bladder	11	12	27	87	137	37
Uterine cervix	—	28	—	172	200	31

Table 2
Frequency of Micronucleated Cells by Smoking Status and Tissue

	Mean % micronucleated cells (SE)[a]			
	Buccal mucosa	Bronchus	Urinary bladder	Uterine cervix
Smoker	0.24 (0.07)[b] n = 23	0.31 (0.05)[c] n = 58	0.30 (0.04)[d] n = 67	0.36 (0.04)[d] n = 98
Nonsmoker	0.07 (0.05) n = 20	0.12 (0.04) n = 32	0.05 (0.02) n = 65	0.07 (0.02) n = 101

[a]Standard T-test, smoker versus nonsmoker
[b]$P < 0.05$
[c]$P < 0.005$
[d]$P < 0.001$

shows the frequencies of micronucleated epithelial cells from the oral cavity and from the bladder. Similar frequencies of micronucleated cells were found for smokers only and for persons who both smoked and consumed alcohol: buccal mucosa, 0.23 (0.12) versus 0.24 (0.08); urinary bladder, 0.35 (0.08) versus 0.29 (0.05).

The effect of the number of cigarettes smoked on the prevalence of micronucleated cells was examined, and results are displayed in Table 4. No statistical difference was observed in the frequency of micronuclei for smokers according to the amount smoked for any of the tissues examined. Similar values are seen for the two smoking levels shown, a pack per day or less and more than one pack per day. Finer stratification of cigarette consumption likewise failed to show a dose-response.

Table 3
Frequency of Micronucleated Cells by Current Smoking Status, Alcohol Use and Tissue Type

	Mean % micronucleated cells (SE)[a]			
	Nonsmoker nondrinker[b]	Current smoker only	Current drinker only	Current smoker and drinker
Buccal mucosa	0.00 (-) n = 7	0.23 (0.12) n = 6	0.11 (0.08) n = 13	0.24 (0.08)[c] n = 17
Urinary bladder	0.02 (0.01) n = 44	0.35 (0.08)[d] n = 19	0.11 (0.05) n = 21	0.29 (0.05)[d] n = 48

[a]Standard T-test, referent nonsmoker-nondrinker
[b]Drinker refers to alcohol
[c]$P < 0.005$
[d]$P < 0.001$

Table 4
Frequency of Micronucleated Cells by Number of Cigarettes Smoked Per Day

No. of cigarettes per day:	Mean % micronucleated cells (SE)[a]		
	0	1-20	≥ 21
Buccal mucosa	0.07 (0.05)	0.24 (0.08)	0.24 (0.14)
	n = 20	n = 18	n = 5
Bronchus	0.12 (0.04)	0.28 (0.05)	0.36 (0.09)
	n = 32	n = 39	n = 19
Urinary bladder	0.05 (0.02)	0.29 (0.04)	0.29 (0.12)
	n = 65	n = 55	n = 12
Uterine cervix	0.07 (0.02)	0.37 (0.04)	0.12 (0.09)
	n = 101	n = 91	n = 7

[a]Standard T-test, 1-20 cigarettes versus ≥ 21; all $P > 0.05$, NS

Passive smoke exposure by nonsmokers was evaluated. No significant elevation of the frequency of micronucleated epithelial cells from any of the four organs was seen for nonsmokers married to smokers. The results are shown in Table 5.

DISCUSSION

Epidemiologic studies have linked cigarette smoking to increased risk of cancer in a number of human organs. The effect seems to be strongest for the oral cavity, larynx, and lungs, which come into direct contact with the broad range of compounds in cigarette smoke. Consistent epidemiologic associations have been demonstrated, however, between cigarette smoking and increased risk of cancer at more distant sites which do not have direct contact with cigarette smoke, such as the

Table 5
Frequency of Micronucleated Cells among Nonsmokers Married to Smokers by Specimen Type

	Mean % micronucleated cells (SE)[a]			
	Buccal mucosa	Bronchus	Urinary bladder	Uterine cervix
Spouse smokes	0.05 (0.05)	0.15 (0.09)	0.06 (0.03)	0.05 (0.03)
	n = 8	n = 5	n = 13	n = 26
Nonsmoking spouse	0.20 (0.20)	0.18 (0.08)	0.14 (0.08)	0.09 (0.05)
	n = 5	n = 12	n = 11	n = 26

[a]Standard T-test, smoking versus nonsmoking spouse; all $P > 0.05$, NS

bladder, kidney, pancreas, and esophagus (U.S. Department of HEW 1979). More recently, an association between cigarette smoking and cervical cancer risk has been reported, and there is a need to determine whether the relationship is etiological or indirect, i.e., due to confounding factors (Lyon et al. 1983).

One way to address the biologic plausibility of presumed etiologic associations is provided by the micronucleus test, a short-term in vivo test which detects cytogenetic damage. Utilizing this technique, we found evidence of tobacco-induced nuclear damage in cells of four different organs. The results are particularly noteworthy for the cervix. Morphologic studies have indicated that cervical dysplasia is first seen in the endocervical region, which led to the hypothesis that the endocervical mucus provides a carcinogenic stimulus to the surface epithelium of the endocervix (Duque et al. 1979). Sasson et al. (1985) recently reported high levels of nicotine and its major metabolite, cotinine, in the cervical mucus of a group of smokers compared to nonsmokers. This evidence supports their hypothesis that cervical epithelial cells of smokers are exposed to primary and secondary constituents of tobacco smoke that may exert a clastogenic effect. A study to examine the mutagenicity of cervical mucus using the Ames/Salmonella microsomal assay relative to the woman's current smoking status reported a greater proportion of positive tests among current smokers compared to nonsmokers (Holly 1985). Our data support the possibility of a causal association between cigarette smoke and cervical cancer.

Unlike Stich and Rosin (1983b), who found the frequency of micronucleated buccal cells elevated only in those individuals smoking at least one package of cigarettes per day and also consuming at least 150 ml of ethanol daily, we found significantly elevated frequencies for smokers compared to nonsmokers regardless of the amount smoked. The lack of tobacco dose-response effect in our material needs further investigation. The sensitivity of the test as we use it (without counterstain) may be low. In addition, the population of smokers was relatively homogeneous. Only 17% smoked more than one pack per day and ten of 246 smokers consumed over 40 cigarettes per day. The dose-response findings, therefore, may reflect the small number of subjects who were heavy smokers. Nor did we find any enhancement of the tobacco effect by alcohol use. However, the two study populations may not be comparable in alcohol consumption since the previous study utilized subjects from alcohol detoxification centers and we screened a general hospital population.

CONCLUSION

The micronucleus test is a valuable tool which can be utilized to evaluate human exposure to environmental carcinogens. Our data demonstrate tobacco-induced chromosome damage in buccal, bronchus, bladder, and cervical tissues consistent with increased risk of cancer at these sites among smokers.

ACKNOWLEDGMENTS

This work was supported by a grant from the Board of Regents of the State of Louisiana.

REFERENCES

Duque, E., C. Cuello, N. Aristizabal, W. Haenszel, S. Botero, and P. Correa. 1979. Premalignant lesions of the cervix in women of Cali, Colombia. *J. Natl. Cancer Inst.* **63**: 953.

Holly, E., N. Petrakis, N. Friend, D. Sarles, R. Lee, and L. Flander. 1985. Mutagenic cervical mucus in women smokers. *Am. J. Epidemiol.* **122(3)**: 518.

Lyon, J.L., J.W. Gardner, D.W. West, W.M. Stanish, and R.M. Hebertson. 1983. Smoking and carcinoma in site of the uterine cervix. *Am. J. Public Health* **73(5)**: 558.

Sasson, I.M., N.J. Haley, D. Hoffmann, E.L. Wynder, D. Hellberg, and S. Nilsson. 1985. Cigarette smoking and neoplasia of the uterine cervix: Smoke constituents in cervical mucus. *N. Engl. J. Med.* **312**: 315.

Schmid, W. 1973. Chemical mutagen testing on *in vivo* somatic mammalian cells. *Agents Actions* **3/2**: 77.

Stich, H.F. and M.P. Rosin. 1983a. Micronuclei in exfoliated human cells as an internal dosimeter for exposures to carcinogens. In *Carcinogens and mutagens in the environment, Vol. II, Naturally occurring compounds: Endogenous formation and modulation* (ed. H.F. Stich), p. 17. CRC Press, Boca Raton, Florida.

――――. 1983b. Quantitating the synergistic effect of smoking and alcohol consumption with the micronucleus test on human buccal mucosa cells. *Int. J. Cancer* **31**: 305.

――――. 1984. Micronuclei in exfoliated human cells as a tool for studies in cancer risk and cancer intervention. *Cancer Lett.* **22**: 241.

U.S. Department of Health, Education and Welfare. 1979. *Smoking and health. A report to the Surgeon General.* DHEW Publ. No. (PHS) 79-50066. U.S. Government Printing Office, Washington, D.C.

Wargovich, J. and W.R. Bruce. 1983a. Early histopathologic events to evaluation of colon cancer in C57BL/6 and CF-1 mice treated with 1,2-dimethyl-hydrazine. *J. Natl. Cancer Inst.* **71**: 125.

Wargovich, J., T. Goldberg, H. Newmark, and W.R. Bruce. 1983b. Nuclear aberrations as a short-term test for genotoxicity to the colon: Evaluation of 19 agents in mice. *J. Natl. Cancer Inst.* **71**: 133.

COMMENTS

BRUNNEMANN: I notice that your backgrounds are much lower than Drs. Rosin and Stich.

CORREA: We base our assays on counts per 500 cells. If you were to see these slides, there are many things that look like fragments of nuclei; but they have to have the right color and the right size and the right position for us to call it a micronucleus. Therefore, we have a conservative estimate of the total number of micronuclei.

TANNENBAUM: What is the significance of these details?

CORREA: The significance is that we're using this as a validation for the status of smokers. For instance, I think it is significant that in the cervix we find an excess of micronuclei in the smokers. I think that is an indication that there has been some genotoxic damage in women who smoked.

TANNENBAUM: Is that a tissue at risk?

CORREA: Yes. We will be reporting more about it in another session. We also found in a study that we did in Colombia some years ago that the topography of lesions did not favor the current theories about cervical cancer causation's being mostly viral. The viruses suspected of producing this disease are in the ectocervix. But the dysplasias, which are the first indication of carcinogenesis, are not in the exocervix, but in the endocervix. So some years ago we speculated that the endocervical mucus brought down some carcinogens.

YOAKUM: One possible interpretation of your results is that these micronuclei rarely or seldom respond to a rather heavy dose of DNA damage. Have you attempted to correlate some of your very sensitive measurements for micronuclei production with some sensitive assays using other ways of measuring DNA damage?

CORREA: No, we have not. We don't have the facilities, but we would be very interested in collaborative work.

Mutagens in the Urine of Cigarette Smokers

EDMOND J. LA VOIE,* ISAAC M. SASSON,* DIETRICH HOFFMANN,*
MILTON V. MARSHALL,† AND WALTER ROGERS**
*Division of Environmental Carcinogenesis
American Health Foundation
Valhalla, New York 10595
†Cardiopulmonary Department
Southwest Foundation for Biomedical Research
San Antonio, Texas 78284
**Department of Bioengineering
Southwest Research Institute
San Antonio, Texas 78285

OVERVIEW

Several investigators have reported an association between urinary mutagens and cigarette smoking, yet in some instances mutagens have also been detected in the urine of nonsmokers. The excretion of mutagens in urine of smokers and nonsmokers was investigated in this study with volunteers on strictly defined daily dietary protocols. The diet regimens consisted of either a typical western diet high in meat and fat content or a vegan diet. The results indicated that smokers' urine has an elevated level of mutagenic activity in *S. typhimurium*. The effect of diet on the excretion of mutagens was also pronounced and could readily confound any effort to obtain a clear correlation on the mutagenicity of urine and cigarette smoking. The cigarette-smoking baboon was used as an animal model which allowed for control of most of the environmental factors. Cigarette-smoking baboons were shown to have more mutagenic activity in their urine than sham puffers. The baboon model is currently being explored as an effective means for isolating and structurally elucidating the mutagens in urine associated with cigarette smoking.

INTRODUCTION

The association between cigarette smoking and bladder cancer has been documented by several epidemiological studies (Public Health Service 1982). It has been assumed that etiologic agents responsible for the increased incidence of bladder cancer among cigarette smokers are present in the urine. Yamasaki and Ames (1977) were the first to report the presence of mutagens in the urine of cigarette smokers, thus suggesting a correlation between an elevated risk for bladder cancer and mutagens in smokers' urine. Since publication of these initial data, several other investigators have also reported a similar association between the presence of mutagens in urine and cigarette smoking (Sirtori et al. 1978; Van Doorn et al. 1979; Aeschbacher and Chappuis 1981; Dolara et al. 1981; Recio et al. 1982). The urine of smokers participating in these studies generally contained mutagens. However, a dose-response correlation between the urinary excretion of mutagens and cigarette consumption or cigarette smoke yields and uptake has not been established (Jaffe et al. 1983).

The confounding influence of health status, diet, and other environmental factors on the detection of mutagens in urine has been observed by several investigators (Gelbart and Sontag 1980; Garner et al. 1982; Sasson et al. 1985; Sousa et al. 1985). In several instances, nonsmokers were found to have mutagenic urine. Although some investigators have suggested that environmental smoke exposure may contribute to the observed urine mutagenicity among nonsmokers (Puzrath et al. 1981; Bos et al. 1983), the influence of diet on the urinary excretion of mutagens has been documented to be quite pronounced (Baker et al. 1982; Sasson et al. 1985; Sousa et al. 1985).

The association between mutagens in urine and cigarette smoking is most appropriately studied with adequate diet control. In our laboratories the influence of smoking and different diets on the excretion of mutagenic agents in urine was investigated in a study with volunteers who adhered to strictly defined diet protocols and provided 24-hour urine specimens. Individual variations in inhalation of or exposure to cigarette smoke, as well as urinary pH and urinary creatinine concentrations, were carefully monitored for both cigarette smokers and nonsmokers.

The cigarette-smoking baboon represents one of the more suitable animal models to determine the association between the presence of urinary mutagens and the exposure to tobacco smoke since dietary and environmental variables can be strictly controlled. In the baboon animal model, cigarette smoke is delivered to the lungs in a manner simulating human smoking (Rogers et al. 1981). Therefore, we used this model in our evaluation of the relationship between smoke exposure and occurrence of urinary mutagens. We also instilled cigarette smoke condensate directly into the lungs of a baboon and determined the excretion of mutagens in urine with time. In both studies a direct comparison of the mutagenic activity in urine was made with that of control baboons.

RESULTS

Comparison of Smokers and Nonsmokers

We examined the effects of cigarette smoking and diet on the excretion of mutagens in human urine by having smokers and nonsmokers adhere to strictly defined daily diets. Our initial study included five smokers and five nonsmokers. These volunteers consisted of men and women over 18 years of age who were in apparent good health and not taking any medication. For 5 days, all ten volunteers consumed a western diet (Table 1) which contained large amounts of meat and was high in fat content. Urine (24-hour specimens) was collected on days 3, 4, and 5 in polyethylene bottles and stored in a freezer prior to extraction. Following a procedure modified from that by Yamasaki and Ames (1977), thawed urine (pH adjusted to 7.0) was gravity-filtered through Amberlite XAD-2 resin (3 g per 100 ml of urine). The resin was washed with distilled water (10 ml per 100 ml urine) and eluted with acetone (10 ml per 100 ml urine). To ensure that histidine and other highly water soluble urine constituents were completely removed, the acetone eluate was concentrated and partitioned between methylene chloride and brine. The organic layer was washed with brine and concentrated.

Mutagenicity assays were performed using *S. typhimurium* TA1538 with activation by Aroclor-induced Fischer rat liver S9 mix (Ames et al. 1975). The method of linear regression was used to determine the mutagenicity of the urine samples. In this study the mean levels of urinary mutagens were expressed as histidine revertants per 20-ml sample. The linear portion of the dose-response curves generated from 0-, 6.26-, 12.5-, and 25-ml equivalents of urine per average of 2 plates each was employed to determine the mutagenicity of a 20-ml sample. After subtracting the control values, the results are divided by the creatinine contents of 1.0 ml of urine as a means to adjust for differences in the concentrations of the initial

Table 1
Diet Regimen A

Meat diet (days 1–5)
Breakfasts	Eggs, ham, sausages, waffles, butter, toast, juice, coffee, tea
Lunches	Tuna fish, roast beef, pastrami, turkey, chicken, rye bread, lettuce and tomatoes, soda, coffee, tea
Dinners	Steak, veal cutlet, lamb chop, pork chop, chicken, rice, potatoes, string beans, carrots, broccoli, ice cream, coffee, tea

Vegan diet (days 6–10)
Breakfasts	Granola, raisins, corn or bran muffin, preserves, soy milk, juice, herbal teas, coffee substitute
Lunches	Peanut butter, tofu, sprouts, sunflower or sesame seeds, soyburgers, canned fruits, packaged tabboule (burgul or cracked wheat), lettuce, fruits, rye or whole wheat bread or pita, herbal teas, coffee substitute
Dinners	Packaged or canned dinners (frozen tofu lasagna, vegetable patties, legume tofu ravioli, macaroni, soyburgers), frozen broccoli, spinach, string beans, cauliflower, rye or whole wheat bread or pita, sunflower or sesame seeds, iceberg lettuce, tomatoes, cucumbers, carrots, sprouts, radishes, chickpeas, dried fruits, jello, granola bars, nondairy ice cream, herbal teas, coffee substitute

urine specimens. The mutagenic activity observed in the urine concentrates obtained on days 3 and 5 from nonsmokers (*1-5*) compared to those from smokers (*6-10*) is illustrated in Figure 1A, B.

On the sixth day, all volunteers were placed on a vegan diet (Table 1) for 5 additional days. Urine was collected on days 8, 9, and 10. The urine concentrate of each 24-hour urine specimen was obtained as previously outlined and assayed for mutagenic activity in *S. typhimurium* TA1538 in the presence of rat liver homogenate. The mutagenic activity, expressed as histidine revertants per 20-ml sample for the nonsmokers and smokers in this study, is outlined in Figure 2A, B.

Urinary cotinine levels were determined by radioimmunoassay using a modification (Haley et al. 1983) of the procedure by Langone et al. (1973). The levels of

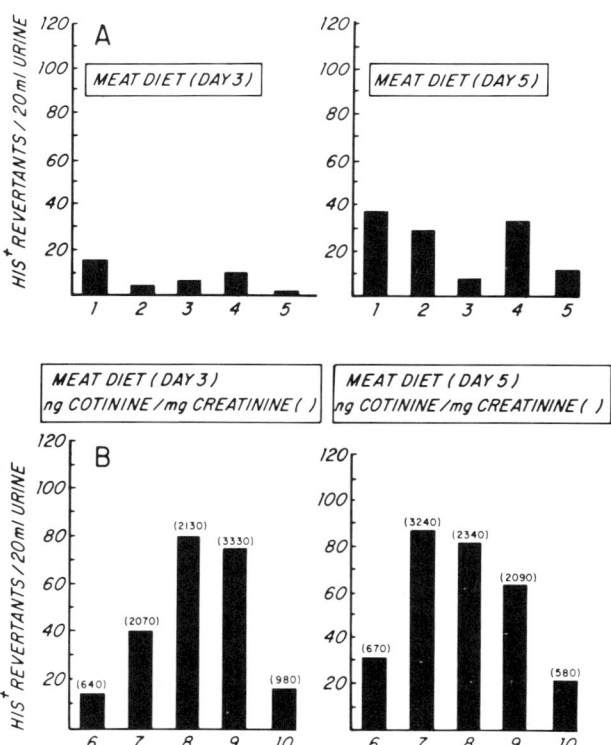

Figure 1
The mutagenic activity of urine concentrates obtained from nonsmokers (*A*) and smokers (*B*) on a western diet

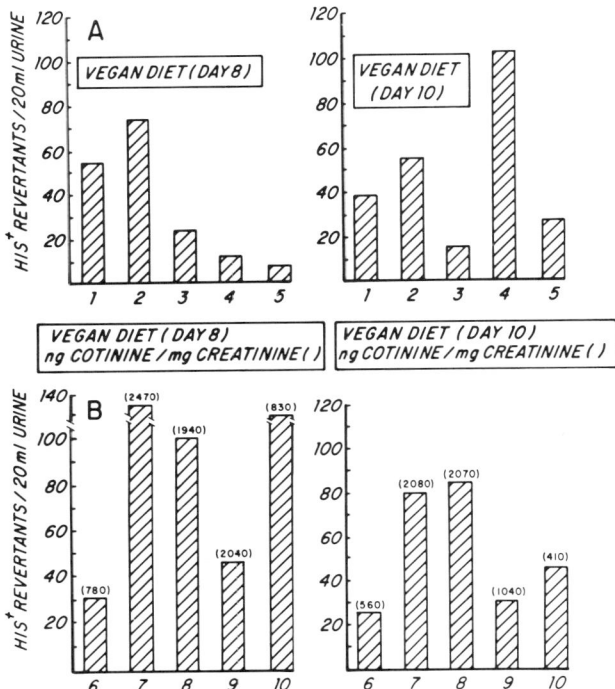

Figure 2
The mutagenic activity of urine concentrates of nonsmokers (A) and smokers (B) on a vegan diet

cotinine detected among nonsmokers in this study ranged from 0–40 ng per mg creatinine, which might be expected by exposure to passive smoking (Hoffmann et al. 1984). The levels of cotinine detected in the urine of smokers ranged from 410 ng per mg to 3240 ng per mg of creatinine. There is evidence of a general pattern of increasing mutagenic potency in the urine of cigarette smokers with an increase in the smoking habit as measured by the urinary cotinine levels. Of the five smokers in this study, the three volunteers who exhibited the highest cotinine levels also had the greatest mutagenic potency of all participants on the western diet (volunteers 7, 8 and 9; Fig. 1A and 2B). The obvious influence of the vegan diet on mutagenic activity of the urine concentrates, however, precluded the observation of a similar correlation in the second phase of this study. Although individual variations in urinary pH ranged from 5.4 to 7.2, urinary pH did not seem to be related to mutagenic activity.

A second control diet study with five smokers and five nonsmokers was set up and in this case a normal western diet was followed for 3 days and a 24-hour urine sample was collected on the third day. The participants then followed a macrobiotic diet regimen for 5 days providing 24-hour urine specimens on the last 2 days (Table 2). The results of assays of the urine concentrates in this study expressed in revertants per 1% of the total 24-hour specimen for days 3 and 8 of this study are illustrated in Figure 3A, B. There were no consistent differences in this diet study in the mutagenic activity of urine excreted by those on the western diet versus those on the macrobiotic diet. It is evident, however, that two of the five nonsmokers on either diet were found to have mutagenic activity in the urine concentrate.

Assays with Baboons

The various methods employed in assays with cigarette-smoking baboons in a controlled laboratory setting have been previously detailed by Marshall et al. (1983). In these settings, cigarette-smoking baboons had significantly greater urinary mutagenicity in *S. typhimurium* TA1538. In addition, a greater proportion of the cigarette-smoking animals exhibited measurable mutagenic activity in their urine concentrates (Table 3). In these studies no significant increase in mutagenic activity was observed with urine concentrates following glucuronidase treatment, an observation previously reported for mutagens in human urine (Aeschbacher and Chappuis 1981; Connor et al. 1983). Extensive studies comparing the relative mutagenic activity of the urine of cigarette-smoking baboons with that of sham-puffers were performed to determine which factors actually correlated with mutagenic activity. Mutagenic activity was not significantly different in the urine of male and female cigarette-smoking baboons. Although age and smoking history did not correlate with mutagenic activity, mean carboxyhemoglobin levels did. Under these

Table 2
Diet Regimen B

Meat diet (days 1–3)	
Breakfasts	Eggs, cereal, bread rolls, milk, juice, coffee, tea
Lunches	Tuna fish, roast beef, turkey, bread rolls, juice, coffee, tea
Dinners	Steak, lamb chop, chicken, rice, baked potatoes, string beans, broccoli, ice cream, coffee, tea
Macrobiotic diet (prepared fresh daily) (days 4–8)	
Breakfasts	Oatmeal, butternut squash, brown rice cream, baked apple, sourdough bread, barley tea
Lunches and Dinners	Brown rice, beans, millet, barley, seaweed, steamed fresh carrots, broccoli, onions, scallions, squash, turnips, romaine lettuce, spinach, tofu, rice cakes, barley tea

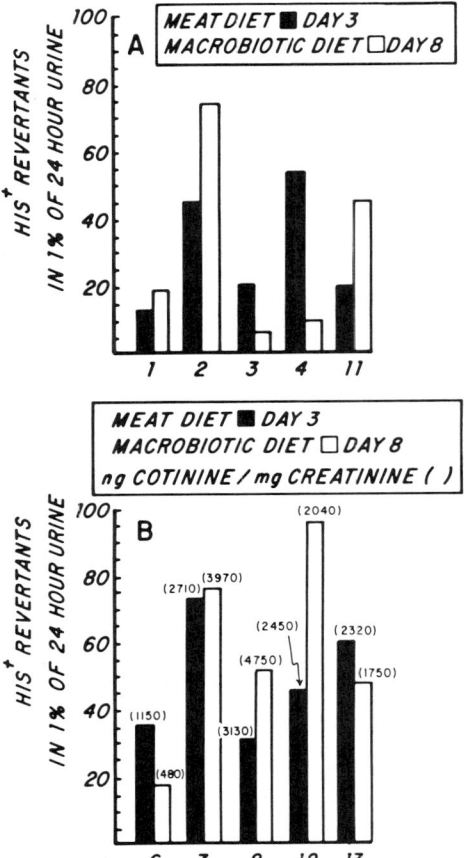

Figure 3
The mutagenic activity of urine concentrates of nonsmokers (A) and smokers (B) on a western diet (■) and a macrobiotic diet (□)

controlled experimental conditions, these data clearly demonstrate the underlying association of cigarette smoking and the excretion of urinary mutagens.

A group of ten sham-puffing baboons was monitored for the effects of the depth of inhalation of cigarette smoke on the production of urinary mutagens. During the initial 28 weeks of smoking, a positive correlation was observed between the following indices of cigarette smoke exposure: blood carboxyhemoglobin (COHb), urinary nicotine and cotinine, and plasma nicotine and cotinine (Table 4). When

Table 3
Mutagenic Activity of Urine Concentrates from Cigarette-smoking Baboons and Sham Puffers

		No. of animals	Smoking (pack-yrs)[a]	Blood COHb (%)	TA 1538 revertants/100 ml
Smokers	All	17	7.3 ± 0.5[b]	2.6 ± 0.3[c]	22 ± 1.3
	Males	10	7.9 ± 0.7	3.0 ± 0.4	26 ± 1.9
	(range)		(0.4 – 12.5)	(0.3 – 5.9)	(<1 – 119)
	Females	7	6.5 ± 0.6	2.0 ± 0.4	16 ± 1.6
	(range)		(3.7 – 12.5)	(0.9 – 4.3)	(<1 – 52)
Sham puffers	All	12		1.0 ± 0.1	0.8 ± 0.4
	(range)			(0.7 – 1.3)	(<1 – 6)

[a] Each animal routinely smoked 30 cigarettes/day, 7 days a week.
[b] Mean ± standard error
[c] Mean ± standard error of four samples prior to mutagenicity testing

Table 4
Correlation Between Urine Revertants and Cigarette Smoking

Urine revertants comparison	Mean pack-years of smoking[a]	Correlation coefficient (r)	Stat. Sign.
Plasma COHb	12	0.86	$P < 0.01$
Plasma COHb	1.2	0.78	$P < 0.01$
Urine nicotine	0.8	0.68	$P < 0.05$
Urine cotinine	0.8	0.57	$P < 0.10$
Plasma nicotine	0.8	0.75	$P < 0.02$
Plasma cotinine	0.8	0.89	$P < 0.01$

[a]Each animal routinely smoked 30 cigarettes/day, 7 days a week.

this group of animals was compared with a group of ten established smokers with a 12 pack-year smoking history (average COHb blood levels of 4.6% with a range of 2.1-12.5%), a positive correlation with levels of present COHb and urinary mutagens was also observed. The correlation between urinary mutagens and nicotine or cotinine was not as good as that observed between urinary mutagens and blood COHb.

When mutagenic activity is assessed in smokers versus nonsmokers, the difficulties encountered by the confounding variables, diet and environment, are likely to be compounded in any effort to isolate and structurally elucidate the tobacco-related urinary mutagen(s). Comparative analyses of the urine from cigarette-smoking baboons and urine from sham-puffers provide an ideal setting in which experimental variables can be carefully controlled. Despite these advantages, sufficient material for obtaining spectral data on suspect mutagenic components has in our initial studies been hindered by their trace amounts. In order to provide some direction for such analytical studies, we have extended the use of the baboon animal model to include the instillation of cigarette smoke condensate (CSC) into the lung. Cigarette smoke condensate ($\simeq 3.3g$) from which the nicotine had been largely removed by steam distillation was dissolved in 10% propylene glycol and 100 μM dipalmitoyl lecithin solution and instilled in each of the five major lobes of the lung via fiberoptic bronchoscope. In contrast to the urine collected 2 days prior to the instillation of the CSC, there was a sharp and pronounced increase in the excretion of mutagens in the urine within the first 24 hours after instillation. The excretion of mutagens in the urine rapidly declined 24 hours after instillation (Fig. 4). Chemical fractionation of the urine voided during the first 24 hours after instillation demonstrated that the mutagenic activity which persisted was in both the neutral and basic subfractions (Fig. 5). The capillary gas chromatography (GC) profiles of these subfractions as compared to urine collected prior to instillation clearly reveal chemical differences in composition. Currently we are using this animal model to identify those urinary mutagens that are associated with both the instillation of CSC and eventually with cigarette smoking.

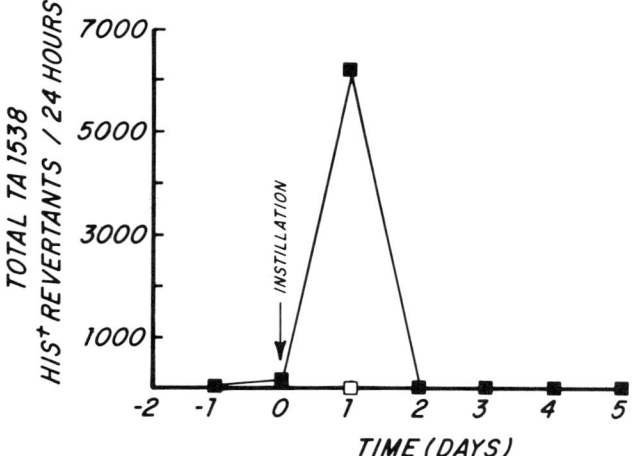

Figure 4
Mutagenic activity of the urine concentrate and its acidic, basic, and neutral fractions obtained from a baboon in which cigarette smoke condensate was instilled into the lungs. These results were obtained on the urine collected during the first 24 hrs after administration of the nicotine-reduced cigarette smoke condensate. (□) Vehicle control; (■) cigarette smoke condensate.

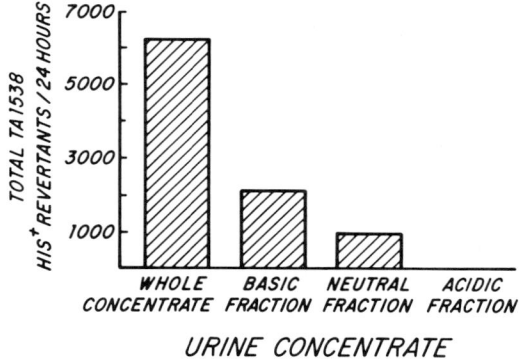

Figure 5
The mutagenic activity of the unfractionated urine concentrate obtained 24 hrs after administration of cigarette smoke condensate and its basic, neutral, and acidic fractions

DISCUSSION

Cigarette smoking has clearly been shown to be a contributing factor in the development of bladder cancer (Public Health Service 1982). Thus, there has been intense interest in the presence of mutagens in the urine of cigarette smokers.

Experimental data suggest that the urine concentrate of smokers is more likely to have significant mutagenic activity than that of nonsmokers. As is evident from a comparison of Figures 1 and 2, dietary factors also have a profound effect on the mutagenic potency of urine concentrates. In the case of the nonsmoker 2 on the vegan diet (Fig. 2), it is evident that the mutagenic activity of the urine concentrate is greater than that of several smokers (6 and 10) on the western diet (Fig. 1). These results indicate that cigarette smoking may not be the only factor associated with mutagens in urine and it also may not be the dominant factor in human studies without a suitable diet control.

The agents responsible for the mutagenicity of urine from individuals on the initial vegan diet are not known. Processed foods and food additives have been found to contain mutagens (Pariza et al. 1979; Weisburger and Spingarn 1979; Sugimura and Sato 1983; Krone and Iwaoka 1984). Plants also contain flavonoids, some of which are mutagens (White et al. 1973; MacGregor and Jurd 1978; Brown and Dietrich 1979; Ames 1983; Stavric 1984). There are, in addition, other as yet unidentified mutagens in food products derived from plants (Van der Hoeven et al. 1982). Potent mutagens have also been reported to be formed from protein pyrolysates (Nagao et al. 1977; Sugimura et al. 1977; Wakabayashi et al. 1978). Any one of these agents are likely to confound a clear correlation between the presence of urinary mutagens and cigarette smoking.

Studies performed using cigarette-smoking baboons have shown that there is a positive correlation between blood COHb levels and urinary mutagens. The correlation between physiological levels of nicotine and cotinine and the levels of mutagenicity in urine of cigarette-smoking baboons was not as significant as that observed between urine mutagens and blood COHb. Some of the circulating levels of nicotine and cotinine arise from buccal absorption. In contrast blood COHb levels arise primarily by the absorption of tobacco upon inhalation. The correlation between COHb levels and urinary mutagens suggests that urinary mutagens associated with cigarette smoking may be absorbed primarily from the lung rather than the oral cavity. This correlation is particularly interesting in view of the fact that an elevated risk for bladder cancer has not been observed in the majority of the epidemiological studies on pipe and cigar smokers (Wynder and Goldsmith 1977; Hartge et al. 1985).

The increased risk for urinary bladder cancer among cigarette smokers has been well established. Our data using the cigarette-smoking baboon animal model demonstrate that under controlled conditions cigarette smoking can elevate the excretion of mutagens. These genotoxic agents may be causally related to the increased risk of bladder cancer among smokers. The identity of these mutagens is, therefore, of major importance. It is critical that those agents associated with cigarette smoking (as opposed to diet or environment) be isolated and identified such that their genotoxic potential to man can be fully assessed. Studies using baboons in which CSC has been instilled into the lung, as well as the cigarette-smoking baboon, represent animal models which are likely to be effective means for advancing tobacco carcinogenesis as it relates to bladder cancer.

CONCLUSION

Our data demonstrate that diet has a pronounced effect upon the level of mutagenic activity as measured in *S. typhimurium* in human urine. Several studies have attempted to relate mutagenic activity in human urine to environmental or occupational factors. Our data suggest that in any such study dietary factors may similarly affect observed results. In any study directed toward isolation and identification of mutagens in human urine related to cigarette smoking, the confounding effect of diet must also be realized. The cigarette-smoking baboon animal model has shown that mutagens excreted in baboon urine are related to cigarette-smoking. The experimentally controlled environment associated with the use of this animal model is likely to provide the necessary experimental controls for successfully isolating and identifying mutagens in urine resulting from cigarette smoking.

ACKNOWLEDGMENTS

We would like to thank Ms. Caryn Axelrad, Mr. Steve Colosimo, and Mrs. Katherine Tilton for their biochemical assistance. We are also grateful to A.J. Noyola for his assistance in performing the mutagenicity assays on baboon urine. This study was supported by American Cancer Society grant SIG-8 and grant CA33069 from the National Cancer Institute.

REFERENCES

Aeschbacher, H.U. and C. Chappuis. 1981. Non-mutagenicity of urine from coffee drinkers compared with that from cigarette smokers. *Mutat. Res.* **89**: 161.

Ames, B.N. 1983. Dietary carcinogens and anticarcinogens. *Science* **21**: 1256.

Ames, B.N., J. McCann, and E. Yamasaki. 1975. Methods for detecting carcinogens and mutagens with the *Salmonella*/mammalian microsome mutagenicity test. *Mutat. Res.* **31**: 347.

Baker, R., A. Arlauskas, A. Bonin, and D. Angus. 1982. Detection of mutagenic activity in human urine following fried pork or bacon meals. *Cancer Lett.* **16**: 81.

Bos, R.P., J.L.G. Theuws, and P.Th. Henderson. 1983. Excretion of mutagens in human urine after passive smoking. *Cancer Lett.* **19**: 85.

Brown, J.P. and P.S. Dietrich. 1979. Mutagenicity of plant flavonoids in the Salmonella/mammalian microsome test. *Mutat. Res.* **66**: 223.

Connor, T.H., V.M.S. Ramanujan, J.B. Ward, Jr. and M.S. Legator. 1983. The identification and characterization of a urinary mutagen resulting from cigarette smoke. *Mutat. Res.* **113**: 161.

Dolara, P., S. Mazzoli, D. Rosi, E. Buiatti, S. Baccetti, A. Turchi, and V. Vanucci. 1981. Exposure to carcinogenic chemicals and smoking increases urinary excretion of mutagens in the humans. *J. Toxicol. Environ. Health* **8**: 95.

Garner, R.C., A.J. Mould, V. Lindsay-Smith, R.A. Cartwright, and B. Richards. 1982. Mutagenic urine from bladder cancer patients. *Lancet* ii: 389.

Gelbart, S.M. and S.J. Sontag. 1980. Mutagenic urine in cirrhosis. *Lancet* i: 894.

Haley, N.J., C.M. Axelrad, and K.A. Tilton. 1983. Validation of self-reported smoking behavior: Biochemical analyses of cotinine and thiocyanate. *Am. J. Public Health* **73**: 1204.

Hartge, P., R. Hoover, and A. Kantor. 1985. Bladder cancer risk and pipes, cigars and smokeless tobacco. *Cancer* **55**: 901.

Hoffmann, D., K.D. Brunnemann, J.D. Adams, and N.J. Haley. 1984. Indoor air pollution by tobacco smoke: Model studies on the update by nonsmokers. In *Indoor air, radon, passive smoking, particulates and housing epidemiology* (ed. B. Berglund, T. Lindvall, and J. Sundell), p. 313, Sweden.

Jaffe, R.L., W.J. Nicholson, and A.J. Garro. 1983. Urinary mutagen levels in smokers. *Cancer Lett.* **20**: 37.

Krone, C.A. and W.T. Iwaoka. 1984. Occurrence of mutagens in canned foods. *Mutat. Res.* **141**: 131.

Langone, J.J., H.B. Gjika, and H. Van Vunakis. 1973. Radioimmunoassay for nicotine and cotinine. *Biochem.* **12**: 5025.

MacGregor, J.T. and L. Jurd. 1978. Mutagenicity of plant flavonoids: Structural requirements for mutagenic activity in *Salmonella typhimurium*. *Mutat. Res.* **54**: 297.

Marshall, M.V., A.J. Noyola, and W.R. Rogers. 1983. Analysis of urinary mutagens produced by cigarette-smoking baboons. *Mutat. Res.* **118**: 241.

Nagao, M., M. Honda, Y. Seino, T. Yahagi, T. Kawachi, and T. Sugimura. 1977. Mutagenicities of protein pyrolysates. *Cancer Lett.* **2**: 335.

Pariza, M.W., S.H. Ashoor, and F.S. Chu. 1979. Mutagens in heat-processed meat, bakery, and cereal products. *Food Cosmet. Toxicol.* **17**: 429.

Public Health Service. 1982. The Health consequence of smoking: A report of the Surgeon General. Publ. No. 82-50179, p. 322. Government Printing Office, Washington, D.C.

Puzrath, R.M., D. Langley, and E. Eisenstadt. 1981. Analysis of mutagenic activity in cigarette smokers' urine by high performance liquid chromatography. *Mutat. Res.* **85**: 97.

Recio, L., H.G. Enoch, and M.A. Hannan. 1982. Parameters affecting the mutagenic activity of cigarette smokers' urine. *J. Appl. Toxicol.* **2**: 241.

Rogers, W.R., B. McCullough, and J.E. Caton. 1981. Cigarette smoking by baboons: In vivo assessment of particulate inhalation using bronchoalveolar lavage to recover (^{14}C)-dotriocontane. *Toxicology* **20**: 309.

Sasson, I.M., D.T. Coleman, E.J. LaVoie, D. Hoffmann, and E.L. Wynder. 1985. Mutagens in human urine: Effects of cigarette smoking and diet. *Mutation Res.* **158**: 149.

Sirtori, C., M. Paganuzzi, C. Lombardo, S. Scalese, and T. Razzon. 1978. Presenza di sostanze mutagene nelle urine di fumatori. *Gaslini* **10**: 18.

Sousa, J., J. Nath, J.D. Tucker, and T.M. Ong. 1985. Dietary factors affecting the urinary mutagenicity assay system. I. Detection of mutagenic activity in human urine following a fried beef meal. *Mutat. Res.* **149**: 365.

Stavric, B. 1984. Mutagenic food flavonoids. *Fed. Proc.* **43**: 2454.

Sugimura, T. and S. Sato. 1983. Bacterial mutagenicity of natural materials, pyrolysis products, and additives in foodstuffs and their association with genotoxic effects in mammals. In *Developments in the science and practice of toxicology*, Proc. 3rd Internat. Congr. on Toxicology, San Diego, Calif. 28 Aug.–3 Sept. 1983, (ed. A.W. Hayes, R.C. Schnell, and T.S. Miya), p. 115. Elsevier Science Publishers B.V.

Sugimura, T., T. Kawachi, M. Nagao, T. Yahagi, Y. Seino, T. Okamoto, K. Shudo, T. Kosuge, and K. Tswi. 1977. Mutagenic principle(s) in tryptophan and phenylalanine pyrolysis products. *Proc. Japn. Acad.* **53**: 56.

Van der Hoeven, J.C.M., W.J. Lagerwey, C.A.J.M. Meeuwissen, P.C.M. Hauwert, A.G.J. Voragen, and J.H. Koeman. 1982. Mutagens in food products of plant origin. In *Mutagens in our environment*, p. 327. Alan R. Liss, New York.

Van Doorn, R., R.P. Box, Ch.-M. Leijdekkers, M.A.P. Wagenaar-Zegers, J.L.G. Theuws, and P.Th. Henderson. 1979. Thioether concentration and mutagenicity of urine from cigarette smokers. *Int. Arch. Occup. Environ. Health* **43**: 159.

Wakabayashi, K., T. Tsuji, T. Kosuge, K. Takeda, K. Yamaguchi, K. Shudo, Y. Iitaka, T. Okamoto, T. Yahagi, M. Nagao, and T. Sugimura. 1978. Isolation and structure determination of a mutagenic substance in L-lysine pyrolysate. *Proc. Japn. Acad.* **54B**: 569.

Weisburger, J.H. and N.E. Spingarn. 1979. Mutagens as a function of the model of cooking meals. In *Naturally occurring carcinogens–Mutagens and modulators of carcinogenesis* (ed. E.C. Miller, J.A. Miller, I. Hirono, T. Sugimura, and S. Takayama) p. 177. Japan Soc. Press, Tokyo, Japan.

White, R.D., P.H. Krumperman, P.R. Cheeke, and D.R. Buhler. 1973. An evaluation of acetone extracts from six plants in the Ames mutagenicity tests. *Toxicol. Lett.* **15**: 25.

Wynder, E.L. and R. Goldsmith. 1977. The epidemiology of bladder cancer. A second look. *Cancer* **40**: 1246.

Yamasaki, E. and B.N. Ames. 1977. Concentration of mutagens from urine by adsorption with the non-polar resin XAD-2; cigarette smokers have mutagenic urine. *Proc. Natl. Acad. Sci. U.S.A.* **74**: 3555.

COMMENTS

LAVOIE: All of the results that I have presented on the mutagenic activity of human urine concentrates were performed in the presence of rat liver homogenate. We removed any residual histidine from these urine concentrates by dissolving the residue from the acetone eluent in methylene chloride and washing the methylene chloride layer with saturated saline. In this manner we felt that we removed any trace amounts of histidine from the urine concentrate.

TANNENBAUM: Did you deconjugate?

LAVOIE: We did deconjugate human urine to see if there was an increase in mutagenic activity. In studies with human urine samples, we observed, as have others, that there is an increase in toxicity to the bacteria without an increase in mutagenic activity when the urines are treated with deconjugating enzymes. With regard to studies on urines from smoking baboons, a similar effect was observed using both sulfatase and β-glucuronidase enzymes to deconjugate the urine specimens from smoking and nonsmoking baboons.

BELAND: What happens to urinary pH in light of the relationship between urinary pH and bladder tumor induction?

LAVOIE: This is a critical point, so let me give you the ranges. Throughout the study, urinary pH values ranged from 5.4-7.2. Urinary pH did not seem to be related at all to mutagenic activity. We were very concerned about urinary pH because of the impact this can have on the stability of certain components in urine.

BELAND: Do baboons get tumors? If they don't, is there any advantage to using the baboon when you already seem to have a good model—man?

LAVOIE: Well, the advantage is quite simple. We can control all situations. With the baboon animal model not only can we control dietary factors, but we can control the entire environment and activity of the baboon. Our studies on human urine have shown that diet can influence the mutagenic activity of urine concentrates. The baboon animal model provides an excellent starting point to determine the chemical nature of those urinary mutagens related to smoking. We do not want to spend a great deal of time isolating and structurally elucidating a urinary mutagen which may be related to the diet or to some chance occupational or environmental exposure. Our goal is specifically related to the identification of urinary mutagens associated with cigarette smoking.

BELAND: However, unless you can demonstrate tumor formation, you may be chasing something that has nothing to do with the carcinogenesis process.

LAVOIE: We are a long way from saying that we are attempting to isolate a urinary bladder carcinogen. As in any systematic study, we will evaluate the carcinogenic potential of those mutagens we identify in the urine of cigarette smokers. The purpose of the baboon animal model is to focus our analytical studies on certain likely agents.

BELAND: Aren't you obliged to use an animal model in which you can get tumors?

LAVOIE: It should be noted that no one has clearly shown the development of urinary bladder tumors from the administration of either cigarette smoke or cigarette smoke condensate to laboratory animals. The intention of using the baboon animal model is to determine what mutagens related to cigarette smoking or cigarette smoke condensate are ultimately excreted in the urine. We would then further examine its genotoxic potential. The idea at this time is to narrow our focus to a few specific components in the rather complex mixture commonly observed in these urine concentrates.

BARTSCH: I have a comment on the value of urinary mutagenicity. I think as long as the nature of urinary mutagenic metabolites has not been identified, the usefulness of such data as an indicator of exposure to carcinogens or the eventual health risk resulting thereof is rather limited. I should draw your attention to a study that was organized by the International Program on Chemical Safety in which our laboratory participated. Rats were given pairs of carcinogens and noncarcinogens, i.e., 2- and 4-acetylaminofluorene or benzo[a]pyrene and pyrene. When we compared the amount of excreted mutagenicity, the rats who received the noncarcinogens excreted as many mutagens as those receiving the same dose of carcinogens. In other words, urinary mutagenicity assays did not distinguish the carcinogenic compounds from the noncarcinogenic analogs. I'm surprised that such validation studies have not been done since 1974 when the assay was described for the first time.

LAVOIE: It has been over 9 years since the first report of mutagenic agents in the urine of cigarette smokers. I think the complexity of the problem was initially underestimated. The fact that diet and other variables can contribute to the mutagenic activity of human urine has, I believe, hampered efforts by chemists to isolate and structurally elucidate mutagens associated with cigarette smoking.

Endogenous Formation of *N*-Nitrosoproline in Smokers and Nonsmokers

GERHARD SCHERER AND FRANZ ADLKOFER
Council on Smoking and Health
Harvestehuder Weg 88
2000 Hamburg 13, West Germany

INTRODUCTION

The tobacco smoke-related nitrosamine burden of smokers and passive smokers may be of exogenous and endogenous origin. The *N*-nitrosoproline (NPRO) test, first introduced by Ohshima and Bartsch (1981), is a convenient method of estimating the endogenous nitrosamine formation in humans under various conditions. Hoffmann and Brunnemann (1983) and Ladd et al. (1984) reported higher NPRO formation rates in smokers compared to nonsmokers. Hoffmann et al. (1984) have found no indication of an increased urinary excretion of NPRO in nonsmokers exposed to tobacco smoke. In order to contribute to the assessment of tobacco smoke in endogenous nitrosamine formation, we have investigated the urinary NPRO excretion of smokers and nonsmokers.

MATERIALS AND METHODS

Experiment 1

The outline of the first experiment is given in Table 1. Twenty male subjects aged 18 to 40 years (ten smokers and ten nonsmokers) received daily oral applications of 500 mg proline dissolved in 20 ml water on three consecutive days. A 24-hour urine was sampled in flasks supplemented with 17.6 g ascorbic acid (E. Merck, Darmstadt, W. Germany) and 0.4 g merthiolate (thimerosal) (C. Roth KG, Karlsruhe, W. Germany) in order to prevent artefactual nitrosamine formation and to stabilize the urine. The sampling period lasted from the afternoon of the third day until the afternoon of the fourth day. The diet was not controlled in this experiment, but the subjects were asked to protocol their food, beverages, and tobacco consumption. The aim of this experiment was to find out whether or not a difference between smokers and nonsmokers in endogenous NPRO formation could be observed under real-life conditions, as was found in two controlled studies (Hoffmann and Brunnemann 1983; Ladd et al. 1984).

Table 1
Timetable for Experiment 1 (with Ten Smokers and Ten Nonsmokers)

Day	Time	
First	4:00 pm	Oral application of 500 mg proline; distribution of forms to protocol food, beverages, and tobacco consumption during the following 24 hours
Second	4:00 pm	Return of completed protocol forms; oral application of 500 mg proline; distribution of forms (see above)
Third	4:00 pm	Return of completed protocol forms; oral application of 500 mg proline; distribution of forms (see above); distribution of sampling flasks for 24-hr urine
Fourth	4:00 pm	Return of completed protocol forms and urine flasks

Experiment 2

In a second experiment five smokers and ten nonsmokers (partly identical with subjects of the first experiment) received daily oral applications of 500 mg proline on three consecutive days (Table 2). On the second day (control day) the subjects were served a controlled diet, avoiding coffee, black tea, beer, and dietary ascorbic acid. Any exposure to tobacco smoke (smoking or passive smoking) was avoided

Table 2
Timetable for Experiment 2 (with Five Smokers and Ten Nonsmokers)

Day	Time	
First	8:30 am	Oral application of 500 mg proline
Second	8:30 am	Oral application of 500 mg proline; drawing of blood samples for COHb measurement; distribution of sampling flasks for 8-hr urine
	9:00 am	Stay in a test room for 8 hours without exposure to cigarette smoke. Breakfast, lunch, tea, and cookies were served.
	5:00 pm	Return of urine flasks with an 8-hr urine; drawing of blood samples for COHb measurement; distribution of urine flasks for the following 16 hours and protocol forms. Subjects were asked to avoid smoking and passive smoking, coffee, black tea, beer, and orange juice
Third	8:30 am	Exactly as on day 2 except heavy cigarette smoke exposure in the test room for 8 hours
	9:00 am	
	5:00 pm	Exactly as on day 2, but restrictions on smoking were abolished
Fourth	8:30 am	Return of completed protocol forms and urine flasks

on the control day. The third day (exposure day) followed exactly the same pattern as the second except that smokers were allowed to smoke while the nonsmokers were heavily exposed to tobacco smoke in a test room for a period of 8 hours. On both the control and exposure day 24-hour urine was sampled.

Analytical Methods

NPRO in urine was measured by Prof. PreuBmann (Deutsches Krebsforschungszentrum, Heidelberg, W. Germany) as follows: to urine aliquots of 15 ml each were added 200 ng nitrososarcosine and 200 ng nitrosopipecolinic acid as internal standards. To precipitate urinary proteins, 1 ml $K_4Fe(CN)_6$ solution (106 g $K_4Fe(CN)_6 \times 2\ H_2O$/liter water) and 1 ml $ZnSO_4$ solution (219 g $ZnSO_4 \times 7H_2O$/liter 3% acetic acid) were added. The mixture was filtered off under suction after 20 minutes. The filtrate was saturated with $(NH_4)_2SO_4$ and acidified with 1ml 50% H_2SO_4 (pH 1.2-1.4). The sample was poured on an Extrolut column and eluted 20 minutes later with 60 ml ethyl acetate. The organic phase was concentrated to 1 ml by means of a rotation evaporator, transferred to a receiver by flushing with 2 ml ethyl acetate, and concentrated to 1 ml by a stream of N_2. Then 2 ml of diazomethane dissolved in ether were added. After 20 minutes the mixture was concentrated to 1 ml (N_2 stream). The analysis was performed with gas chromatography (GC) and thermal energy assay (TEA) (column OV 275, 6%, 2 м, 140-210°C). The detection limit for NPRO under these conditions was 2.5 ppb. The results were not corrected for recovery rates, which amounted to 80% at a minimum.

Nitrate in urine was detected colorimetrically (Sen and Donaldsen 1978). COHb was determined immediately after taking the blood samples using a CO-oximeter (Instrumentation Laboratories Ltd., Model 182). Carbon monoxide, nitric oxide, and nitrogen dioxide were continuously measured in the test room in the passive smoking study (experiment 2) on both the control day and the exposure day by means of an infrared CO analyzer (Model 867, Beckman Instruments Inc., Fullerton, California) and a nitric oxide analyzer (Model 8840, Monitor Labs, supplied by Kontron Analytik GmbH, Munich, W. Germany).

RESULTS

The results of the first experiment are presented in Table 3. Smokers excreted significantly higher amounts of NPRO when compared to nonsmokers (6.1 vs. 1.6 μg/24 hr; $P < 0.05$). Both groups excreted about the same amount of nitrate (18.6 and 18.1 mg/24 hr for smokers and nonsmokers, respectively). Urine volumes were significantly higher in smokers than in nonsmokers (1785 vs. 950 ml; $P < 0.05$). An analysis of the self-reported beverage consumption data revealed that the smokers drank significantly more beer and coffee than the nonsmokers. The self-reported

Table 3
Urinary Excretion of NPRO and Nitrate in Smokers and Nonsmokers under Uncontrolled Conditions (Experiment 1)

Subject no.	Smoking during sampling period (cig/24 hr)	Urine volume (ml/24 hr)	Nitrate (mg/24 hr)	NPRO (µg/24 hr)
		Smokers		
1	10	1000	10.1	5.4
7	39	2760	23.2	9.4
9	21	2080	29.5	ND[a]
10	24	2500	15.0	ND
11	15	1300	13.7	6.7
13	17	1040	21.8	9.4
15	24	1820	21.5	ND
16	26	1350	17.7	19.6
17	25	2000	15.6	ND
18	25	2000	17.6	10.9
Mean ± SD	22.6 ± 7.8	1785 ± 600	18.6 ± 5.6	6.1 ± 2.1
		Nonsmokers		
2		950	13.0	5.1
3		610	6.1	ND
4		1060	8.6	2.8
5		700	29.1	2.3
6		1230	23.6	3.4
8		670	11.3	2.6
12		710	11.1	ND
14		1040	25.3	ND
19		1880	37.4	ND
20		650	15.5	ND
		950 ± 390	18.1 ± 10	1.6 ± 0.6

[a]ND = Not detectable; detection limit: 2.5 ppb

intake of fruit juices, tea, soft beverages, vegetables, and meat was not different in the two groups.

The passive smoking exposure conditions during the second experiment are illustrated in Figure 1. The carbon monoxide level in the test room was less than 3 ppm on the control day and increased to more than 20 ppm during the 8-hour exposure period. Nitric oxide changed from about 10 ppb on the control day to about 400 ppb on the exposure day. Nitrogen dioxide increased from about 20 ppb on the control day to about 40 ppb on the exposure day. The tobacco smoke exposure is also reflected in the differences in the subjects' carboxyhemoglobin levels

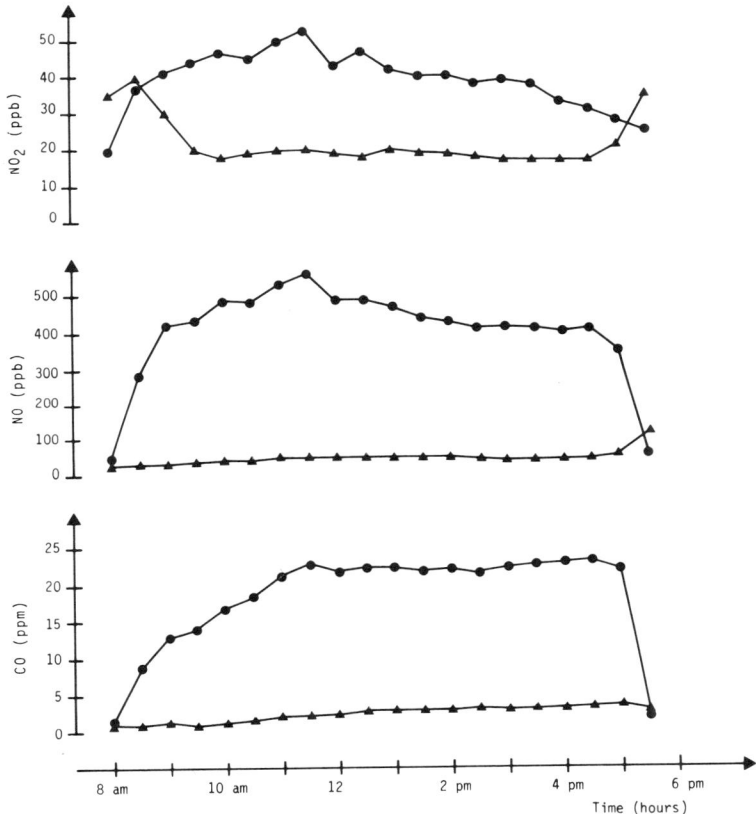

Figure 1
Levels of CO, NO, and NO_2 in the test room (experiment 2). On the exposure day 149 cigarettes were smoked between 8 am and 5 pm. The window was opened at 5 pm on both the control and exposure day. (▲——▲) Control day; (●——●) exposure day.

before and after the 8-hour stay in the test room on either the control or exposure day (Table 4).

On both the control and exposure day there was no difference between smokers and nonsmokers with respect to their NPRO formation. Furthermore, the urinary NPRO excretion did not increase in either smokers or nonsmokers as a result of the tobacco smoke exposure. Most of the subjects exhibited urinary NPRO concentrations below the detection limit.

Table 4
Urinary Excretion of NPRO and Nitrate in Smokers and Nonsmokers under Controlled Conditions (Experiment 2)

Subject no.	Control day ΔCOHb[a] (%)	Control day Urine volume (ml/24 hr)	Control day Nitrate (mg/24 hr)	Control day NPRO (μg/24 hr)	Exposure day ΔCOHb[a] (%)	Exposure day Smoking during sampling period (cig/24 hr)	Exposure day Urine volume (ml/24 hr)	Exposure day Nitrate (mg/24 hr)	Exposure day NPRO (μg/24 hr)
				Smokers					
13	−1.6	1450	19.4	13.1	+7.0	19	2200	20.0	10.3
9	−2.7	720	17.6	5.0	+12.0	28	1850	40.3	ND
7	−3.1	750	15.4	ND[b]	+5.3	36	2500	21.8	ND
16	−1.4	1300	32.0	6.0	+4.7	17	1600	17.3	ND
18	−0.1	750	18.5	3.8	+7.3	35	1650	21.0	ND
Mean ± SD	−1.6 ± 1.3	994 ± 352	20.6 ± 6.5	5.6 ± 4.3	+7.3 ± 2.9	27.0 ± 8.8	1960 ± 383	24.1 ± 9.3	
				Nonsmokers					
3	−1.0	750	7.7	2.1	+3.0		(240[c])	0.3	(ND[c])
5	−1.2	1600	19.5	8.2	+2.2		1650	14.6	ND
21	−1.3	1000	11.4	3.2	+3.3		1690	13.5	ND
6	−0.8	1220	59.5	10.4	+2.9		760	44.6	4.8
8	−1.1	1250	9.5	5.4	+3.2		1450	14.7	12.9
12	−0.7	750	10.5	ND	+2.7		750	4.1	2.9
22	−0.7	1370	14.1	5.5	+2.1		1060	12.2	4.8
23	−0.8	2140	14.3	ND	+3.3		2250	16.4	ND
19	−0.2	770	11.1	ND	+3.1		1170	12.3	ND
24	−0.3	1880	12.4	ND	+2.8		1600	10.9	ND
Mean ± SD	−0.7 ± 0.4	1273 ± 485	17.0 ± 15.3	3.5 ± 3.8	+2.7 ± 0.8		1376 ± 488	16.0 ± 11.3	

[a] Difference before and after the 8-hr control or exposure period
[b] ND = Not detectable; detection limit: 2.5 ppb
[c] Return of an incomplete 24-hr urine

Under both conditions smokers tended to excrete higher amounts of nitrate. However, this difference is not statistically significant. The NPRO levels did not correlate with the urinary nitrate levels when the data of both experiments were pooled.

Five smokers (subjects 7, 9, 13, 16, 18) and six nonsmokers (subject 3, 5, 6, 8, 12, 19) participated in both experiments so that three NPRO and nitrate measurements for each of these individuals are available. Analysis of these data revealed that intraindividual variations were high with respect to urinary nitrate excretion (average coefficient of variance $\bar{c}v = 33\%$ and extremely high with respect to urinary NPRO excretion ($\bar{c}v = 102\%$).

DISCUSSION

The results of our first experiment performed without dietary control confirm those of other authors (Hoffmann and Brunnemann 1983; Ladd et al. 1984) who reported a higher NPRO formation in smokers compared to nonsmokers. However, none of our smokers excreted an extraordinarily high amount of NPRO (> 20 $\mu g/24$ hr) as, for example, Hoffmann and Brunnemann (1983) observed in their study. In four subjects of the smoking group and five subjects of the nonsmoking group, NPRO concentrations were below the detection limit. Since smokers had significantly higher urine volumes than nonsmokers, the difference in NPRO excretions between smokers and nonsmokers might be even higher due to a more pronounced urine dilution effect in smokers that could decrease the NPRO concentration below the detection limit. On the other hand, we observed a positive correlation between NPRO excretion and urine volume ($r = 0.56, P < 0.02$) which suggests that the increased NPRO in smokers might partly be attributed to their higher urine volume. It is a well-known phenomenon that urinary excretion of foreign compounds increases with elevated diuresis. Thus, increased NPRO excretions coupled with increased 24-hour urine volumes do not necessarily implicate higher NPRO formation rates. It may well be that other excretion routes, for example, sweat, (Bogovski et al. 1984), are inversely related to diuresis. However, more data are needed to substantiate this speculation.

The self-reported higher beer and coffee intake by smokers could further increase the difference in NPRO formation between smokers and nonsmokers, since beer is reported to contain nitrosation-inhibiting substances (Pignatelli et al. 1983). Polyphenols in coffee may both catalyze and inhibit the endogenous NPRO formation (Pignatelli et al. 1980).

The second experiment was designed in order to investigate the NPRO formation possibly caused by passive smoking. In spite of an extremely high passive smoke exposure, documented in the indoor air concentrations of carbon monoxide, nitric oxide, and nitrogen dioxide (Figure 1) as well as in the increase of the COHb level (Table 4), we were unable to find an increase in the NPRO formation as a result of the passive smoke exposure. This is in line with findings by Hoffmann et al. (1984), who did not see an increase in the urinary NPRO excretion after passive smoke exposure either.

Unexpectedly, we could not confirm the results of our first experiment nor those by Hoffmann and Brunnemann (1983) showing increased NPRO excretions in smokers compared to nonsmokers. The results of our second study, however, are in agreement with that of Ladd et al. (1984), who found no difference in NPRO formation between smokers and nonsmokers when the diet was not supplemented with nitrate. It should also be mentioned that, due to the control of the diet, no significant difference in urine volume was found between smokers and nonsmokers in experiment 2, so that a volume effect as discussed for experiment 1 is not to be expected.

Three hypotheses on the mechanism by which smoking might enhance the urinary NPRO excretion could be discussed:

(1) Compounds from tobacco smoke, probably nitrite derived from nitric oxide, act as nitrosating agents in stomach, oral cavity, lungs, or blood. A comparison of the uptake of the potentially nitrosating agent, nitric oxide, by cigarette smoking (40-200 μmole NO) (Williams 1980) or passive smoking (15-100 μmole NO) (Weber and Fisher 1980) and nitrite by diet (90 μmole nitrite) (Committee on Nitrite and Alternative Curing Agents in Food 1981) suggests that at least in the case of passive smoking, nitrosating agents from dietary sources may outweigh those from tobacco smoke. Furthermore, the data of Ladd et al. (1984) and Ohshima and Bartsch (1981) indicate that nitrate intake has to exceed a certain amount before the urinary NPRO excretion significantly increases. The urinary nitrate excretion in our subjects is low compared to those reported by other authors (Radomski et al. 1978; Tannenbaum et al. 1978), suggesting that in our volunteers this threshold might not be exceeded.

(2) Elevated salivary thiocyanate in smokers catalyses the NPRO formation. This hypothesis is favored by Ladd et al. (1984). The diet was supplemented with nitrate. Since thiocyanate levels in plasma, saliva, and urine of passive smokers do not exceed those in unexposed subjects (Jarvis and Russell 1983), an increased NPRO excretion as a result of passive smoking is unlikely. These data are in accordance with those of Hoffmann and Brunnemann (1984) as well as with our results in passive smokers. Our findings on smokers at least do not contradict this hypothesis.

(3) NPRO excretion increases with increasing urine volume. This is a well-known phenomenon with xenobiotics but has not been reported for NPRO. This hypothesis has to be validated by systematic investigations.

CONCLUSIONS

Smokers were found to excrete higher amounts of NPRO than nonsmokers in an uncontrolled study. Since smokers exhibit higher urine volumes, a volume-dependent effect could have contributed to this result. In a controlled study no differences between smokers, nonsmokers, and passive smokers, with respect to their NPRO excretion, were observed. In both experiments the volunteers had relatively low urinary nitrate levels, possibly insufficient to raise the urinary NPRO excretion above the background level.

Our results demonstrate that smoking or passive smoking may not contribute substantially to the uptake of agents capable of nitrosating proline. They would, however, be compatible with the hypothesis that tobacco smoke-derived thiocyanate may by its catalyzing effect increase the endogenous NPRO formation. Further research is needed to elucidate the role of tobacco smoking in the endogenous nitrosamine formation.

REFERENCES

Bogovski, P. A., M. A. Rooma, and J. M. Kann. 1984. Studies on the excretion of endogenously formed N-nitrosoproline. I. Percutaneous excretion of N-nitrosoproline in humans. In *N-Nitroso compounds: Occurrence, biological effects and relevance to human cancer* (ed. I.K. O'Neill, R.C. von Borstel, C.T. Miller, J. Long, and H. Bartsch). IARC Scientific Publications no. 57, p. 199. IARC, Lyon, France.

Committee on Nitrite and Alternative Curing Agents in Food. 1981. *The health effects of nitrate, nitrite, and N-nitroso compounds.* National Academy Press, Washington, D.C.

Hoffmann, D. and K. D. Brunnemann. 1983. Endogenous formation of N-nitrosoproline in cigarette smokers. *Cancer Res.* **43**: 5570.

Hoffmann, D., K. D. Brunnemann, J. D. Adams, and N. J. Haley. 1984. Indoor air pollution by tobacco smoke: Model studies on the uptake by nonsmokers. In *Indoor air* (ed. B. Berglund, T. Lindvall, and J. Sundell), vol. 2, p. 313. Swedish Council for Building Research, Stockholm, Sweden.

Jarvis, M. J. and M. A. H. Russell. 1983. Measurement and estimation of smoke dosage to non-smokers from environmental tobacco smoke. In *ETS-environmental tobacco smoke. Report from a workshop on effects and exposure levels.* (ed. R. Rylaw, Y. Peterson, and M.-C. Snella), p. 68. University of Geneva, Switzerland.

Ladd, K. F., H. L. Newmark, and M. C. Archer. 1984. N-Nitrosation of proline in smokers and nonsmokers. *J. Natl. Cancer Inst.* **73**: 83.

Ohshima, H. and H. Bartsch. 1981. Quantitative estimation of endogenous nitrosation in humans by monitoring N-nitrosoproline excreted in the urine. *Cancer Res.* **41**: 3658.

Pignatelli, B., M. Friesen, and E. A. Walker. 1980. The role of phenols in catalyses of nitrosamine formation. In *N-nitroso compounds: Analysis, formation and occurrence* (ed. L. Griciute, M. Castegnaro, M. Börzsöng, and W. Davis), IARC Scientific Publications no. 31, p. 95. IARC, Lyon, France.

Pignatelli, B., R. Scriban, G. Descotes, and H. Bartsch. 1983. Inhibition of endogenous nitrosation in rats by lyophilized beer constituents. *Carcinogenesis* **4**: 491.

Radomski, J. L., C. Palmiri, and W. L. Hearn. 1978. Concentrations of nitrate in normal human urine and the effect of nitrate ingestion. *Toxicol. Appl. Pharmacol.* **45**: 63.

Sen, N. P. and B. Donaldsen. 1978. Improved colorimetric method for determining nitrate and nitrite in foods. *J. Assoc. Off. Anal. Chem.* **61**: 1389.

Tannenbaum, S. R., D. Fett, V. R. Young, P. D. Land, and W. R. Bruce. 1978. Nitrite and nitrate are formed by endogenous synthesis in the human intestine. *Science* **200**: 1487.

Weber, A. and T. Fisher. 1980. Passive smoking at work. *Int. Arch. Occup. Environ. Health* **47**: 209.

Williams, T. B. 1980. The determination of nitric oxide in gas phase cigarette smoke by non-dispersive infrared analysis. *Beitr. Tabakforsch. Int.* **10**: 91.

COMMENTS

BRUNNEMANN: What is your detection limit for nitrosoproline in urine?

SCHERER: The detection limit for NPRO in urine must be about 0.5 ppb and this is better than ours. It is therefore not surprising that we found quite a large number of subjects in our study with NPRO levels below the detection limit.

BRUNNEMANN: But maybe then you didn't really see the fine print, if the detection wasn't adequate.

SCHERER: Yes, I agree, but I believe that NPRO urine levels around or below 2.5 ppb are quite common in subjects obviously not exposed to nitrosating agents. Levels of biological significance should be clearly above 2.5 ppb.

MAGEE: You spoke of possible nitrosation by NO_2 which would take place in the lungs rather than in the stomach. Is there any evidence for this happening?

SCHERER: It has been shown in a number of animal experiments that in vivo nitrosation takes place after inhalation of NO_2. However, it is an open question whether these kind of experiments will help to determine the site of nitrosation.

HOFFMANN: Klaus [Brunnemann], could you briefly discuss your study on the endogenous formation of *N*-nitrosomorpholine in mice?

BRUNNEMANN: In cooperation with the NIEHS, we gavaged mice with morpholine, and then let them inhale NO_2. Subsequently, various sections of the mice were analyzed for nitrosomorpholine, and it was only found in the stomach. However, I must point out that when the mice, or parts of them, were analyzed, they were skinned and beheaded. As you know, Mirvish found some nitrosating agents in the skin and in the hair of mice. But our mice were skinned; therefore we found nitrosomorpholine only in the stomachs.

SUMMARY DISCUSSION

HOFFMANN: Would anyone like to discuss some of the topics presented so far?

WINKELSTEIN: Ed [LaVoie], your colleagues recently reported cotinine and nicotine in the cervical fluid of smokers. Did you do mutagenic tests on that material?

LAVOIE: Yes. We used a pooled sample from among all of the smokers in that study versus the nonsmokers; and we did not find any mutagenic activity when we attempted a dose-response. But there has been a report. N.L. Petrakis and coworkers analyzed the cervical fluid for mutagenicity.

RANDERATH: We need to find out which subfractions of cigarette smoke condensate give the adducts observed by us; and these experiments are planned.

HOFFMANN: I think that one of the purposes of this meeting is for us to communicate with each other. The molecular biologist should speak with the tobacco scientist. I think that to advance we should apply our methodology there, where it's most urgently needed. There is no question in my mind that smoking is *the* major environmental factor for cancer in humans. On the other side, we in tobacco science may not have advanced sufficiently; we should also apply the elegant molecular biological methodology.

MAGEE: I think, Dr. Randerath, that you did say that you were starting to apply your methods to the tobacco-specific nitrosamines.

HECHT: Did it give a spot?

RANDERATH: NNK gave several spots.

HECHT: Where were they?

E. RANDERATH: They were located in the upper left quarter of the chromatograms.

HECHT: What kinds of compounds move in that portion of the chromatogram?

RANDERATH: They were in an unusual location.

LAVOIE: Did you find DNA adducts in your chromatographs following application of aza-arenes?

RANDERATH: Yes, we have. Schurdak, in my laboratory, has studied adducts from several dibenzocarbazoles and dibenzacridines. Some of them run in proximity to NNK adducts in our TLC systems.

HOFFMANN: No, carbazols are neutral compounds and acridines are basic compounds.

Session 2:
New Aspects of Tobacco Carcinogenesis

Chemical Analysis of the Major Constituents in Clove Cigarette Smoke

MARCUS B. WISE AND MICHAEL R. GUERIN
Analytical Chemistry Division
Oak Ridge National Laboratory
Oak Ridge, Tennessee 37831

OVERVIEW

The smoke of clove-containing cigarettes has been potentially linked to a variety of acute toxicological effects in humans. A lack of information with respect to the chemical constituents present in the smoke has made it difficult to determine the cause of the reported health problems. This research has focused on the identification and quantitation of the major components unique to clove cigarettes. Conventional chromatographic methods as well as combined gas chromatography/mass spectrometry (GC/MS) were utilized for analysis of the gas-phase, whole-smoke, and total particulate matter (TPM) constituents. The smoke composition profiles were found to be similar to those of conventional tobacco cigarettes, but with the addition of significant quantities of the major clove oil components including eugenol, eugenol acetate, beta-caryophyllene, alpha-humulene, and caryophyllene-epoxide. Particularly significant is the delivery of up to 15 mg of eugenol per cigarette when smoked under standard Federal Trade Commission (FTC) conditions. Deliveries of the other constituents range from 2 mg for beta-caryophyllene and eugenol acetate to less than 200 μg per cigarette for alpha-humulene and caryophyllene-epoxide. Tar and nicotine deliveries are also somewhat higher than for domestic tobacco cigarettes.

INTRODUCTION

Clove-flavored cigarettes (kreteks) imported from Indonesia have become a growing fad among young adults in North America during recent years (T.L. Guidotti et al., in prep.). These cigarettes are actually a blend of 35-40% clove material with 60-65% tobacco by weight (Hirs 1984) and have possibly been associated with cases of moderate to severe acute illnesses (Anderson 1985). According to a report by the Centers for Disease Control (CDC) (Schechter et al. 1985), some of the symptoms potentially linked to clove cigarette smoke include pulmonary edema, hemoptysis, and bronchospasm. Other effects include angina, nausea, vomiting, and chronic cough. Even though kreteks are smoked by most adult males in Indonesia, the health effects there have not been extensively studied (Schechter et al. 1985).

Growing concern about the potential dangers of clove cigarettes has led to the need to establish a sound cause-effect relationship between kreteks and the reported illnesses. This, however, has been hindered by a lack of information regarding the chemical nature of clove-cigarette smoke. Eugenol, for instance, has long been known to be the major ingredient in clove oil (Guenther 1950; Masada 1976), but the fate of this compound during the burning of a cigarette was uncertain. In particular, it was not known whether or not eugenol (or the other clove oil constituents), when pyrolyzed or burned in the presence of tobacco material, produced significant quantities of unusual or highly toxic compounds.

This research has centered on the chemical analysis of the major constituents present in the smoke of Indonesian kreteks. Because cigarette smoke is a highly complex mixture of thousands of compounds, emphasis was placed predominantly on the determination of constituents that could be readily identified as clove oil-related and thus unique to kreteks. To accomplish this, clove oil, clove extracts, and the smoke and TPM from experimental 100% clove cigarettes were analyzed. This enabled the identification of the principal clove oil distillate and pyrolysis products in the absence of tobacco-related products. The deliveries of these constituents were then quantitated in the TPMs of several popular brands of Indonesian kreteks. The initial findings indicate that the primary pyrolysis and combustion products in the gas phase of clove smoke are predominantly the same as those in tobacco smoke except for the absence of nitrogen-containing species. The TPM of 100% clove cigarettes, however, consists almost entirely of clove oil that is distilled directly into the smoke.

RESULTS

Analysis of Clove Oil and Clove Extracts

Prior to the analyses of clove cigarette smoke, clove oils and clove extracts were analyzed using combined capillary gas chromatography/mass spectrometry (GC/MS). This enabled the determination of chromatographic retention times and mass spectral characteristics of the volatile and extractable clove constituents in the absence of interferring pyrolysis and combustion products. The compounds identified in clove oil are summarized in Table 1. Pure samples of the major constituents were also obtained and used to confirm initial assignments. Eugenol (2-methoxy, 4-allyl-phenol) was the most abundant component in each of the samples studied, comprising approximately 80–85% by weight. Other significant compounds include beta-caryophyllene, alpha-humulene (both are $C_{15}H_{24}$ sesquiterpenoids), eugenol acetate, and beta-caryophyllene-epoxide. Several additional terpenoids, phenols, and organic acids were also found in minor concentrations. These findings are in agreement with those reported in the literature on essential oils (Masada 1976).

Table 1
Constituents in Clove Oils and Clove Extracts

Constituent	(%) Approximate
Major	
Eugenol	80–85
Eugenol acetate[a]	3–5
Beta-caryophyllene	3–5
Alpha-humulene	1
Beta-caryophyllene epoxide	1
Minor	(less than 1%)
Iso-eugenol	
Isomeric sesquiterpenoids	
Benzyl-acetate	
Benzyl-benzoate	
Methyl-salicylate	
Methyl-eugenol	
Palmitic acid	
Stearic acid	
Lineolic acid	

[a] Eugenol acetate is not found in clove-leaf oil.

Clove Cigarette Smoke Characteristics

Smoke composition profiles were generated for two brands of popular unfiltered kreteks, a commercial domestic tobacco cigarette, a 2R1 Kentucky reference tobacco cigarette, and an experimental 100% clove cigarette. Both gas-phase and whole-smoke profiles were characterized for each cigarette. The gas phase is considered to consist of the volatile, low molecular weight combustion, pyrolysis, and distillate products, whereas the whole smoke consists of the higher boiling, higher molecular weight "particulate phase" or aerosol material (Wynder and Hoffmann 1967; Guerin 1980).

Material for profile analysis was collected by trapping the smoke of a 2-second (mid-cigarette) puff on Tenax sorbant. Gas phase constituents were selectively isolated by placing a Cambridge filter pad between the cigarette butt and Tenax to remove the particulates from the effluent. Whole smoke was collected similarly except the Cambridge filter pad was removed from the sampling device (Higgins et al. 1984). Analyses were performed by transferring a portion of the Tenax material to the inlet of a gas chromatograph (GC) where the components were thermally desorbed, separated, and analyzed. Conventional chromatographic analyses were performed with capillary columns (DB-5 phase), flame ionization, and nitrogen-specific detectors. Compound identifications were made via retention time matching with known compounds in a standard mixture. GC/MS was also performed on all samples. A capillary GC column (DB-5) and quadrupole mass spectrometer were utilized. Identifications were based on GC retention times, mass spectrometric fragmentation patterns, and comparison with authentic samples of pure compounds whenever possible.

Gas-phase Profiles

Representative gas-phase profiles for a 2R1 tobacco cigarette, a 100% clove cigarette, and an Indonesian kretek are shown in Figure 1. Despite the dramatically different nature of the materials burned in the tobacco cigarette versus the 100% clove cigarette, the gas-phase profiles are surprisingly similar. Although a quantitative study of the gas-phase constituent deliveries was not performed, an effort was made to analyze approximately the same quantity of smoke in each case, thus providing some information on relative deliveries between cigarette types. For instance, de-

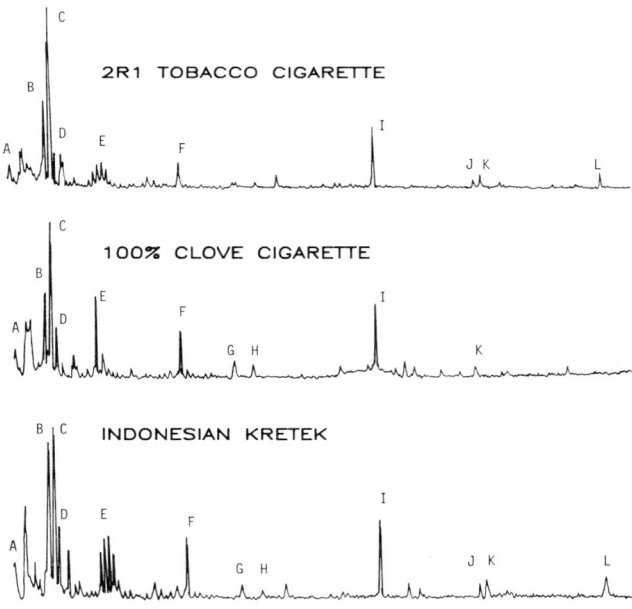

Figure 1
Gas phase smoke composition profiles for a 2R1 tobacco cigarette, a 100% clove cigarette, and an Indonesian kretek. (A) Carbon dioxide; (B) acetone; (C) isoprene; (D) methyl-butene; (E) pentadiene; (F) benzene; (G) dimethyl-cyclopentane; (H) ethyl-pentane; (I) toluene; (J) ethylbenzene; (K) xylene; (L) limonene.

liveries of acetone, isoprene, benzene, toluene, and xylene appear to be similar for all of the cigarettes studied.

A detailed analysis of the gas phase by GC/MS showed the presence of C_3-C_9 hydrocarbons (alkanes and alkenes), low molecular weight aldehydes and ketones, aromatic hydrocarbons, and furans for each type of cigarette. The most noticeable difference is the lack of nitrogen-containing compounds in the smoke of the 100% clove cigarette. This deficiency was confirmed by GC/MS as well as conventional gas chromatography with a nitrogen-specific detector. Additionally, the clove cigarette smoke (100% clove and kretek) showed elevated deliveries of hydrocarbons such as methyl pentene relative to the 2R1 tobacco cigarette.

Since most of the compounds identified in the gas phase of the 100% clove cigarette were not found to be present in the clove oils and clove extracts, it is assumed that they are combustion and pyrolysis products of clove oil and the fiberous clove-bud material (cellulose). Isoprene, for instance, is a reasonable pyrolysis product of the sesquiterpenoids present in clove oil.

Whole-smoke Profiles

Typical whole-smoke profiles (from toluene to neophytadiene) for the three types of cigarettes studied are shown in Figure 2. Both the 2R1 tobacco cigarette and Indonesian kretek have highly complex profiles with hundreds of constituents. Some of the major compounds common to these two types of cigarettes include toluene, xylenes, limonene, nicotine, and neophytadiene. It is interesting (and quite diagnostic) that the profile for the 100% clove cigarette is amazingly simple. The principal components are those of clove oil: eugenol, beta-caryophyllene, alpha-humulene, beta-caryophyllene-epoxide, and eugenol acetate. There does not appear to be a significant amount of pyrolysis products which elute between toluene and eugenol, thus the complexity of the kretek profile can be attributed primarily to the presence of the tobacco constituents. As can be seen from Figure 2, superposition of the 100% clove cigarette profile upon the tobacco cigarette profile accounts for most of the peaks observed in the profile of the kretek. The kretek does, however, show an elevated delivery of phenol relative to the 2R1 and 100% clove cigarettes, as well as the presence of an unidentified constituent (molecular weight 210?) which elutes between caryophyllene-epoxide and neophytadiene. These anomalies may be due to the different types of tobaccos used in the kretek.

Quantitation of the Major Constituents

Tar, nicotine, and the major clove oil constituents were quantitatively analyzed in the TPMs of several brands of filtered and unfiltered kreteks, 2R1 tobacco cigarettes, commercial tobacco cigarettes, and 100% clove cigarettes. In addition, commercial tobacco cigarettes painted with clove oil (approximately 30 mg each) were also analyzed.

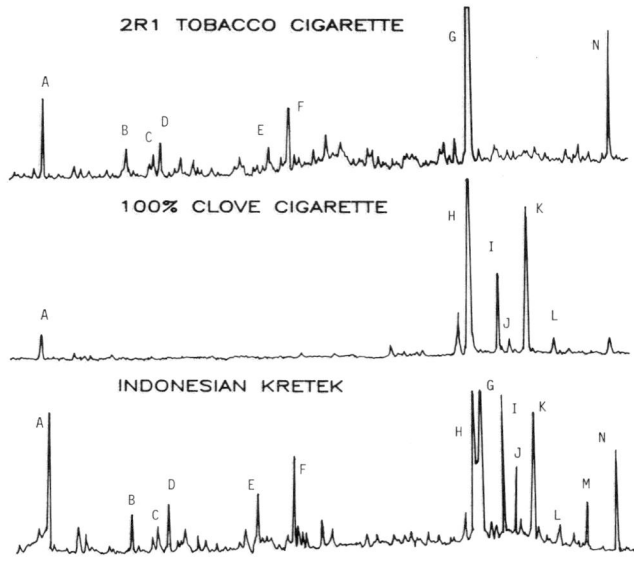

Figure 2
Whole-smoke composition profiles for a 2R1 tobacco cigarette, a 100% clove cigarette, and an Indonesian kretek. (A) Toluene; (B) furfural; (C) ethyl-benzene; (D) xylene; (E) phenol; (F) limonene; (G) nicotine; (H) eugenol; (I) beta-caryophyllene; (J) alpha-humulene; (K) eugenol acetate; (L) caryophyllene-epoxide; (M) unidentified (MW 210); (N) neophytadiene.

Packed column GC as well as capillary column GC/MS were utilized for this phase of the study. All cigarettes were smoked using standard FTC conditions (1 puff/min, 2 second puff, 35 ml volume) and were conditioned for 24–48 hours at 60% humidity in individual humidors prior to smoking. Some experiments with kreteks were also performed using more severe smoking conditions (3 puff/min, 2.5 second puff, 75 ml volume) to approximate deliveries to humans under abusive conditions.

Deliveries of the major constituents are summarized in Table 2. Values reported for the unfiltered and filtered kreteks are actually average deliveries for three different brands each.

Due to the wide range of component concentrations as well as the limited dynamic range of the equipment used, it was not possible to accurately quantitate both eugenol and the low concentration constituents (alpha-humulene, caryophyllene-epoxide) at the same time. Additionally, an interferring component co-eluting with caryophyllene epoxide, further complicated quantitation. More work

Chemical Analysis of Clove Cigarette Smoke / 157

Table 2
Average Deliveries per Cigarette of Major Constituents in the Total Particulate Matter (mg/cigarette)

Constituent	Unfiltered kretek	Unfiltered[a] kretek	Filtered kretek	100% Clove cigarette	Tobacco with clove oil	2R1 Tobacco cigarette
Tar	54	113	48	62	33	38
Nicotine	2.2	4.5	2.2	ND	1.8	2.6
Eugenol	13	23	10	25	6	0.005
Eugenol acetate	0.6	1.2	0.5	2.7	0.3	ND
Beta-caryophyllene	1.2	2.1	1.0	2.1	1.4	ND
Alpha-humulene[b]	0.16	0.27	0.13	0.27	0.18	ND
Caryophyllene-epoxide[b]	<0.1	[c]	<0.1	<0.1	<0.1	ND

[a] Unfiltered kreteks smoked under severe conditions. All other cigarettes smoked under FTC conditions.
[b] Values for alpha-humulene and caryophyllene-epoxide are estimated by relative responses to beta-caryophyllene using a total-ion GC-mass spectrum.
[c] Not determined in this sample
ND = not detected

will be required to provide accurate deliveries of caryophyllene-epoxide; however, GC/MS studies suggest that deliveries are in the range of 10-50 µg per cigarette.

For all of the cigarettes that contained cloves or clove oil, eugenol was found to be the single most abundant constituent in the TPMs. Average delivery was 13 mg/cigarette for unfiltered kreteks and found to be as high as 15 mg/cigarette for certain brands (smoked using FTC conditions). Interestingly, filtered kreteks showed only about a 20% reduction in clove oil delivery per cigarette. For both filtered and unfiltered kreteks, tar and nicotine deliveries were found to be higher than those for corresponding domestic tobacco cigarettes. These data are in agreement with an earlier study (White et al. 1982).

Experiments with the tobacco cigarettes painted with clove oil also showed high eugenol deliveries with approximately 25% of the applied clove oil recovered in the TPM. Significant quantities of the clove oil components were not found in the conventional tobacco cigarettes studied. Eugenol was identified; however, the delivery was only 5 µg/cigarette for the 2R1 (over 1000 times less than for the kreteks). For those kreteks smoked using severe puff conditions, the deliveries of tar, eugenol, and nicotine were found to double.

Finally, to determine whether or not iso-eugenol (2-methoxy-4-propenylphenol) could be determined in the presence of eugenol, a mixture of pure eugenol and iso-eugenol was chromatographed and found to be well separated. It was determined that iso-eugenol was not a significant constituent in kreteks (compared with eugenol).

DISCUSSION

Overall, it appears that the major chemical difference between the smoke of tobacco cigarettes and that of Indonesian kreteks is the presence of significant quantities of eugenol and the other clove oil constituents. No unusual pyrolysis or combustion products have yet been identified that can be directly attributed to the cloves as is particularly well illustrated by the whole-smoke profiles in Figure 2. It is emphasized, however, that due to the extreme complexity of the kretek smoke profile, additional research will be required before the minor clove-related constituents can be determined. It may be that some of the minor constituents are responsible for, or at least contribute to the observed toxicological effects in humans.

On the surface it may seem surprising that so much clove oil is transferred directly to the smoke as opposed to decomposing via pyrolysis or combustion. This is quite reasonable, however, considering the volatile nature of clove oil and the conditions favorable for distillation in the inner region of the cigarette's fire cone (Wynder and Hoffmann 1967).

Although the toxicological effects of eugenol and the other clove oil constituents on the respiratory system have not yet been established, the anesthetic properties of eugenol (and clove oil) are well known (Sell and Carlini 1976; Kozan 1977).

It has been suggested that eugenol anesthetizes the backs of smokers' throats, allowing deeper inhalation (Schechter et al. 1985). Eugenol has also been reported to cause dermatitis among health care workers (T.L. Guidotti, et al., in prep.). Although many epoxides are known to be carcinogenic, the chronic health effects of caryophyllene epoxide have not been established.

SUMMARY

Indonesian clove cigarettes have been found to have high deliveries of eugenol, tar, and nicotine. Clove oil is apparently transferred very efficiently directly to the mainstream smoke via distillation. This transfer results in deliveries of five times as much eugenol as nicotine per kretek. Qualitative studies of the gas-phase constituents indicate that the pyrolysis and combustion products of cloves and clove oil are similar to those for tobacco except for the lack of nitrogen compounds. Additional work will be required to determine the minor constituents related to clove combustion.

ACKNOWLEDGMENT

The authors thank Susan K. Holladay, Cecil E. Higgins, and Roger A. Jenkins of Oak Ridge National Laboratory for their help with this research. We also thank Arthur Vaught of the University of Kentucky Tobacco and Health Research Institute for manufacturing the experimental 100% clove cigarettes. This research was sponsored by the National Cancer Institute (NCI) under Interagency Agreement No. Y01-CP-30508 under Martin Marietta Energy Systems, Inc., contract DE-AC05-84OR21400 with the U.S. Department of Energy.

REFERENCES

Anderson, I. 1985. Deaths follow U.S. craze for clove cigarettes. *New Sci.* **105**: 7.

Guenther, E. 1950. Oil of cloves. In *The essential oils*, vol. 4, p. 396. D. Van Nostrand Company, New York.

Guerin, M. 1980. Chemical composition of cigarette smoke. In *Banbury Report 3: A safe cigarette* (ed. G. Gori et al.), p. 191. Cold Spring Harbor Laboratory, Cold Spring Harbor, New York.

Higgins, C., W. Griest, and M. Guerin. 1984. *Sampling and analysis of cigarette smoke using solid adsorbent tenax, ORNL/TM-9167.* Oak Ridge National Laboratory, Oak Ridge, Tennessee.

Hirs, A. 1984. Sales of clove cigarettes gain in U.S., health questions emerge. *Tob. Int.* **186**: 57.

Kozam, G. 1977. The effect of eugenol on nerve transmission. *Oral Surg.* **44**: 799.

Masada, Y. 1976. *Analysis of essential oils by gas chromatography and mass spectrometry*, p. 124. John Wiley and Sons, New York.

Schechter, F., P. Hackett, Q. Rodriguez, A. D. Dauer, N. A. Sagle, L. W. Wilson, S.A. Kerley, B. Sanger et al. 1985. Illnesses possibly associated with smoking clove cigarettes. *Morbidity and Mortality Weekly Report.* **34**: 297.

Sell, A. and E. Carlini. 1976. Anesthetic action of methyl eugenol and other eugenol derivatives. *Pharmacology* **14**: 367.

White, S., G. Henderson, and R. Jenkins. 1982. Selected constituents in the smokes of two brands of Indonesian cigarettes sold in the United States: Tar, nicotine, carbon monoxide, and carbon dioxide. *Topical Report NCI/S&HP/ORNL #124.* Oak Ridge National Laboratory, Oak Ridge, Tennessee.

Wynder, E. and D. Hoffmann. 1967. *Tobacco and tobacco smoke*, p. 85. Academic Press, New York.

COMMENTS

HOFFMANN: These cigarettes appear to have filter tips with low efficiency. Would you expect the selective filtration of volatiles and semivolatiles by these filter tips?

WISE: I don't know exactly what types of filter materials are used for kreteks; however, substantial deliveries of triacetin are typically found in the smoke of the filtered variety.

HOFFMANN: Yes, the filter tips are treated with triacetin as plasticizer, but don't you know whether the filter material was cellulose or cellulose acetate? Did you check whether there was increased epoxide formation with aging of the cigarettes?

WISE: We have not tried an aging study to look for increased epoxide formation.

HOFFMANN: But the occurrence of the epoxide could reflect aging of the tar. I would be surprised if the plants produce the epoxide.

WISE: The presence of caryophyllene-epoxide in clove bud oil has been known for many years, but its origin is uncertain. There is some evidence that suggests it is formed by oxidation of caryophyllene and is not a natural biological constituent.

HOFFMANN: You demonstrated that the smoke of a kretek cigarette can contain several milligrams of eugenol. Do we know anything about the metabolism of eugenol? One may be able to determine a metabolite in the urine and could thereby measure the smoking intensity of a kretek smoker. Do you have any information regarding this aspect?

WISE: At this time I don't know of any metabolites that are characteristic of kretek smoke. It might be worth investigating. Thank you.

HECHT: Your compound of molecular weight 210? I think that that might be about the molecular weight of the nitrosated musk from the Indian tobacco.

WISE: It is an unusual compound and I would be interested in talking with you about its possible structure.

HARRIS: What is known, if anything, about smoking patterns among people who are actually using this product? Do they tend to inhale more than with other cigarettes?

WISE: Reports in the literature suggest that kretek smokers do inhale deeper. This has been attributed by some to the anesthetic effect of eugenol on the throat.

HALEY: Kretek use by adolescents in this country generally resembles inhalation patterns seen with marijuana rather than with tobacco cigarettes. When comparisons are made with regard to toxicity in Indonesia and the United States, this difference in dosing should be taken into account.

ENZELL: You said that the gas chromatograms of these cigarettes and regular cigarettes were quite similar. I thought you showed only the very top of the chromatogram. Were they also similar at the lower level?

WISE: We have not looked in detail at the lower level constituents. However, the expanded chromatograms, showing a comparison of a kretek and tobacco cigarette, do indicate that they are basically similar even for constituents at the low microgram level per cigarette.

ENZELL: There should be many clove constituents; and the gas chromatograms, I think, should be quite different.

WISE: At first it is surprising that the differences are not that significant; but considering the high volatility of clove oil, this may not be unreasonable. The reducing atmosphere in the fire cone of the kretek may actually favor distillation of the volatile components enabling them to be transferred efficiently to the mainstream smoke without extensive pyrolysis or combustion.

LAVOIE: I have a brief comment regarding the type of toxicological evaluation that we've done. Again, using the data from Oak Ridge National Laboratory, we have evaluated some of the major constituents in cloves by intratrachial installation into the lung. Our studies have shown that these compounds, particularly eugenol, are extremely toxic when administered by intratrachial installation, giving rise to lung hemorrhaging—certainly at doses well below those that one might have expected on the basis of either i.u. or s.c. injections. Basically these data suggest that the major compound in a clove cigarette—eugenol—may be directly responsible for most of the acute toxic effects that have been reported from individuals smoking clove cigarettes.

HOFFMANN: Did you find polycyclic aromatic hydrocarbons in the smoke of kreteks?

WISE: I have identified several of the smaller polycyclic aromatic hydrocarbons, but I have not yet attempted to quantitate the deliveries.

MAGEE: You said that the toxicity of eugenol was much greater by intratrachial than by intravenous tests. It's a little surprising to me since when an intravenous injection is given, the capillary blood vessels are the first major thing to be hit.

LAVOIE: Yes, and it is very interesting in the sense that when we actually did one particular intratrachial installation, the compound got into one lobe of the lung and not the other. That lobe was hemorrhagic and almost destroyed; the other lobe was intact. The animal did survive for several hours, indicating that it was not a systemic effect, but almost a contact phenomena. Again, the doses were extremely low, and we've done this diluted in vehicles as well. So it does seem to be almost a contact phenomena with the lung tissue.

Isoprenoid Flavor Components of Tobacco and Their Formation

CURT R. ENZELL
Research Department
Swedish Tobacco Company
S-104 62 Stockholm, Sweden

OVERVIEW

Isoprenoids constitute an essential part of the aroma of tobacco. A large number of these constituents can be viewed as the result of biodegradation of carotenoids and diterpenoids of the cembrane and labdane type. Considerable insight into these transformations has been gained through the isolation and determination of stereostructures of several hundred tobacco isoprenoids. Further information has been obtained through biomimetic experiments, which have involved singlet oxygen reactions, epoxidations, and rearrangements. The results allow a deeper understanding of the chemistry and importance of the postharvest processes and provide a means to attain better control of the taste and aroma of tobacco.

INTRODUCTION

The typical aroma of the tobacco leaf is created during the postharvest treatment, which involves air-, heat-, fire-, or air-curing, and aging. It leads to very substantial chemical changes, the consequences of which amount not only to the generation of flavorants but also of precursors furnishing odoriferous components on thermolysis. A more detailed understanding of the chemistry of the postharvest treatments is therefore a prerequisite for clarifying their influence on the aroma of tobacco and smoke. Since elucidation of the genetic and chemical relationships of tobacco constituents frequently reveals the underlying reactions and also provides a means to influence and simulate their action, attention shall be focused on these. Moreover, the paper will be restricted to isoprenoids, which organoleptically are the single most important group of the tobacco aroma constituents as well as the chemically best elucidated one.

RESULTS AND DISCUSSION

Studies over the last two decades involving separation, isolation, elucidation of stereostructures, and biomimetic syntheses have revealed that the isoprenoid-derived aroma constituents of tobacco mainly stem from three types of precursors (Fig. 1), carotenoids (A), cembranoids (B), and labdanoids (C) (Enzell et al. 1977;

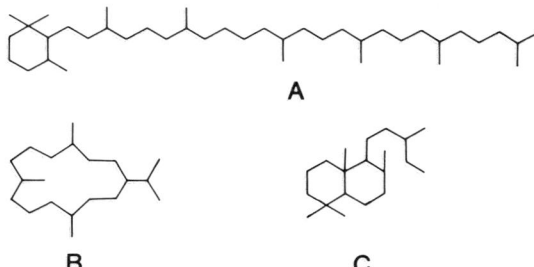

Figure 1
Carbon skeletons of monocyclic carotenoids (A), cembranoids (B), and labdanoids (C)

Enzell and Wahlberg 1980). Each of these provide specific and highly interesting chemistry and they shall therefore be treated separately, although briefly.

CYCLIC CAROTENOIDS

The carotenoids of tobacco are degraded on maturation, senescence, curing, and aging. Although the majority of the carotenoid metabolites are most abundant at and subsequent to the time of cell wall degradation, many are present in the green plant prior to and during the time of the most rapid growth (Wahlberg et al. 1977; Burton and Kasperbauer 1982). These reactions are probably effected in the intact plant by oxygenase systems and during the postharvest treatment by photo-oxygenation and other nonenzymatic oxidations. Although there is a certain preference for attack on the 9,10 double bond of cyclic carotenoids yielding C_{13} constituents, C_9, C_{10}, and C_{11} tobacco constituents are also formed by routes such as those indicated in Figure 2.

On the grounds of the end groups present in cyclic tobacco carotenoids, we would expect to find, solely as a result of 9,10 double bond cleavage, six C_{13} methyl ketones. Four of these (1-4) have been encountered in tobacco (Fig. 3).

Whether they are detected in tobacco or not, it is convenient to regard these primary C_{13} methyl ketones as precursors of the other representatives of the series, now amounting to some 50 compounds (Enzell 1985). Many of these secondary metabolites can be viewed as arising by simple reactions, such as those shown in Figure 4, which illustrates probable routes of interconversion of a few known tobacco constituents. Some of them have outstanding flavor properties, e.g., the megastigmatrienones (11, 12), regarded by some (Wilson et al. 1982) as the heart of tobacco aroma.

Many of these C_{13} compounds are clearly formed by more complex routes, which make the precursor-product relationships less obvious, and in the absence of

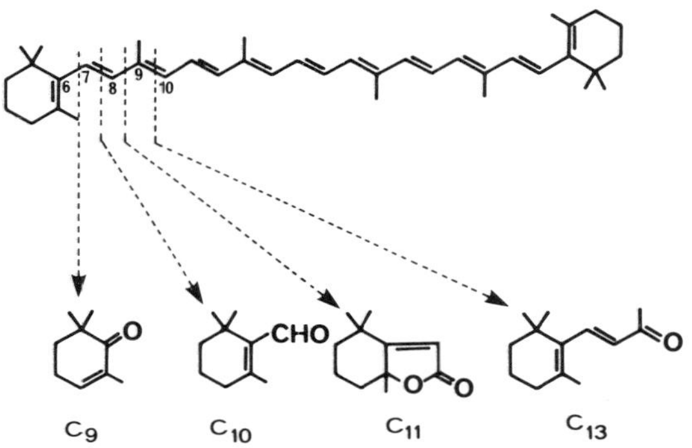

Figure 2
Degradation of carotenoids

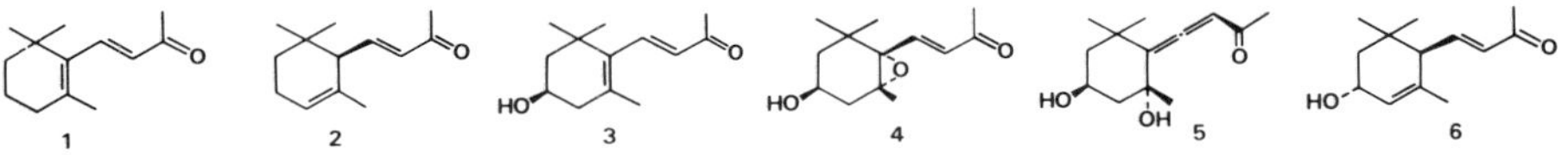

Figure 3
Primary C_{13} tobacco carotenoid metabolites

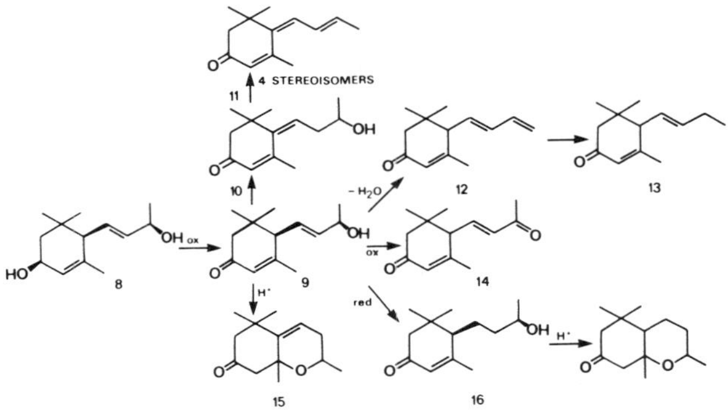

Figure 4
Routes of formation proposed for some secondary carotenoid metabolites

isotopic experiments, leave the stereochemical information and the numerous chemical studies as the sole source of information about these relationships. A pertinent example is provided by the damascones, which are all oxygenated at C-7 and whose importance as tobacco flavorants equals that of the megastigmatrienones. Thus, damascenone (*17*) can be viewed as arising from the primary precursor (*5*), the grasshopper ketone, or from the primary precursor (*3*) via this ketone (*5*), which is able to yield damascenone (*17*) on reduction, rearrangement, and dehydration. Damascenone (*17*) can, in turn, give rise to the bicyclodamascenones A (*21*) and B (*22*) by the reactions shown in Figure 5, which have been accomplished experimentally (Demole and Enggist 1976). Acid treatment leads initially to a stereospecific cyclization of the *trans*-hydroxyallyl cation (*18*), which in turn furnishes a bicyclic intermediate (*19*) and a protonated cyclobutanone (*20*). On deprotonation accompanied by cleavage of the 5,8- or 5,6-bond, this produces bicyclodamascenone A (*21*) and B (*22*), respectively.

The recent isolation of glucosides such as the glucosides of 3-oxo-α-ionol and 5,6-epoxy-5,6-dihydro-3-hydroxy-β-ionol (Kodama et al. 1984) from green leaf shows that the carotenoid metabolites can be generated and transformed in the intact cell since glucosidation must occur after cleavage of the 9,10 double bond in the precursor.

DITERPENOIDS

Dependent upon the genetic background, tobacco cultivars produce cembranes, labdanes, or both types of cyclic diterpenoids (Colledge et al. 1975; Reid 1974). These compounds, which are present in high concentrations in the gummy exudate of the tobacco leaf and flower, readily undergo degradation with the formation of a very large number of metabolites, many of which influence the aroma of the final product (Enzell et al. 1977; Enzell and Wahlberg 1980; Burton et al. 1983).

Cembranoids

Extensive chemical studies have provided considerable insight into the biological transformations of the tobacco cembranoids. Nearly sixty C_{20} cembranoids are known and their formation from the two major cembratrienediols (*23,24*) accounted for by biomimetic reactions, which in most cases have been verified experimentally (Wahlberg and Enzell 1984). Of these reactions, the ring cleavages are of particular interest in this context since they serve to explain the formation of a series of key metabolites which have 18, 15, 14, 13, or 12 carbon atoms and whose formation is indicated in structure 25 (Fig. 6).

The cleavages of the 7,8 and 11,12 double bonds are likely to occur in an oxidative manner, either by way of an enzyme-assisted reaction or one involving singlet oxygen. Singlet oxygen attack is initiated by an ene reaction leading to the forma-

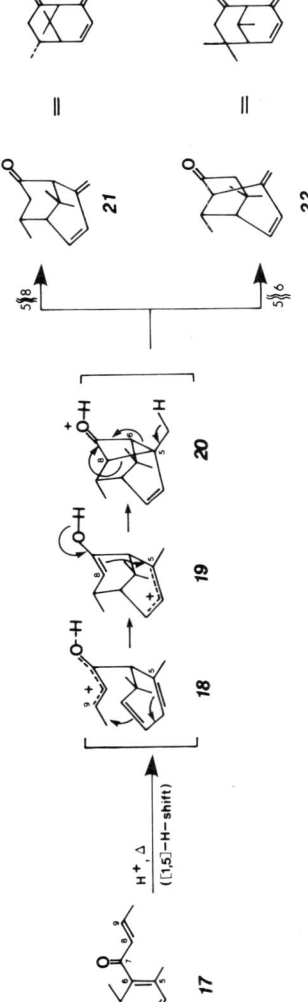

Figure 5
Formation of bicyclodamascenone A (*21*) and B (*22*)

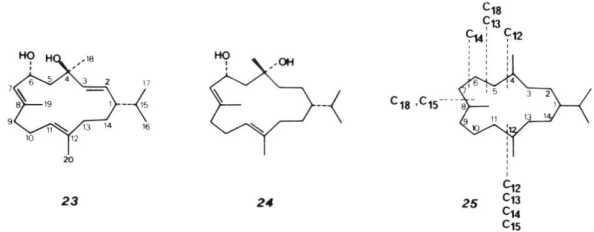

Figure 6
The two major cembratrienediols of tobacco (23,24) and routes of formation of C_{18}, C_{15}, C_{14}, C_{13}, and C_{12} cembranoid metabolites (25)

tion of a hydroperoxide, which under acidic conditions is amenable to Hook-Criegee rearrangement involving rupture of the original double bond.

In the two major cembratrienediols (23,24), the proneness of the double bonds to react with singlet oxygen can on account of the differences in substitution be predicted to be in the order 11,12; 7,8; 2,3. Consistent with this, the 4S,6R-diol (23) reacted smoothly with singlet oxygen at the 11,12 double bond. The reaction is not only quite site-specific but surprisingly stereospecific, as shown by the proportionate yields of the four triols resulting on reduction with triethyl phosphite (Wahlberg et al. 1984).

It could be concluded, therefore, that the reactions proceed predominantly by way of conformer *a* and that this conformation is more densely populated or more prone to react than that of conformer *b* (Fig. 7). It also follows from Figure 7 that the generation of the 12S-hydroperoxide from conformer *a* involves transfer of the

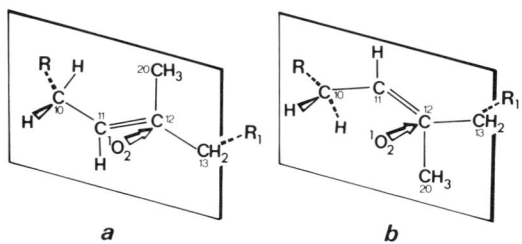

Figure 7
Proposed mechanism for $^1O_2$ attack at the 11,12 double bond of (1S,2E,4S,6R,7E,11E)-2,7,11-cembratriene-4,6-diol

pro-R-hydrogen at C-10, whereas the formation of the 12R-hydroperoxide from conformer b requires migration of the pro-S-hydrogen at C-10.

The most direct evidence of the occurrence of these reactions in tobacco comes from the recent isolation from this source of the five hydroperoxydiols 26-30. It should be noted, however, that their presence does not exclude agents other than singlet oxygen, since enzyme-assisted reactions may also lead to the formation of hydroperoxides (Wahlberg et al. 1983) (Fig. 8).

The cleavages of the 5,6 bond and of the 4,5 bond are readily accounted for by the reactions shown in Figure 9. The former involves an acid-catalysed, essentially irreversible 1,3-diol fragmentation leading in the case of the two predominant diols (23,24) to the seco-aldehyde 31, first reported as a constituent of tobacco flower. The cleavage of the 4,5 bond is easily explained as a result of retroketol condensation of the tobacco ketols 32 and 33, derivable from the same two diols (23,24) by oxidation of the secondary hydroxyl group; the resulting seco-diketone 34 is a constituent of dark-fired tobacco (Enzell et al. 1977).

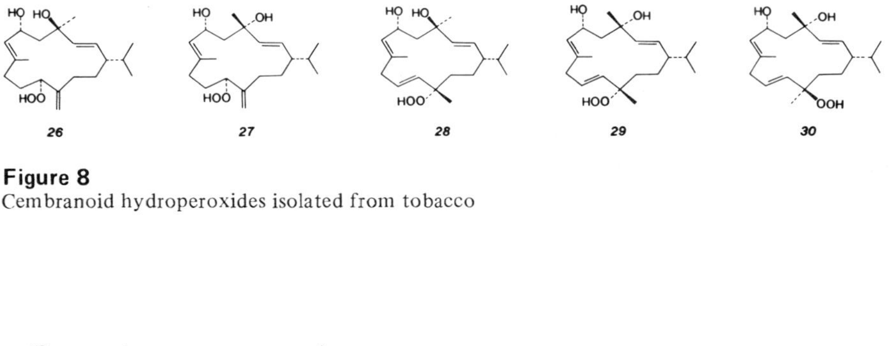

Figure 8
Cembranoid hydroperoxides isolated from tobacco

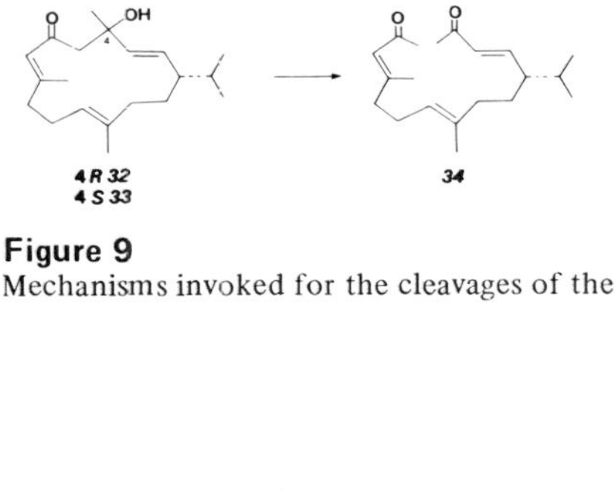

Figure 9
Mechanisms invoked for the cleavages of the 5,6 and 4,5 bonds of cembranoids

Rupture of the 7,6 bond was initially proposed to occur by acid-catalysed rearrangement of the 7S, 8S- and/or 7R, 8R-epoxides derived from either or both of the major diols (23,24) by the mechanism outlined for 35 in Figure 10 (Enzell et al. 1977). However, attempts to carry out this reaction on either of the four possible stereoisomeric precursors have so far not been successful in our hands. An alternative pathway involving fragmentation of 7-hydroperoxides by a route such as shown for 36 is therefore presently being considered, but up to now only supported by circumstantial evidence including the isolation of tobacco cembranols possessing appropriate oxygenation patterns, e.g., the tetrol 37 (Wahlberg and Enzell 1984).

The key metabolites derived in this fashion by cleavage of two of the ring bonds undergo further reactions, including loss of carbon atoms. Some 60 representatives have hitherto been found in tobacco, many of which are important flavorants. They are recognized by their irregular terpenoid skeletons and by possessing the 1S, 2E-configuration of the parent cembranoids (Enzell and Wahlberg 1980; Enzell 1981). It has been estimated that they constitute some 10% of the total volatile material of Burley tobacco (Demole 1974).

Of the five predicted key metabolites, solanone (38) and norsolanadione (39) are predominant constituents of the tobacco volatiles and important contributors to the flavor of tobacco smoke (Fig. 11). Although both are probable precursors of a series of secondary metabolites, it will suffice to consider the formation of those viewed as arising from solanone (38).

Most of these reactions, which are outlined in Figure 12 and which involve oxidation, reduction, hydration, or rearrangement, are straightforward and only the formation of dioxabicyclo (3.2.1) octane (40) and dioxabicyclo (3.3.1) nonane (41) require further comment. The mechanisms invoked for these reactions, which have been carried out experimentally, are shown in Figure 13 (Demole and Demole

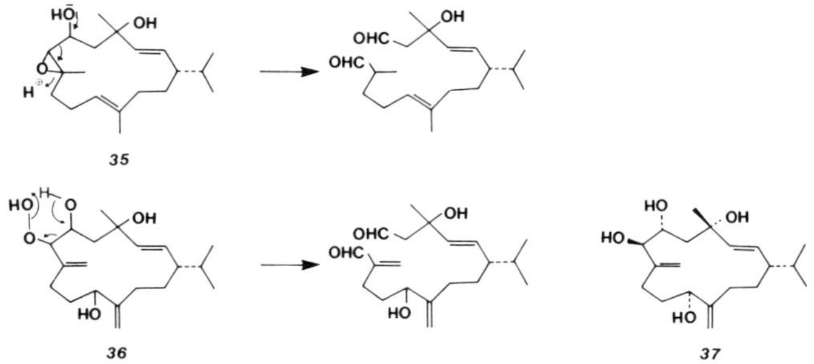

Figure 10
Mechanisms invoked for the cleavage of the 6,7 bond of cembranoids

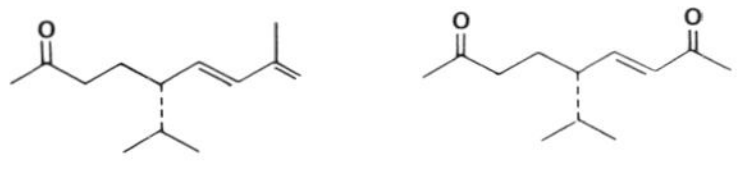

Figure 11
Solanone (38) and norsolanadione (39)

1975). The absolute configurations have been assigned on the basis of the assumption that (5S)-solanone (38) is the precursor and that only the 6S, 7R-epoxide (42) could yield the dioxabicyclo (3.2.1) octane (40), because in the isomeric 6R, 7S-epoxide steric hindrance between the isopropyl and hydroxyisopropyl groups would prevent bond formation between the oxygen atom of the epoxide and C-2 (Enzell et al. 1977). Moreover, the high stereospecificity encountered in

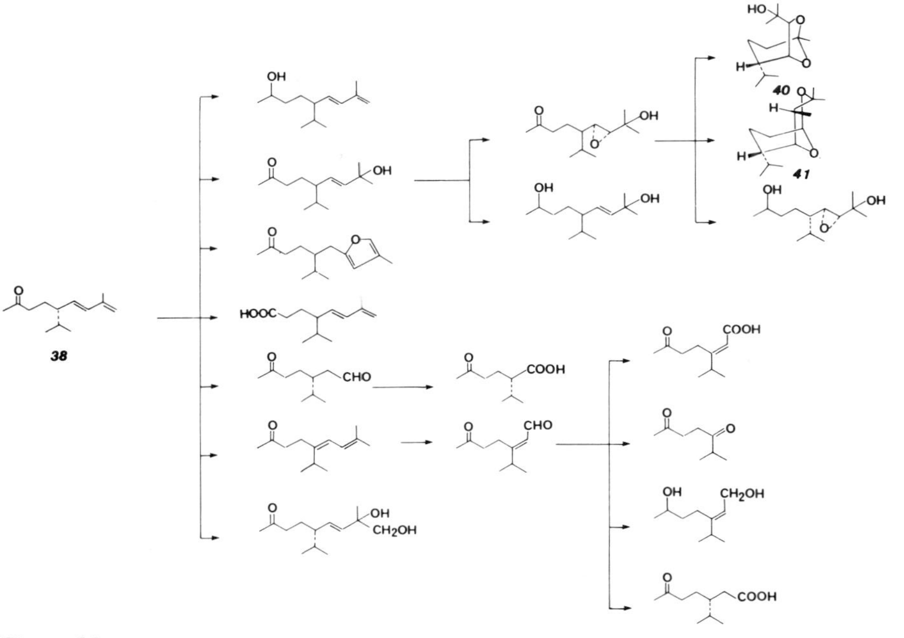

Figure 12
Pathways proposed for the degradation of (5S)-solanone (38)

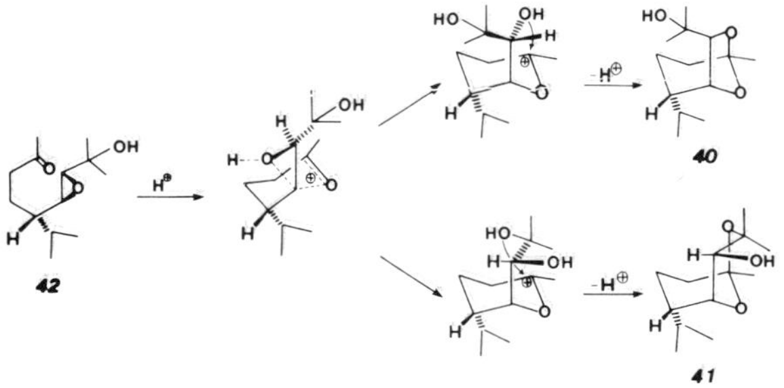

Figure 13
Mechanisms proposed for the formation of dioxabicyclo (3.2.1) octane *(40)* and dioxabicyclo (3.3.1) nonane (41)

the epoxidation leading to *42* infers the absolute configuration shown for the dioxabicyclo(3.2.1)octane *(40)* and dioxabicyclo(3.3.1)nonane *(41)* (Demole and Demole 1975).

Labdanoids

The C_{20} labdanoids known to date as constituents of tobacco are detailed in Figure 14. Of these, those boxed are derivable by singlet oxygen oxidation from Z-and/or E-abienol, the former being the major constituent of green leaf and flower, while the E-isomer is present in small quantities only (Enzell and Wahlberg 1980). The biogenesis of several of the other compounds may also be rationalized by further or other types of oxidation of abienol, which vanishes on curing.

The first step in these processes involves attack on the side chain double bonds and parallels the reactions of acyclic olefins towards singlet oxygen (Turner and Herz 1977; Schulte-Elte et al. 1978; Schulte-Elte and Rautenstrauch 1980) in some conformers, while in others the hydroxyl group at C-8 provides anchimeric assistance and the reaction can be envisaged to occur via the peroxirane intermediate shown in Figure 15 (Wahlberg et al. 1978, 1979).

All three routes lead to C_{20} compounds—the ene reaction to *49-52*, the peroxirane to *45-48* and *54-57*, and the 1,4-addition to *63-65, 71*, and *72*. However, all tobacco labdanoids having less than 20 carbon atoms can be viewed as derived solely from the hydroperoxides formed in the ene reaction. Thus, initial Hook-Criegee cleavage followed by a set of simple reactions account for the formation of all known C_{18} and C_{17} tobacco labdanoids from the 13-hydroperoxide *73* (Fig. 16) and all known C_{16} and C_{15} representatives from the 12-hydroperoxide *85* (Fig. 17). It is obvious that many alternative routes exist in addition to those shown.

Many of the degraded tobacco labdanoids are of interest both per se and as precursors of other odoriferous compounds. Thus, most of the C_{14} and C_{15}

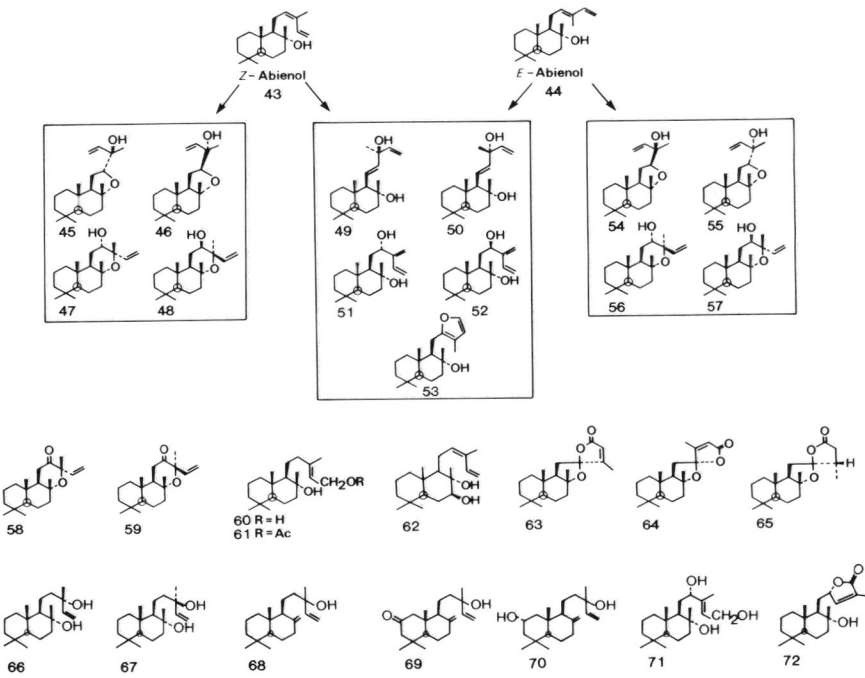

Figure 14
Tobacco-derived C_{20} labdanoids (*43-72*)

labdanoid-derived tobacco constituents possess a characteristic cedarwood type of aroma, while the odorless C_{18} ketone 14,15-bisnor-8(17)-labden-13-one (*96*) has been demonstrated (Ohloff et al. 1976) to furnish on UV-irradiation an ambergris-smelling product, whose major components are shown in Figure 18.

Of the two primary products (*97,76*), the diene (*97*), which is formed by a Norrish type II fragmentation and partly converted by a thermally reversible reaction to the odorless cyclobutane (*98*), has a woody resinous smell whereas the tobacco ketone (*76*) is odorless. On prolonged irradiation, however, the tobacco ketone (*76*) gave rise to two odorless compounds (*101,102*) and two substances having an ambergris type of smell, the cyclopentanol (*100*) and the tetracyclic ether (*99*), the latter of which is reconverted to the parent ketone (*76*) above 190°C. It follows from these results that both irradiation and mild thermolytic conditions, well below those encountered close to the glowing zone of a burning cigarette, may convert odorless compounds to odiferous and vice versa.

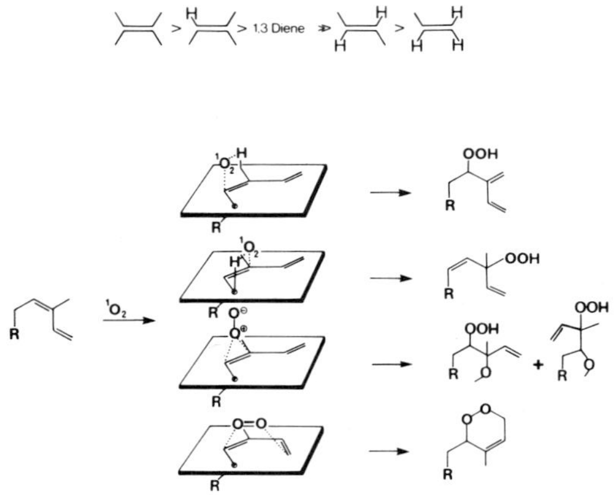

Figure 15
Mechanisms proposed for singlet oxygen reactions with abienol

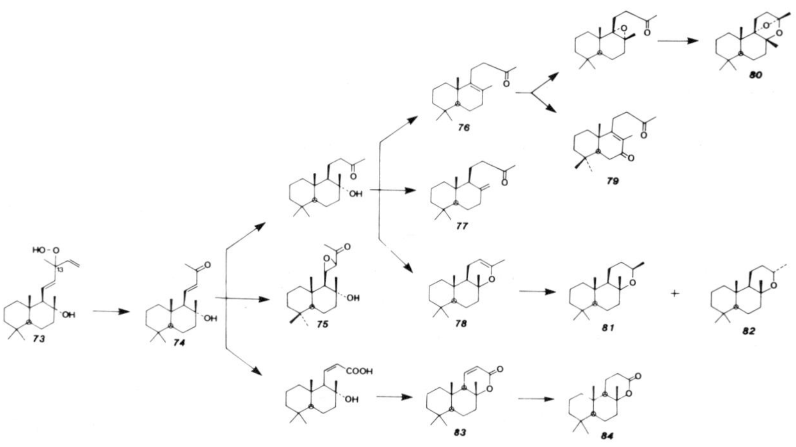

Figure 16
Proposed genesis of C_{18} (74–82) and C_{17} (83, 84) labdanoids of tobacco

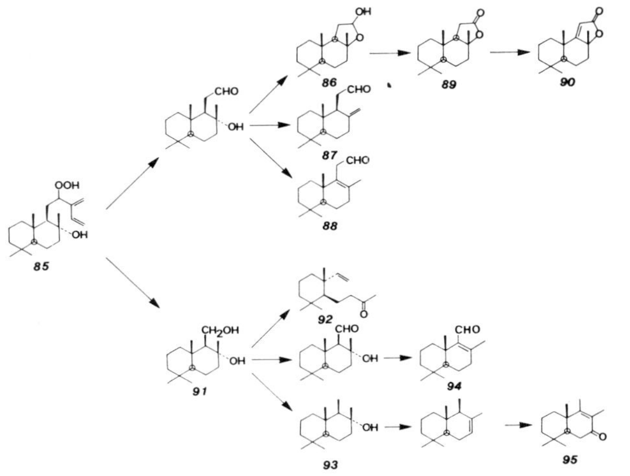

Figure 17
Proposed genesis of C_{16} (*86-90*) and C_{15} (*91-95*) labdanoids of tobacco

SUMMARY

Present knowledge about the biodegradation of tobacco isoprenoids provides a means of comprehending many of the reactions occurring in tobacco, especially during the postharvest processing. Although our overall understanding of these reactions and their organoleptic implications is still very limited, and tracer ex-

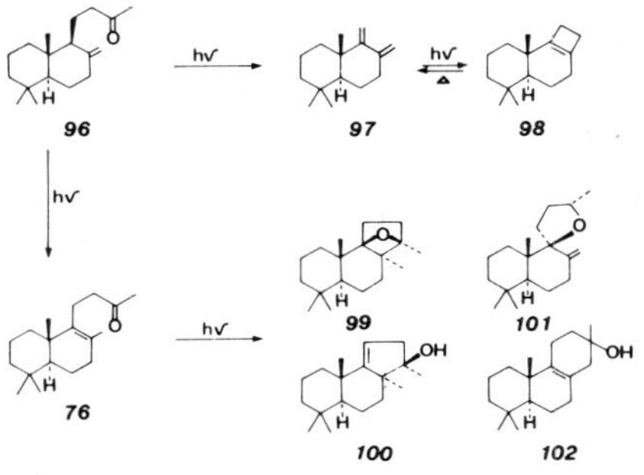

Figure 18
Major components obtained on UV-irradiation of 14,15-bisnor-B(17)-labden-13-one (*96*)

periments, as well as further in vitro studies are urgently required, we are now in a much better position to judge what isoprenoid constituents to expect in tobacco and how to influence and simulate their formation. Some of this information also has a bearing on the transformations of other types of tobacco constituents during the postharvest treatment.

REFERENCES

Burton, H.R. and M.J. Kasperbauer. 1982. Chemical changes during air-curing of Burley tobacco. *Coresta symposium.* Winston-Salem, North Carolina.

Burton, H.R., L.P. Bush, and J.L. Hamilton. 1983. Effect of curing on the chemical composition of Burley tobacco. *Recent Adv. Tob. Sci.* **9**: 91.

Colledge, A., W.W. Reid, and R. Russel. 1975. The diterpenoids of *Nicotiana* species and their potential technological significance. *Chem. Ind.* **13**: 570.

Demole, E. 1974. Chemistry of Burley tobacco flavor (*Nicotiana tabacum* L.). Novel constituents and newer syntheses. VI. *International Congress of Essential Oils.* San Francisco, California.

Demole, E. and C. Demole. 1975. Identification and synthesis of twelve irregular terpenoids related to solanone, including 7,8-dioxabicyclo(3.2.1)octane and 4,9-dioxabicyclo(3.3.1)nonane derivatives. *Helv. Chim. Acta* **58**: 1867.

Demole, E. and P. Enggist. 1976. A chemical study of Virginia tobacco flavour (*Nicotiana tabacum* L.) I. Isolation and synthesis of two bicyclodamascenones. *Helv. Chim. Acta* **59**: 1938.

Enzell, C.R. 1981. Influence of curing on the formation of tobacco flavour. In *Flavour 81* (ed. P. Schreier), p. 449. Walter de Gruyter, Berlin, West Germany.

———. 1985. Biodegradation of carotenoids–An important route to aroma compounds. *Pure Appl. Chem.* **57**: 693.

Enzell, C.R. and I. Wahlberg. 1980. Leaf composition in relation to smoking quality and aroma. *Recent Adv. Tob. Sci.* **6**: 64.

Enzell, C.R., I. Wahlberg, and A.J. Aasen. 1977. Isoprenoids and alkaloids to tobacco. *Progr. Chem. Organic N.* **34**: 1.

Kodama, H., T. Fujimori, and K. Kato. 1984. Glucosides of ionone-related compounds in several *Nicotiana* species *Phytochemistry* **23**: 583.

Ohloff, G., Ch. Vial, H. Wolf, and O. Jeger. 1976. Neue Ambra-Riechstoffe durch photochemische Reaktionen von 15,16-Dinorlabd-8(20)-en-13-on. *Helv. Chim. Acta* **59**: 75.

Reid, W.W. 1974. The phytochemistry of the genus *Nicotiana. Ann. Tab. SEITA* **2**: 145.

Schulte-Elte, K.H. and V. Rautenstrauch. 1980. Preference for the syn ene additions of $^1O_2$ to 1-methyl-cycloalkenes. Correlation with ground-state geometry. *J. Am. Chem. Soc.* **102**: 1738.

Schulte-Elte, K.H., B. Muller, and V. Rautenstrauch. 1978. Preference for syn ene additions of $^1O_2$ to trisubstituted, acyclic olefins. *Helv. Chim. Acta* **61**: 2777.

Turner, J.A. and W. Herz. 1977. Fe(II)-induced decomposition of unsaturated cyclic peroxides derived from butadienes. A simple procedure for synthesis of 3-alkylfurans. *J. Org. Chem.* **42**: 1900.

Wahlberg, I. and C.R. Enzell. 1984. Tobacco cembranoids. *Beitr. Tabakforsch. Int.* **12**: 93.

Wahlberg, I., K. Karlsson, M. Curvall, T. Nishida, and C.R. Enzell. 1978. Sensitized photo-oxygenation of (12Z)-abienol. Biomimetic synthesis of tobacco labdanoids. *Acta Chem. Scand.* **B32**: 203.

Wahlberg, I., K. Nordfors, M. Curvall, T. Nishida, and C.R. Enzell. 1979. Synthesis of tobacco labdanoids by sensitized photo-oxygenation of (12E)-abienol. *Acta Chem. Scand.* **B33**: 437.

Wahlberg, I., K. Nordfors, C. Vogt, T. Nishida, and C.R. Enzell. 1983. Five new hydroperoxycembratrienediols from tobacco. *Acta Chem. Scand.* **B37**: 653.

Wahlberg, I., R. Arndt, I. Wallin, C. Vogt, T. Nishida, and C.R. Enzell. 1984. Six new cembratrienetriols from tobacco. *Acta Chem. Scand.* **B38**: 21.

Wahlberg, I., K. Karlsson, D.J. Austin, N. Junker, J. Roeraade, C.R. Enzell, and W.H. Johnson. 1977. Effects of flue-curing and aging on the volatile neutral and acidic constituents of Virginia tobacco. *Phytochemistry* **16**: 1217.

Wilson, R.A., B.D. Mookherjee, and J.F. Vinato. 1982. A comparative analysis of the volatile constituents of Virginia, Burley, Turkish and Black Tobacco. Chemistry of tobacco smoke. *American Chemical Society National Meeting.* Kansas City, Missouri.

COMMENTS

HECHT: I noticed that many of your compounds were of a class of alpha-beta unsaturated ketones. Since these kinds of compounds seem to react with DNA, I wonder to what extent many of them have been quantified in tobacco? What are their relative levels?

ENZELL: We made some quantification in the case of Virginia tobacco. Most of them are present at very low levels, and, of course, the amount that is present in any particular tobacco is dependent on all the factors I mentioned. Since it is difficult to quantify them, I don't think I could give you any general clue to their occurrence in cigarettes. However, there are compounds, such as solanone and norsolanadione, which can, of course, be quantified quite readily since they are present in high concentrations.

HECHT: Is there an isomer of solanone which is an alpha-beta unsaturated carbonyl compound? Is that a major constituent of tobacco?

ENZELL: No, I don't think it's a major constituent. However, we have looked at a number of terpenoids from smoke, and, as you say, many are very active. In fact, they form a most active group.

HOFFMANN: Let me congratulate you on your outstanding studies. I am always amazed at the tremendous progress in organic chemistry during the last decades. Your studies reflect such advances. My specific question is, have you, or has someone at your laboratory, tried to correlate the structure of tobacco-specific terpenoids with their potential as flavor components? Are there special structural entities which are specifically recognized by the receptors in the olfactory organ? Can one correlate the structure of compounds with their strength as flavor component?

ENZELL: It has been done, but not on tobacco compounds.

HOFFMANN: You have never tried this?

ENZELL: We have not tried it, because I think that the whole issue is too complex to be approached in this fashion. There are people looking at selected groups of compounds, trying to find out what the structure-activity relationships are. It has always been found to be of limited general validity. There are a few exceptions, but very local ones, such as Ohloff's 1,2,4-triaxial rule for decalines, which relates the arrangement of the substituents to the organoleptic properties of the molecule. It seems to work to a certain extent, which is very nice, but it is not adequate for establishing relationships between the structure and aroma of tobacco constituents.

HOFFMANN: In other words, you will continue with the organic chemistry and will identify certain types of components that will contribute to the flavor bouquet of tobacco smoke. You don't envision that one day all these data can be computerized to help define specific structures of organic compounds that have a high affinity for the receptors in the olfactory organs?

ENZELL: No, I don't think that this will be possible in the foreseeable future.

Perinatal Disposition and Metabolism in Mice and Hamsters of Some N-Nitrosamines Present in Tobacco and Tobacco Smoke

HANS TJÄLVE,* BOËL LÖFBERG,* ANDRE CASTONGUAY,†
NEIL TRUSHIN,† AND STEPHEN S. HECHT†
*Department of Pharmacology and Toxicology
Swedish University of Agricultural Sciences
S-751 23 Uppsala, Sweden
†Naylor Dana Institute for Disease Prevention
American Health Foundation
Valhalla, New York 10595

OVERVIEW

The potential noxious effects of maternal smoking during pregnancy and nursing on the health of the fetuses and the newborn babies have not been fully elucidated. In addition to adverse effects on the fetal and infant development, some tobacco chemicals may act as transplacental carcinogens and/or induce cancer in the offspring by exposure via sidestream smoke or breast milk during neonatal life. Perinatal exposure of animals to compounds present in tobacco and tobacco smoke have been shown to induce tumors, but the chemical nature of the tobacco carcinogens which might cause similar effects in man is not known. In the present study, the perinatal metabolism of the tobacco-specific N-nitrosamines 4-(methylnitrosamino)-1-(3-pyridyl)-1-butanone (NNK) and N'-nitrosonornicotine (NNN) and the volatile N-nitrosamine N-nitrosodiethylamine (NDEA), also present in tobacco and tobacco smoke, have been studied in C57B1 mice and Syrian golden hamsters. These N-nitrosamines are potent organ-specific carcinogens in adult animals and NDEA has been shown to induce tumors transplacentally or by exposure during neonatal life. Our results indicated that these three N-nitrosamines pass the placental membranes to the fetuses and that they are bioactivated by some fetal tissues during the latest phase of pregnancy as well as by tissues of infant animals. For NDEA our results correlate with previously reported carcinogenicity data. For the tobacco-specific N-nitrosamines, the carcinogenic effects at transplacental or neonatal exposure have not been examined. However, our results indicate that the enzyme systems necessary for the activation of these procarcinogens are operative during the late phase of pregnancy and during neonatal life, and exposure to NNK or NNN during these periods could therefore result in the development of tumors.

Concerns regarding the possible deleterious effects of tobacco smoke inhalation during pregnancy and nursing have repeatedly been expressed, and increased research in this area is warranted.

INTRODUCTION

Several epidemiological studies have linked maternal tobacco smoking during pregnancy to adverse effects, such as fetal growth retardations, spontaneous abortions, and neonatal deaths (U.S. Department of Health, Education and Welfare 1979; U.S. Department of Health and Human Services 1980). There are also suggestive evidences that tobacco smoke inhalation may be related to transplacental carcinogenesis, resulting in increased risks of tumor development during childhood or adult life (Neutel and Buck 1971; Everson 1980; Preston-Martin et al. 1982; U.S. Department of Health and Human Services 1982). A number of agents in tobacco and tobacco smoke have been identified as transplacental carcinogens in animals. Among these are N-nitrosamines, hydrazines, and benzo[a]pyrene (Everson 1980; Rice 1981; U.S. Department of Health and Human Services 1982).

Our interest has focused on the N-nitrosamines present in tobacco and tobacco smoke. These compounds are formed during tobacco processing and during tobacco smoking from amines reacting with nitrite or nitrogen oxides. When they are given to animals, most N-nitrosamines exhibit strong organ-specific carcinogenic effects (Magee et al. 1976). The N-nitrosamines derived from the tobacco-alkaloids (tobacco-specific N-nitrosamines) are the most prevalent ones in tobacco and tobacco smoke (Hoffmann et al. 1984). Several volatile N-nitrosamines may also be present in tobacco products and tobacco smoke (Hoffmann et al. 1984), and some of these are potent transplacental carcinogens in animals (Mohr et al. 1980).

There is evidence that the enzymatic capacity of organs to activate the N-nitrosamines to alkylating agents is a determining factor in the organ-specific carcinogenicity (Magee et al. 1976). The short-lived electrophilic reactive species which are formed would react with cellular macromolecules close to the site of their formation. It is known that procarcinogens induce tumors only during the late phase of gestation (Mohr et al. 1980; Rice 1981). It can be assumed therefore that the fetal enzyme systems necessary for the activation of these carcinogens become operative only during late pregnancy, as suggested by Mohr and coworkers (1979).

The tissue distribution and the ontogeny of metabolism of the tobacco-specific N-nitrosamine 4-(methylnitrosamino)-1-(3-pyridyl)-1-butanone (NNK) was studied in pregnant and newborn C57B1 mice. We studied the tissue-distribution of the tobacco-specific N-nitrosamine N'-nitrosonornicotine (NNN) in the mice and NNK in pregnant Syrian golden hamsters. Finally, we have examined the ability of various tissues of fetal and infant Syrian golden hamsters to metabolize N-nitrosodiethylamine (NDEA) and the fate of this N-nitrosamine in pregnant hamsters has been studied in vivo. NDEA, which regularly is found in the gas phase of tobacco smoke

(Hoffmann et al. 1984), has been shown to induce transplacental tumors of the respiratory tract in Syrian golden hamsters (Mohr et al. 1975).

RESULTS

Whole-body autoradiography, performed according to Ullberg (1977), with [carbonyl-^{14}C] NNK in 13-, 16-, and 18-day pregnant C57B1 mice showed a passage of NNK and/or its metabolites across the placental barrier to the fetuses. The levels of radioactivity in the fetuses increased slowly after injection of the NNK and at 1 and 4 hours' survival the labeling of fetal tissues exceeded that of many maternal tissues (Fig. 1A,B). The radioactivity in the fetal eye melanin, kidney, and urinary bladder was higher than in other fetal tissues. There was a slow accumulation of radioactivity in the amniotic fluid. In order to trace organs accumulating bound metabolites, sections were extracted with trichloroacetic acid and organic solvents before the autoradiographic procedure. It was found that in 16- and 18-day pregnant mice tissue-bound radioactivity was retained in the fetal nose and eye melanin, whereas in the 13-day pregnant mice bound radioactivity was found only in the eye melanin (Fig. 2A,B). Autoradiograms of 1-, 3-, and 6-day-old mice showed a homogeneous radioactivity in most tissues and a labeling, which exceeded the homogeneous radioactivity, in the nose, the tracheobronchial mucosa, the liver, the pigmented tissues, the gastrointestinal contents, the kidney, and the urinary bladder. After washing, there was a marked retention of radioactivity in the nose and the pigmented tissues and also some labeling of the liver and tracheobronchial mucosa (Fig. 3A,B). In the mothers, tissue-bound metabolites were found in the nose, the tracheobronchial mucosa and the liver.

The evolution of the metabolic pathways of NNK in the nose, the lung, and the liver of fetal and newborn mice and the metabolism of NNK by the same maternal tissues, as revealed by in vitro incubations and quantifications by high-performance liquid chromatography (Castonguay et al. 1984a), are shown in Table 1. The results indicate that the reductive pathway leading to the formation of 4-(methylnitrosamino)-1-(3-pyridyl)butan-1-ol (NNA1) (Fig. 4) is developed in the tissues of fetal and newborn mice to an extent comparable to that in the maternal tissues. The products of α-carbon-hydroxylations of NNK (the keto alcohol *12* and the keto acid *13*) were not observed in the 13-day-old fetuses. However, the ontogeny of these metabolic pathways began in the tissues of 16- to 18-day-old fetuses and then increased with the age of the newborn mice. At all ages of the fetuses and the infants and in the mothers the amounts of *12* and *13* formed in the nose were higher than in the lung and the liver. Other variations in the metabolism of NNK among the tissues were also observed. For example, NNK-N-oxide (*1*) was found in the lung, but not in the nose or the liver, of 16- and 18-day-old fetuses, and this metabolite was more prevalent in the lung than in the nose and the liver also in the infants and the mother.

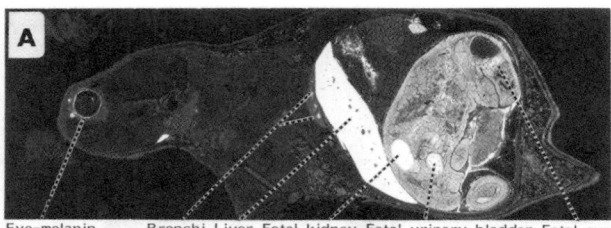
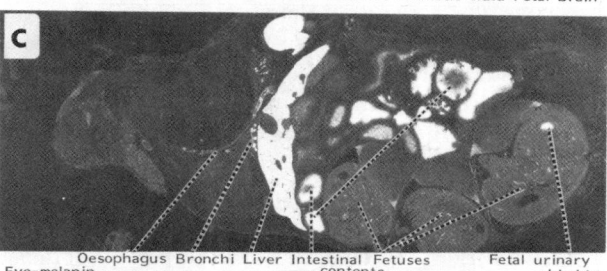
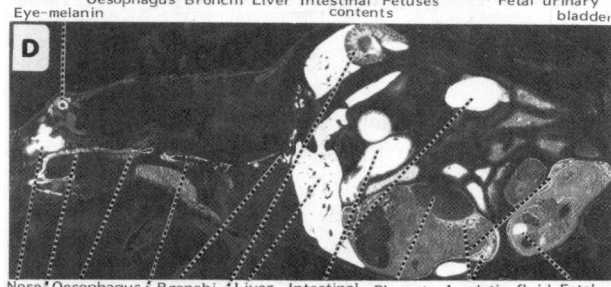

Figure 1
Whole-body autoradiograms of C57B1 mice on day 18 of gestation after i.v. injection of [carbonyl-^{14}C]NNK (5 µCi; 7.0 mg/kg) or [2'-^{14}C]NNN (5 µCi; 1.4 mg/kg). (*A*) [carbonyl-^{14}C]NNK, 1 hour's survival; (*B*) [carbonyl-^{14}C]NNK, 4 hours' survival; (*C*) [2'-^{14}C]NNN, 1 hour's survival; (*D*) [2'-^{14}C]NNN, 4 hours' survival.

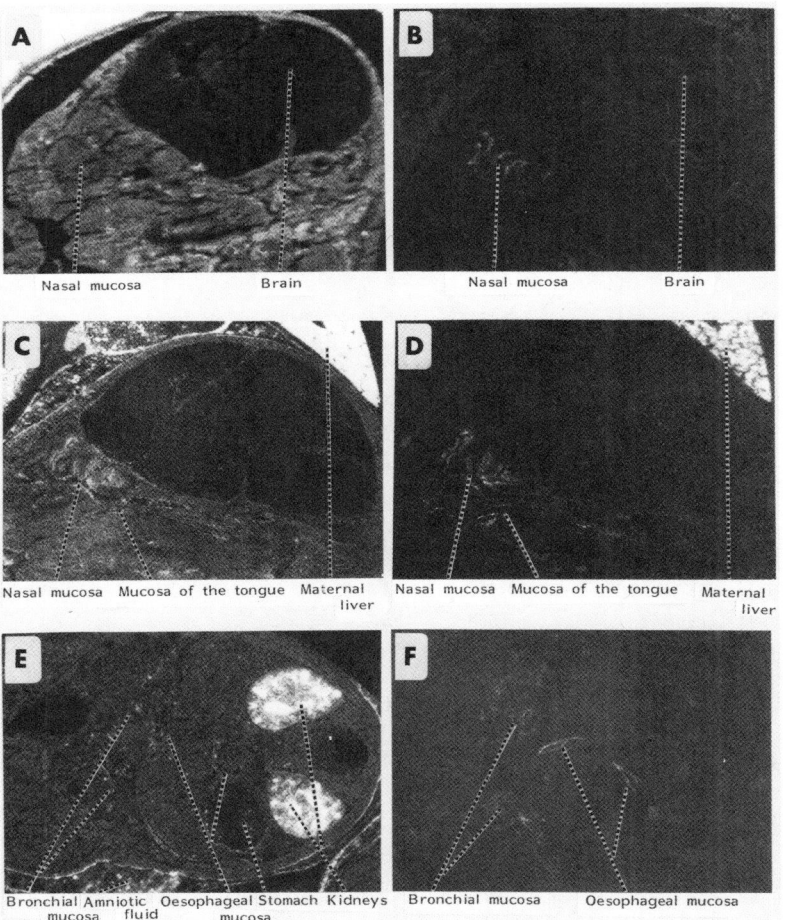

Figure 2
Enlargements of whole-body autoradiograms showing parts of fetuses of C57B1 mice on day 18 of gestation 4 hours after i.v. injection of [carbonyl-^{14}C]NNK (5 µCi; 7.0 mg/kg) or [2'-^{14}C]NNN (5 µCi; 1.4 mg/kg). (*A, B*) [carbonyl-^{14}C]NNK; (*C-F*) [2'-^{14}C]NNN; (*A, C,* and *E*) autoradiograms of freeze-dried nonextracted tissue sections; (*B, D,* and *F*) autoradiograms of tissue sections adjacent to *A, C,* and *E*, respectively, that were extracted with trichloroacetic acid and organic solvents before the autoradiographic exposure.

Extracts from fetuses and placentae of 13-day and 16-day pregnant mice injected with NNK were analyzed by high-performance liquid chromatography, and it was found that NNK, NNA1, and several other metabolites were present in the fetuses and the placentae. Analysis of the amniotic fluid from mice on day 18 of gestation injected with NNK showed the presence of the keto acid *13* and the

Table 1
Formation of Metabolites by Tissues of Fetal, Infant and Maternal C57B1 Mice Incubated with [carbonyl-^{14}C] NNK[a]

Metabolite[b]	Level of metabolites (nmole/g of wet tissue)[c]						
	Nose						
	Fetus			Infant			Mother
	13 days	16 days	18 days	1 day	3 days	6 days	
NNA1	52	48	40	19	28.8	8.7	36
1	ND	ND	ND	2.6	7.3	ND	22
2	ND	ND	ND	ND	4.7	ND	11
12	ND	12	13	30	55.5	51	262
13	ND	31	33	63	162	85	795
14	ND	ND	ND	ND	ND	ND	ND
15	ND	ND	ND	ND	3.1	ND	37
	Lung						
	Fetus			Infant			Mother
	13 days	16 days	18 days	1 day	3 days	6 days	
NNA1	45	66	85	47	78	62	97
1	ND	1.0	3.8	23	28	43	123
2	ND	ND	1.9	2.3	4.1	5.3	23
12	ND	ND	3.3	4.7	6.3	12	29
13	ND	1.3	2.5	16	21.1	30	95
14	ND	ND	ND	ND	0.4	ND	3.4
15	ND	ND	ND	ND	1.1	ND	10
	Liver						
	Fetus			Infant			Mother
	13 days	16 days	18 days	1 day	3 days	6 days	
NNA1	91	100	102	76	90	100	77
1	ND	ND	ND	3.7	3.0	9.1	15
2	ND	1.1	—	—	—	—	—
12	ND	ND	1.1	ND	4.9	16	6.0
13	ND	1.7	2.3	15.2	27.6	37	84
14	ND	ND	ND	4.2	4.9	13.6	46
15	ND	ND	ND	ND	1.6	3.1	ND

[a]Tissue slices were incubated in Krebs-Ringer phosphate buffer containing 33 nmole/ml (0.14 μCi/ml) of [carbonyl-^{14}C]NNK for 2 hours. Metabolites were analyzed by high-performance liquid chromatography.
[b]The structures of the metabolites are shown in Figure 4.
[c]Mean of duplicate values from two mice or from fetuses of two mothers
Modified from Castonguay et al. (1984a) and Tjälve et al. (1984)
ND = not detectable
— = not measured due to interferring peaks

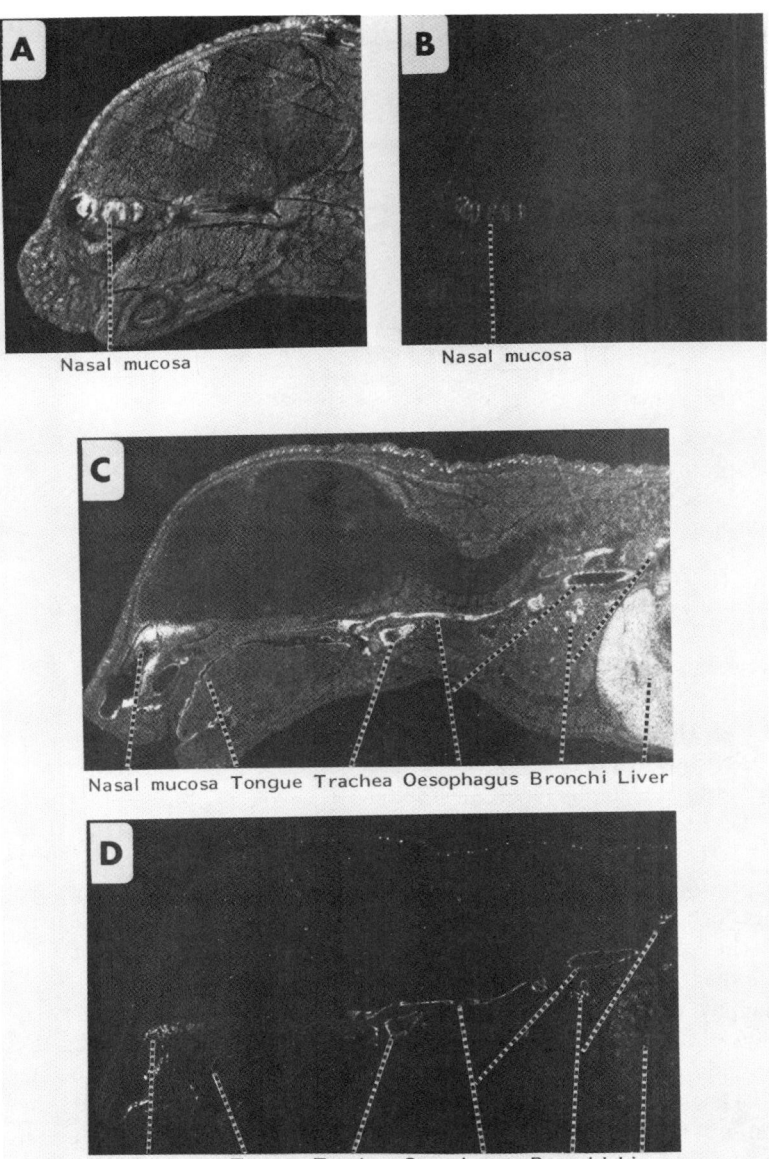

Figure 3
Enlargements of whole-body autoradiograms of 1-day-old C57Bl mice 4 hours after sc injection of [carbonyl-^{14}C]NNK (0.25 μCi; 10.2 mg/kg) or [2'-^{14}C]NNN (0.25 μCi; 2.0 mg/kg). (A, B) [carbonyl-^{14}C]NNK; (C, D) [2'-^{14}C]NNN; (A and C) autoradiograms of freeze-dried nonextracted tissue sections; (B and D) autoradiograms of tissue sections adjacent to A and C, respectively, that were extracted with trichloroacetic acid and organic solvents before the autoradiographic exposure.

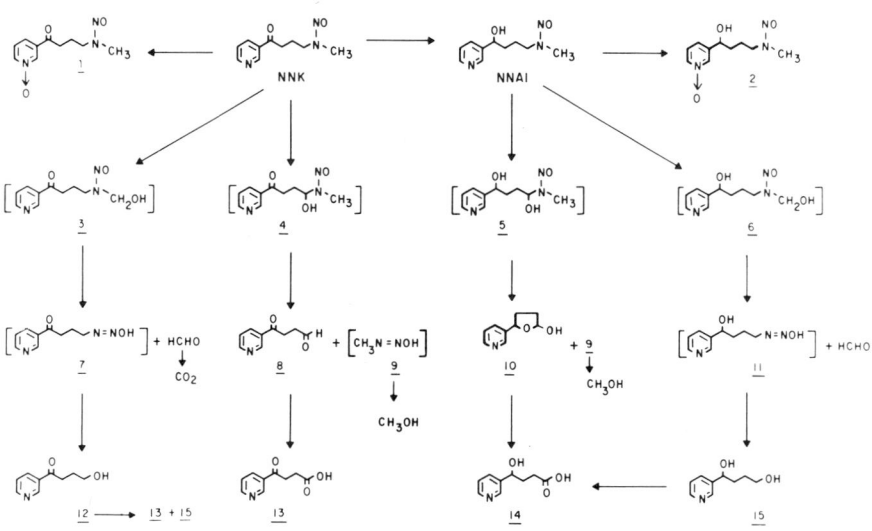

Figure 4
Metabolic transformations of NNK. Structures in brackets are hypothetical intermediates.

hydroxy acid *14*. These metabolites have been shown to be the major urinary metabolites of NNK in Fischer 344 rats (Castonguay et al. 1983).

Whole-body autoradiography with [carbonyl-^{14}C]NNK in 15-day pregnant Syrian golden hamsters also showed an uptake of NNK and/or its metabolites in the fetuses. DNA from fetal nose and liver of 15-day pregnant hamsters injected with NNK was extracted, hydrolysed, and analyzed for methylated guanines by cation-exchange high-performance liquid chromatography-fluorimetry (Castonguay et al. 1984b). The results showed the presence of O^6-methylguanine and 7-methylguanine both in the fetal nose and liver.

Autoradiography with [2'-^{14}C]NNN in 16- and 18-day pregnant mice showed an accumulation of radioactivity in fetuses, placentae, and amniotic fluid (Fig. 1C, D). The distribution pictures were in most respects similar to the ones described in the mice injected with [carbonyl-^{14}C]NNK. Thus, at 1 and 4 hours' survival the labeling of the fetal tissues and the amniotic fluid exceeded that of many maternal tissues. Within the fetuses the radioactivity in the eye melanin, kidney, and urinary bladder was higher than in other fetal tissues. In extracted tissue sections bound radioactivity was detected in the fetal eye melanin and nose and, in addition, at a low level in the tracheobronchial mucosa and the mucosa of the tongue and the esophagus (Fig. 2C-F). The latter tissues were not labeled in the pregnant mice injected with [carbonyl-^{14}C]NNK. Also in the maternal tissues of the mice given

[2'-^{14}C]NNN, a marked radioactivity was observed in the mucosa of the tongue and the esophagus, which was not seen in the mice given [carbonyl-^{14}C]NNK (Fig. 1C,D). The same observation was made in 1-day-old mice given [2'-^{14}C]NNN (Fig. 3C,D). Other maternal tissues and tissues of the young mice were labeled to a similar extent after the injection of [2'-^{14}C]NNN and [carbonyl-^{14}C]NNK.

Whole-body autoradiography of pregnant Syrian golden hamsters, given [1-^{14}C]-NDEA, on day 15 of gestation showed a strong radioactivity in the fetal nasal mucosa, tracheal mucosa, and mucosa of bronchi and bronchioles (Fig. 5). A considerable radioactivity was also present in the fetal liver, whereas other fetal tissues showed a low homogeneously distributed labeling. In 11-day pregnant hamsters there was no specific labeling of the fetal tissues mentioned above. The maternal nasal and tracheobronchial mucosa and liver were strongly labeled.

The ontogeny of NDEA metabolism by the nose, the lung, and the liver in fetuses and young hamsters, and the metabolism of NDEA by the same maternal tissues was studied in vitro, using the formation of $^{14}CO_2$ from the [1-^{14}C]NDEA as an index of metabolism (Löfberg and Tjälve 1984) (Table 2). NDEA is metabolized by α-carbon hydroxylation to acetaldehyde and an ethylating species. Carbon dioxide is probably generated by the degradation of the acetaldehyde and by degradation of ethanol, which is formed from the ethylating species (Phillips et al. 1975). In 11-day-old fetuses, a very low $^{14}CO_2$-formation was detected only in the liver (Table 2). However, the nasal mucosa, the liver, and the lung of the 15-day-old fetuses were found to have a distinct capacity to form $^{14}CO_2$. The fetal lung was very active in this respect and the lungs of 4- and 10-day-old infants were also very efficient in forming $^{14}CO_2$ from the [1-^{14}C]NDEA. A lower activity was observed in the lung of the 20-day-old fetuses and in the adult lung. In the liver a peak activity was observed in the 4- and 10-day-old hamsters. In the nasal mucosa the $^{14}CO_2$-formation was the highest in the 20-day-old hamsters.

DISCUSSION

The results of the present study indicate that NNK, NNN, and NDEA reach the fetuses and are metabolized by a few fetal tissues during the last stages of gestation.

NDEA has been shown to induce nasal, tracheal, and bronchial tumors in the offspring of Syrian golden hamsters, but only when the mothers are treated with the substance during the last 4 days of the pregnancy (Mohr et al. 1975). It was proposed that only at this late stage of pregnancy has the differentiation of the sensitive tissues reached a level at which NDEA can be metabolized to its ultimate carcinogen (Mohr et al. 1975, 1979). Our results in the 11- and 15-day pregnant hamsters are in support of this assumption: An in vitro capacity of the nasal mucosa and the lung to metabolize the NDEA was observed only in the 15-day-old fetuses, and this was correlated to a localization of metabolites in these tissues in vivo. The in vivo autoradiography indicated a metabolism of the substance also in

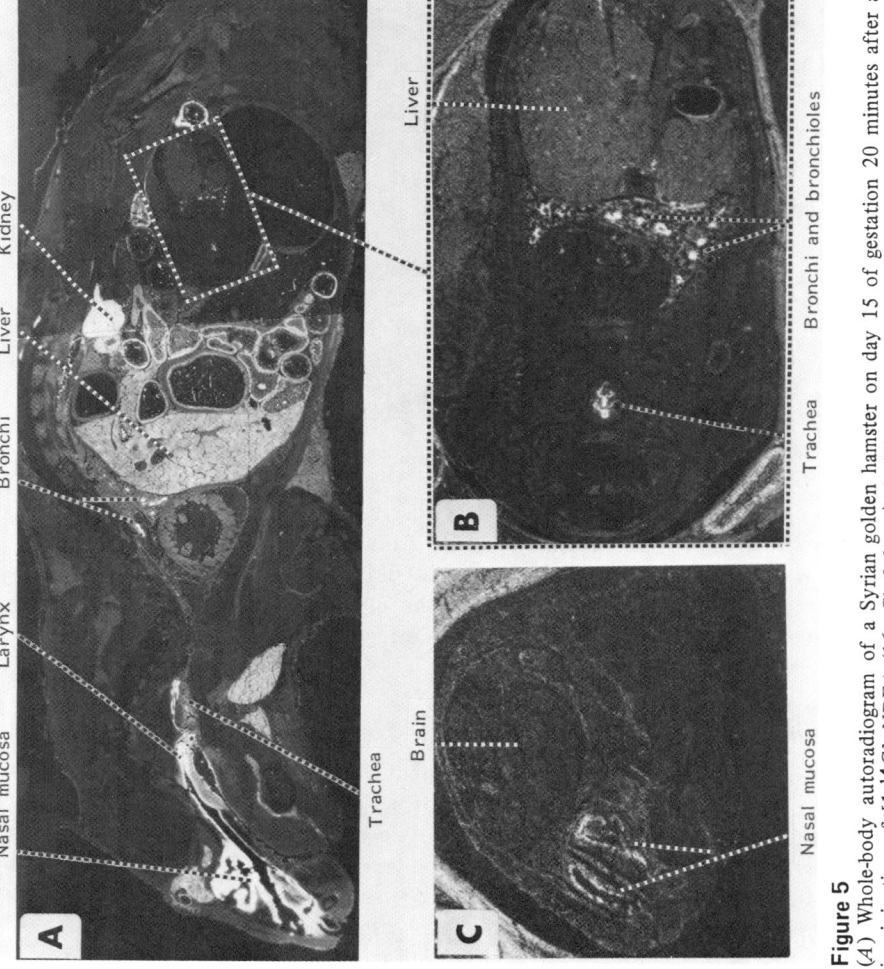

Figure 5
(A) Whole-body autoradiogram of a Syrian golden hamster on day 15 of gestation 20 minutes after an i.v. injection of [1-^{14}C] NDEA (16 μCi; 0.6 mg/kg); (B) enlargement of a fetus, as indicated; (C) enlargement of the head of a fetus from an adjacent whole-body autoradiogram.

Table 2
Formation of $^{14}CO_2$ by Tissues of Fetal, Infant, and Maternal Syrian Golden Hamsters Incubated with $[1-^{14}C]NDEA^a$

Tissue	Level of $^{14}CO_2$-production (dpm/mg of wet tissue)^b				
	Fetus			Infant		Mother
	11 days	15 days	4 days	10 days	20 days	
Nose	ND	35.9 ± 4.9 (3)	288.9 ± 39.6 (3)	813.2 ± 100.1 (3)	1146.9 ± 39.6 (4)	893.0 ± 131.2 (12)
Lung	ND	190.0 ± 7.0 (3)	459.1 ± 33.9 (4)	159.0 ± 8.0 (3)	85.9 ± 5.3 (4)	61.0 ± 13.2 (13)
Liver	1.7 ± 0.3 (3)	34.4 ± 7.7 (4)	606.7 ± 17.5 (4)	605.1 ± 4.4 (3)	429.3 ± 14.5 (4)	396.0 ± 45.1 (8)

^{a}Tissue slices were incubated in Krebs-Ringer phosphate buffer containing 3.8 nmole/ml (0.075 μCi/ml) of $[1-^{14}C]NDEA$ for 1 hour. The $^{14}CO_2$ formed during the incubations was trapped on filter papers moistened with KOH.
^{b}Mean ± SE. The figures within brackets denote the number of incubations.
Modified from Löfberg and Tjälve (1984)
ND = not detectable

the fetal trachea. Reznik-Schüller and Hague (1981) observed an increased labeling of fetal tracheas from day 12 to day 15 of pregnancy in Syrian golden hamsters treated with tritiated NDEA. Metabolic activation of NNK and NNN is presumed to involve α-carbon hydroxylations (Hecht et al. 1984). The keto alcohol *12* and the keto acid *13* are products of α-carbon hydroxylations of NNK (Fig. 4), and these metabolites were formed by the fetal nose, lung, and liver at the latest stages of the mouse pregnancy. In the pregnant hamsters given NNK, O^6-methylguanine was detected in the DNA of the fetal nose and liver. The methylating species is probably the methyldiazohydroxide *9* (Fig. 4). O^6-methylguanine has a potent miscoding efficiency with DNA polymerase and has been associated with neoplastic transformations (Lewis and Swenberg 1980; Eadie et al. 1984).

The whole-body autoradiography of NNN suggests that the fetal mucosa of the tongue and the esophagus, in addition to the nose, lung, and liver, have a capacity to metabolize the substance. The distribution of radioactivity in the maternal tissues of the C57B1 mice injected with [$2'$-^{14}C]NNN was similar to that observed after injection of [carbonyl-^{14}C]NNK: For both N-nitrosamines a labeling was observed in tissues such as the nose, the tracheobronchial mucosa, the liver, and the eye melanin. However, although the mucosa of the mouth and the esophagus was not labeled in the mothers given [carbonyl-^{14}C]NNK, such labeling was observed after administration of [$2'$-^{14}C]NNN. Thus, the ability of the mucosa of the mouth and the esophagus to activate NNN appears to be greater than the ability to activate NNK both in the fetuses and the adults. The autoradiography in the infant mice indicate that the same difference exists during this stage of life. An analogous difference in the labeling of the mouth and the esophagus has also been observed in F344 rats given injections of [carbonyl-^{14}C]NNK and [$2'$-^{14}C]NNN (Brittebo and Tjälve 1981; Castonguay et al. 1983).

Chromatography of the radioactive metabolites present in the amniotic fluid of the mice given [carbonyl-^{14}C]NNK showed that this labeling represented the keto acid *13* and the hydroxy acid *14*. These metabolites are the major urinary metabolites of NNK in F344 rats (Castonguay et al. 1983). Large quantities of urine have been shown to be formed by the fetal kidney in the last stage of gestation and this may contribute considerably to the volume of the amniotic fluid (Vernier and Smith 1968). The autoradiography showed a labeling of the fetal kidney and urinary bladder both in the mice injected with [carbonyl-^{14}C]NNK and [$2'$-^{14}C]-NNN. It is possible, therefore, that the radioactive materials reach the amniotic fluid via the fetal urinary excretion.

The localization of NNK- and NNN-radioactivity in melanin of the eyes can probably be ascribed to the basicity of these N-nitrosamines and some of their metabolites (Larsson and Tjälve 1979). In the fetuses there was evidence of a firm binding of radioactivity to melanin. Some compounds (e.g., thiouracil) (Farishian and Whittaker 1979) can be incorporated into newly synthesized melanin. Conceivably such an incorporation may also take place with NNK and NNN.

Our results indicated a marked metabolism of NDEA, NNK, and NNN in the infant hamsters and mice. The metabolism of NDEA in some tissues of the infant hamsters even exceeded the tissues of the adult animals. Rao and Vesselinovitch (1973) reported that the metabolism of NDEA by livers of 1- to 28-day-old mice exceeded the metabolizing capacity by the livers of 70-day-old mice, and these data were correlated to a higher tumor incidence in young mice than in older mice. It has been shown that NDEA when given to hamsters during nursing will induce cancer in the progeny later in life (Mohr et al. 1972). High levels of cell replication could contribute to the susceptibility of the young animals to the N-nitrosamines.

CONCLUSIONS

Our results have shown that N-nitrosamines present in tobacco and tobacco smoke can cross the placental barrier in pregnant animals and that a metabolism will take place in some fetal tissues at late gestation. Marked N-nitrosamine metabolism was observed in infant animals. For the volatile N-nitrosamine NDEA, the ability of the fetal and infant tissues to metabolize the substance can be correlated to carcinogenic effects. The tobacco-specific N-nitrosamines NNK and NNN have not yet been tested with regard to transplacental carcinogenicity or carcinogenicity at exposure during early life. However, our results suggest that exposure to these N-nitrosamines during the last stages of fetal development or during neonatal life could result in development of tumors.

It is considered that transplacental carcinogenesis as it may relate to cigarette smoking during pregnancy should be investigated more fully. Newborn children of smokers may in addition be exposed to carcinogens present in the breast milk and sidestream smoke and the importance of this exposure in terms of higher risks of cancer should also be examined.

ACKNOWLEDGMENTS

These studies were supported by the Swedish Council for Forestry and Agricultural Research and by U.S. National Cancer Institute grants CA-21393 and CA-32391.

REFERENCES

Brittebo, E.B. and H. Tjälve. 1981. Formation of tissue-bound N'-nitrosonornicotine metabolites by the target tissues of Sprague-Dawley and Fischer rats. *Carcinogenesis* 2: 959.

Castonguay, A., H. Tjälve, and S.S. Hecht. 1983. Tissue distribution of the tobacco-specific carcinogen 4-(methylnitrosamino)-1-(3-pyridyl)-1-butanone and its metabolites in F344 rats. *Cancer Res.* 43: 630.

Castonguay, A., H. Tjälve, N. Trushin, and S.S. Hecht. 1984a. Perinatal metabolism of the tobacco-specific carcinogen 4-(methylnitrosamino)-1-(3-pyridyl)-1-butanone in C57B1 mice. *J. Natl. Cancer Inst.* **72**: 1117.

Castonguay, A., R. Tharp, and S.S. Hecht. 1984b. Kinetics of DNA methylation by the tobacco-specific carcinogen 4-(methylnitrosamino)-1-(3-pyridyl)-1-butanone in F344 rats. In *N-nitroso compounds: Occurrence, biological effects and relevance to human cancer* (eds. I.K. O'Neill, R.C. VonBorstel, C.T. Miller, J. Lone, and H. Bartsch), IARC Scientific Publications no. 57, p. 805. International Agency for Research on Cancer, Lyon, France.

Eadie, J.S., M. Conrad, D. Toorchen, and M.D. Topal. 1984. Mechanism of mutagenesis by O^6-methylguanine. *Nature* **308**: 201.

Everson, R.B. 1980. Individuals transplacentally exposed to maternal smoking may be at increased cancer risk in adult life. *Lancet* **2**: 123.

Farishian, R.A. and J.R. Whittaker. 1979. Tyrosine utilization by cultured melanoma cells: Analysis of melanin biosynthesis using [^{14}C]-tyrosine and [^{14}C]-thiouracil. *Arch. Biochem.* **198**: 449.

Hecht, S.S., A. Castonguay, F.-L. Chung, and D. Hoffmann. 1984. Carcinogenicity and metabolic activation of tobacco-specific nitrosamines: Current status and future prospects. In *N-nitroso compounds: Occurrence, biological effects and relevance to human cancer* (eds. I.K. O'Neill, R.C. VonBorstel, C.T. Miller, J. Lone, and H. Bartsch), IARC Scientific Publications no. 57, p. 793. International Agency for Research on Cancer, Lyon, France.

Hoffmann, D., K.D. Brunnemann, J.D. Adams, and S.S. Hecht. 1984. Formation and analysis of N-nitrosamines in tobacco products and their endogenous formation in consumers. In *N-nitroso compounds: Occurrence, biological effects and relevance to human cancer* (eds. I.K. O'Neill, R.C. VonBorstel, C.T. Miller, J. Lone, and H. Bartsch), IARC Scientific Publications no. 57, p. 743. International Agency for Research on Cancer, Lyon, France.

Larsson, B. and H. Tjälve. 1979. Studies on the mechanism of drug-binding to melanin. *Biochem. Pharmacol.* **28**: 1181.

Lewis, J.G. and J.A. Swenberg. 1980. Differential repair of O^6-methylguanine in DNA of rat hepatocytes and nonparenchymal cells. *Nature* **288**: 185.

Löfberg, B. and H. Tjälve. 1984. The disposition and metabolism of N-nitrosodiethylamine in adult, infant and foetal tissues of the Syrian golden hamster. *Acta Pharmacol. Toxicol.* **54**: 104.

Magee, P.N., R. Montesano, and R. Preussmann. 1976. N-nitroso compounds and related carcinogens. *Am. Chem. Soc. Monogr.* **173**: 491.

Mohr, U., M. Emura, and H.-B. Richter-Reichhelm. 1980. Transplacental carcinogenesis. *Invest. Cell Pathol.* **3**: 209.

Mohr, U., H. Reznik-Schüller, and M. Emura. 1979. Tissue differentiation as a prerequisite for transplacental carcinogenesis in the hamster respiratory system, with special respect to the trachea. *Natl. Cancer Inst. Monogr.* **51**: 117.

Mohr, U., H. Reznik-Schüller, G. Reznik, and J. Hilfrisch. 1975. Transplacental effects of diethylnitrosamine in Syrian hamsters as related to different days of administration during pregnancy. *J. Natl. Cancer Inst.* **55**: 681.

Mohr, U., J. Althoff, A. Emminger, H. Bresch, and R. Spielhoff. 1972. Effects of nitrosamines in nursing Syrian golden hamsters and their offspring. *Z. Krebsforsch.* **78**: 73.

Neutel, C.I. and C. Buck. 1971. Effect of smoking during pregnancy on the risk of cancer in children. *J. Natl. Cancer Inst.* **47**: 59.

Phillips, J.C., B.G. Lake, M.J. Minski, S.D. Gangolli, and A.G. Lloyd. 1975. Studies on the metabolism of diethylnitrosamine in the rat. *Biochem. Soc. Trans.* **3**: 285.

Preston-Martin, S., M.C. Yu, B. Benton, and B.E. Henderson. 1982. N-nitroso compounds and childhood brain tumors: A case-control study. *Cancer Res.* **42**: 5240.

Rao, K.V.N. and S.D. Vesselinovitch. 1973. Age- and sex-associated diethylnitrosamine dealkylation activity of the mouse liver and hepatocarcinogenesis. *Cancer Res.* **33**: 1625.

Reznik-Schüller, H. and B.F. Hague, Jr. 1981. Autoradiography in fetal Syrian golden hamsters treated with tritiated diethylnitrosamine. *J. Natl. Cancer Inst.* **66**: 773.

Rice, J.M. 1981. Effects of prenatal exposure to chemical carcinogens and methods for their detection. In *Developmental toxicology* (eds. C.A. Kimmel and M.A. Buelkesam), p. 191. Raven Press, New York.

Tjälve, H., A. Castonguay, and S.S. Hecht. 1984. Fate of the tobacco-specific carcinogen 4-(methylnitrosamino)-1-(3-pyridyl)-1-butanone in pregnant and newborn C57B1 mice. In *N-nitroso compounds: Occurrence, biological effects and relevance to human cancer* (eds. I.K. O'Neill, R.C. VonBorstel, C.T. Miller, J. Lone, and H. Bartsch), IARC Scientific Publications no. 57, p. 787. International Agency for Research on Cancer, Lyon, France.

Ullberg, S. 1977. The technique of whole body autoradiography. Cryosectioning of large specimens. *Sci. Tools*, special issue, p. 2.

U.S. Department of Health, Education and Welfare. 1979. *Smoking and health. A report of the Surgeon General*, DHEW # (PHS) 79-50066, chp. 8, p. 1. U.S. Government Printing Office, Washington, D.C.

U.S. Department of Health and Human Services. 1980. *The health consequences of smoking for women. A report of the Surgeon General*, p. 1. U.S. Government Printing Office, Washington, D.C.

———. 1982. *The health consequences of smoking. Cancer. A report of the Surgeon General*, DHHS # (PHS) 82-50179, chp. 3, p. 171. U.S. Government Printing Office, Washington, D.C.

Vernier, R.L. and F.G. Smith, Jr. 1968. Fetal and neonatal kidney. In *Biology of gestation* (ed. N.S. Assali), vol. 2, p. 225. Academic Press, New York.

COMMENTS

STELLMAN: The developmental effects of cigarette smoking on human offspring are fairly well known. But what information do you have about actual carcinogenesis—transplacental carcinogenesis—formation of tumors in animal or human offspring, especially human smokers?

TJÄLVE: There are a few epidemiological reports in which tobacco smoking during pregnancy has been correlated with cancer in the offspring during childhood or adult life. Some references to this matter are found in my paper. There is also a report by Correa et al. in which the association of maternal smoking to lung cancer in the progeny has been examined. I don't know how strong the evidence in these studies really is.

TANNENBAUM: But you don't know if it's transplacental or if it just comes from smoking? That's the problem.

HOFFMANN: I think there were a few studies. A few years ago Grufferman from Duke University reported an increased risk for rhabdomyosarcoma in offspring whose fathers were smokers. Recently, Sandler et al. reported an increased risk for hematopoietic cancers in children whose parents were smokers.

BARTSCH: Do you have information on how ethanol affects the distribution of nitrosamines and the binding pattern in fetal and maternal tissues?

TJÄLVE: Yes it is known that ethanol has effects on the metabolism and carcinogenesis of N-nitrosamines in adult animals. I don't think that the possible effect of ethanol on the distribution and metabolism of N-nitrosamines in fetal tissues of pregnant animals has been studied.

HOFFMANN: Do you think that brain tumors in the offspring of smoking mothers could have been induced by N-nitrosamines?

TJÄLVE: I don't think that the N-nitrosamines would induce brain tumors transplacentally, but there may be some other constituents of tobacco smoke which might do that. It is known from animal experiments that some compounds are potent inducers of brain tumors transplacentally.

MAGEE: The most effective transplacental brain tumor inducers are nitrosamides, but not nitrosamines. I think ethylnitrosourea would probably be too unstable; it produces brain tumors in adult rats. However, if it induces brain tumors transplacentally in the offspring, I don't know.

HOFFMANN: So far, chemists have not been able to develop a method for the identification of N-nitrosamides in tobacco products; however, several studies are underway to do just that.

PARSA: But there is something puzzling about the site and diethylnitrosamine transplacental effect. In mice, usually it's the parenchymal cell tumor, such as type 2 aveolar or Clara cells, while you are mainly using the bronchial tree.

TJÄLVE: The cells which are labeled in the lungs are probably the Clara cells in the bronchi and bronchioles. That has been shown by microautoradiography. In the trachea the nonciliated cells are probably the ones that are most strongly labeled. The Clara cells are probably also the ones in the lung which undergo malignant transformations. In the trachea the basal cells may be the ones from which the tumors originate. These cells are also labeled, although to a lower extent than the nonciliated cells. Several factors may determine whether or not a damaged cell will undergo malignant transformation.

PARSA: Usually there are benign nodules in the parenchyma and they arise from the alveolar cells.

TJÄLVE: The labeling of the alveolar cells was low, and this has also been found for other N-nitrosamines we have studied.

WINKELSTEIN: The most prominent effect in humans is weight—fetal weight. Do you have any animal evidence that fetal weight is reduced in mammals in your studies?

TJÄLVE: No, we haven't. Carbon monoxide may be one constituent of tobacco smoke which contributes to the low fetal weight in humans.

HALEY: Children who are born prematurely have been noted to have higher levels of nicotine metabolites circulating in their blood than do larger neonates. However, this does not mean that nicotine is responsible for differences in birth weight.

WINKELSTEIN: Is anything known about the mechanisms of low fetal weight in the premature infants of smoking mothers?

CONNEY: It's very difficult to tell what causes the low body weight in the fetus. Exposure of the fetus to carbon monoxide, nicotine, and polycyclic aromatic hydrocarbons are among the possible causes. Many years ago, it was shown that a single dose of certain polycyclic hydrocarbons inhibit body growth in the rat, but the mechanism(s) has not been worked out.

Laboratory Studies on Oral Cancer and Smokeless Tobacco

KLAUS D. BRUNNEMANN,* BOGDAN PROKOPCZYK,* DIETRICH
HOFFMANN,* JAGADEESAN NAIR,† HIROSHI OHSHIMA,† AND HELMUT
BARTSCH†
*Naylor Dana Institute for Disease Prevention
American Health Foundation
Valhalla, New York 10595
†Division of Environmental Carcinogenesis
International Agency for Research on Cancer
F-69372 Lyon Cedex 08, France

OVERVIEW

This review of the current status of laboratory studies with smokeless tobaccos highlights the nature and quantitative aspects of carcinogenic nitrosamines and examines the possible role of benzo[a]pyrene and polonium-210 as contributors to the carcinogenic potential of orally used tobacco mixtures.

Due to its nitrate content, tobacco has a considerable nitrosation potential which effects the formation of carcinogenic N-nitrosamines from amine precursors in tobacco mixtures. The most potent carcinogens identified in tobacco are nicotine-derived nitrosamines which occur at levels far exceeding concentrations of carcinogenic nitrosamines in other products consumed by humans. Nitrosation of areca alkaloids in betel nut and tobacco mixtures can lead to areca-specific nitrosamines and among these, methylnitrosaminopropionitrile is a very potent animal carcinogen. Concentrations of polonium-210 in smokeless tobacco can reach 1.22 pCi/g and can, therefore, possibly exert long-term carcinogenic effects due to the repeated localized emission of α-radiation from snuff or chewing tobaccos.

One of the synthetic musk additives identified in perfumed chewing tobaccos and in betel nut and tobacco mixtures is mutagenic towards *S. typhimurium* after enzyme activation. Reduction of the levels of carcinogenic and/or mutagenic constituents of smokeless tobacco is urged in view of the extent of oral tobacco use and the magnitude of the oral cancer problem.

INTRODUCTION

Seeking to determine etiologic factors in the high incidence of oral cancer in India and other Asian countries, one is immediately confronted with the observation that chewing of betel quid, both with and without tobacco, has been a widespread habit for several hundred years. Recently, the International Agency for Research on Cancer concluded that "there is sufficient evidence that the habit of chewing betel quid with tobacco is carcinogenic to humans" (IARC 1985). In the United States and in Scandinavian countries, chewing of tobacco has found increasing acceptance as a substitute for cigarette smoking only recently with four kinds of chewing tobacco, i.e., plug tobacco, loose leaf tobacco, twist tobacco, and snuff, available. Currently, the most prevalent form of oral use of tobacco is that of snuff dipping, which has increased, especially among young people. An estimate by Rizio (1983) put the number of snuff dippers in the United States at 7,000,000. In 1984, about 21,600 tons of snuff were consumed in the United States (Maxwell 1985). Upon examination of epidemiological evidence, the International Agency for Research on Cancer affirmed that the oral use of snuff is carcinogenic to humans and that there exists limited evidence that chewing tobacco is carcinogenic (IARC 1985). The association of cancer of the oral cavity and pharynx with snuff dipping is discussed by Winn, this volume. This paper will focus on the current status of laboratory studies with smokeless tobaccos.

RESULTS AND DISCUSSION

Nitrosamines in Smokeless Tobacco

During the processing of tobacco to chewing tobacco and snuff, three types of carcinogenic N-nitrosamines are formed. These are volatile nitrosamines (VNA), nonvolatile nitrosamines (NVNA), and tobacco-specific nitrosamines (TSNA) (Fig. 1). As shown in Table 1, the quantitative aspects of VNA formation do not reveal a specific trend since these compounds are partially lost during aging, curing, and/or fermentation of tobacco because of their volatility. The presence of N-nitrosomorpholine (NMOR) in snuff indicates prior contamination with morpholine due to the additives and/or because of diffusion from packaging materials (Brunnemann et al. 1982). Although up to 690 ppb of NMOR were found in an earlier study, levels in recent analyses have not exceeded 35 ppb (Brunnemann et al. 1985).

Table 2 presents data for NVNA including six nitrosamino acids which have been detected in smokeless tobaccos in recent studies (Brunnemann et al. 1983; Nair et al. 1985a,b; Ohshima et al. 1985; H. Ohshima, pers. comm.). Although some of these acids may not be carcinogenic, their decarboxylation during manufacturing and possibly during aging of tobacco can lead to carcinogenic N-nitrosamines (Brunnemann et al. 1983). In addition, these nitrosamino acids may serve as *trans*-nitrosating agents, leading to the formation of yet other carcinogenic N-nitrosamines. The relatively high levels of the carcinogenic N-nitrosodiethanolamine (NDELA) in some of the smokeless tobaccos are largely due to the presence of residual diethanolamine originating from the treatment of tobacco with the sucker-growth inhibitor maleic hydrazide (MH-30) (Brunnemann and Hoffmann 1981). Due to a government-imposed ban of MH-30 for tobacco cultivation in 1981,

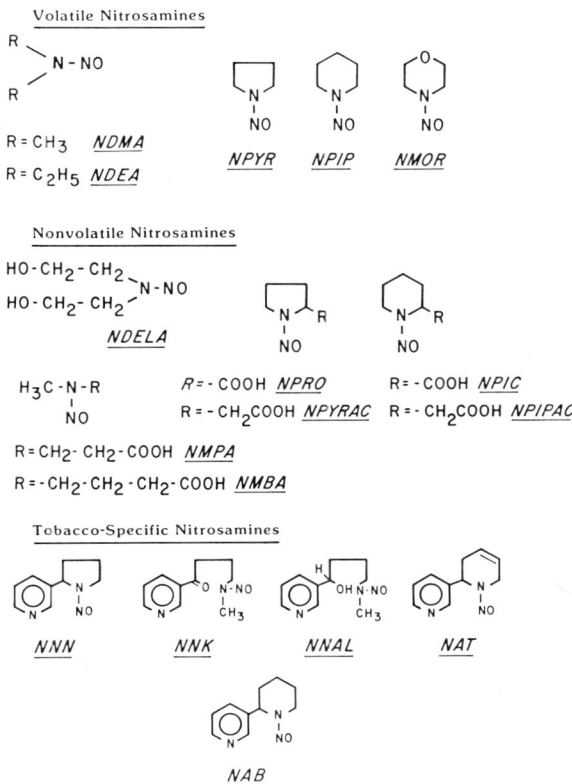

Figure 1
N-Nitrosamines in smokeless tobacco

NDELA levels in smokeless tobacco products have greatly decreased, as shown in Figure 2 for one snuff brand and one loose leaf chewing tobacco brand.

The TSNA are formed from the *Nicotiana* alkaloids by *N*-nitrosation during the preparation of smokeless tobacco products (Hoffmann and Adams 1981; Hoffmann et al. 1982) (Fig. 3). The TSNA occur in high concentrations in most smokeless tobaccos (Table 3). In the case of snuff, TSNA concentrations exceed by at least two orders of magnitude those found in other consumer products and in food (National Research Council 1981; Hoffmann et al. 1982; Brunnemann et al. 1985).

In one study with tobacco-chewing women and in another study with snuff-dipping male college students, we found significant amounts of TSNA in the saliva (Hoffmann and Adams 1981; Palladino et al. 1986) (Table 4). These findings demonstrate that nitrosamines are extracted from the tobacco during chewing and,

Table 1
Volatile Nitrosamines in Smokeless Tobacco (ppb)[a]

Product	NDMA	NPYR	NPIP	NMOR
United States				
Loose leaf[b]	4.1 (1)	ND (1)	ND (1)	ND (1)
Snuff	ND–215 (25)	ND–291 (15)	ND–107 (15)	ND–690 (25)
Sweden				
Chewing tobacco	ND–0.6 (2)	0.9–3.7 (2)		
Snuff	ND–60 (37)	ND–210 (27)	ND–0.5 (37)	ND–0.8 (37)
Canada				
Snuff	23.0–72.8 (2)	321–337 (2)	ND (2)	21.9–32.8 (2)
Denmark				
Chewing tobacco	2.6–3.3 (2)	25.2–25.5 (2)	ND (2)	ND (2)
India				
Chewing tobacco	ND–0.56 (4)	1.55–4.48 (4)	ND (4)	ND (4)
USSR				
Nass[c]	ND (4)	1.74–8.82 (4)	ND (4)	ND (4)

[a] Numbers in parentheses are samples analyzed
[b] One sample also contained 8.6 ppb nitrosodiethylamine (NDEA).
[c] Also contained ND–69.6 NDEA (10)
ND, not detected; NDMA, nitrosodimethylamine; NPYR, nitrosopyrrolidine; NPIP, nitrosopiperidine; NMOR, nitrosomorpholine

Table 2
Nonvolatile Nitrosamines in Smokeless Tobacco (ppb)[a]

Tobacco product	NDELA	NMPA	NMBA	NPRO	NPYRAC	NPIC	NPIPAC
United States							
Loose leaf	224–680 (3)			450–463 (2)			
Snuff	160–6800 (13)	1250–7420 (5)	120–2240 (5)	500–50900 (13)	ND–2000 (5)	ND–6100 (5)	ND–1500 (5)
Sweden							
Snuff	230–390 (8)	510–4400 (12)	ND–260 (12)	890–29500 (12)	100–300 (5)	ND–5560 (12)	100–200 (5)
Canada							
Plug tobacco	110 (1)			100 (1)			
Snuff	1180–2720 (3)			8800–16600 (2)			
Germany							
Plug tobacco	50 (2)			500–700 (2)			
Belgium							
Chewing tobacco		1600 (1)	100 (1)	3300 (1)	200 (1)	100 (1)	200 (1)
USSR							
Nass	40 (4)			ND–180 (4)			
India							
Chewing tobacco	30–110 (4)			190–410 (4)			

[a] Numbers in parentheses are samples analyzed
ND, not detected; NDELA, nitrosodiethanolamine; NMPA, 3-(N-nitroso-N-methylamino)butyric acid; NPRO, nitrosoproline; NPYRAC, nitrosopyrrolidine-acetic acid; NPIC, nitrosopipecolic acid; NPIPAC, nitrosopiperidine acetic acid

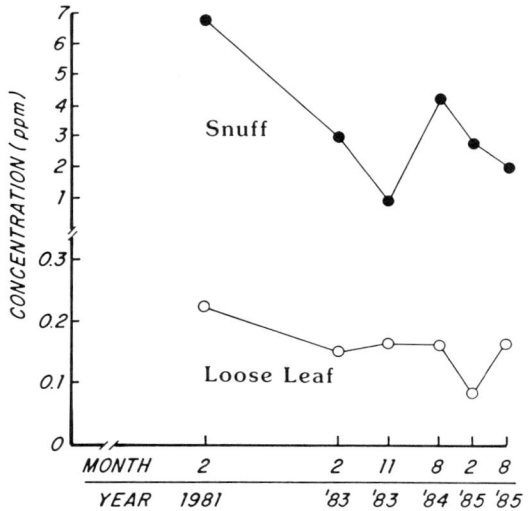

Figure 2
Decrease of *N*-nitrosodiethanolamine since February 1981 in one brand each of snuff tobacco and loose leaf chewing tobacco

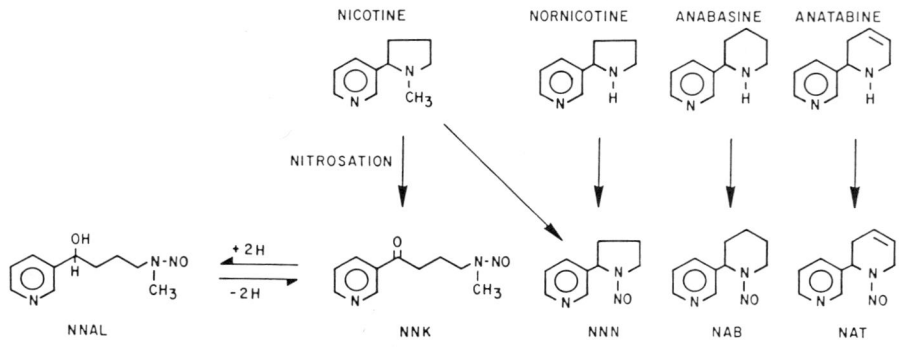

Figure 3
Formation of tobacco-specific *N*-nitrosamines

Table 3
Tobacco-specific N-Nitrosamines in Smokeless Tobacco (ppb)[a]

Product	NNN	NNK	NAT	NAB
United States				
Loose leaf	670–8200 (6)	380 (1)	2300 (1)	140 (1)
Plug tobacco	3400–4300 (3)			
Snuff	3120–135,000 (21)	100–13,600 (20)	1340–339,000 (20)	10–6700 (11)
Sweden				
Snuff	2260–154,000 (18)	870–2950 (18)	1840–21,400 (18)	130–150 (3)
Plug tobacco	2090 (1)	240 (1)	1580 (1)	100 (1)
Canada				
Snuff	50,400–79,100 (2)	3200–5800 (2)	152,000–170,000 (2)	4000–4800 (2)
Denmark				
Snuff	4460–8000 (3)	1350–7030 (3)	2680–6170 (3)	
Germany				
Plug tobacco	1420–2130 (2)	30–40 (2)	330–500 (2)	30–50 (2)
Snuff	6080–6700 (2)	1500–1540 (2)	3920–4370 (2)	
USSR				
Nass	120–520 (4)	20–130 (4)	32–300 (4)	8–30 (4)
India				
Chewing tobacco	470–2400 (5)	130–230 (4)	300–450 (4)	30–70 (4)
Belgium				
Chewing tobacco	7380 (1)	130 (1)	970 (1)	

[a] Numbers in parentheses are samples analyzed
NNN, N'-nitrosonornicotine; NNK, 4-(methylnitrosamino)-1-(3-pyridyl)-1-butanone; NAT, N'-nitrosoanatabine; NAB, N'-nitrosoanabasine

Table 4
Alkaloids and N-Nitrosamines in the Saliva of Snuff Dippers

Saliva component	I (4)[a]	II (8)[a]	III (30)[b]
Nicotine µg/ml		73-1560	
Cotinine µg/ml			0.18-2.48
NNN ng/ml	5-125	25.9-420	37.4-225
NNK ng/ml	7.5-201	<10-96	0-60.6
NAT ng/ml	6.6-147	12.5-470	48.1-555

Numbers in parentheses are saliva samples analyzed
[a]Hoffmann and Adams (1981)
[b]Palladino et al. (1986)
NNN, N'-nitrosonornicotine; NNK, 4-(methylnitrosamino)-1-(3-pyridyl)-1-butanone; NAT, N'-nitrosoanatabine

more importantly, indicate that these powerful carcinogens come in contact with the epithelial tissues of the oral cavity and pharynx, which are the major sites for an increased risk for cancer in snuff dippers (Winn et al. 1981; IARC 1985).

Benzo[a]pyrene and Polonium in Snuff

In cooperation with N. Harley of New York University, we have analyzed the five most popular snuff brands in the United States for benzo[a]pyrene (B[a]P) and polonium-210 (^{210}Po) (Hoffmann et al. 1986). In one sample we found only traces of B[a]P (< 0.1 ppb) and small amounts of ^{210}Po (0.16 pCi); however, the other four samples contained 0.42-63 ppb of B[a]P and up to 1.22 pCi of ^{210}Po. Assuming an average value of 0.5 pCi/g of dry snuff, the average snuff dipper, consuming 10 g of moist snuff daily, will expose a limited area of the oral cavity to about 2.5 pCi per day. This compares with an estimated 1.6 pCi of ^{210}Po for the daily intake of food in Illinois (Watson 1985). B[a]P and other polynuclear aromatic hydrocarbons in these tobaccos most likely derive from the curing process, especially from fire curing, whereas ^{210}Po stems mostly from the phosphate fertilizer (Tso et al. 1966). We consider the presence of ^{210}Po in snuff at these levels as a likely contributing factor for the elevated risk for oral cancer in snuff dippers.

Carcinogenicity of Chewing Tobacco

So far, most bioassays with the extracts of smokeless tobaccos have failed to induce tumors in laboratory animals (IARC 1985). Topical administration of snuff in a surgically created oral canal has induced a few neoplastic lesions in the oral cavity of rats in a study by Hirsch and Thilander (1981). Using the same method we have recently completed a 24-month study in which snuff induced at least two tumors in the oral cavity of 30 rats; the histopathological examination of this assay is currently underway.

Snuff insertion into the surgically created oral canal, in combination with herpes simplex virus type 1 infection, induced squamous cell carcinoma of the oral cavity in rats (Hirsch et al. 1984). The contributory role of herpes simplex virus is also apparent in a study by Park et al. (1985), who reported the induction of squamous cell carcinoma in the buccal pouches of ten out of 25 Syrian golden hamsters that had been infected with the virus and treated with snuff twice daily for 6 months. Treatment with either the virus or snuff alone did not elicit tumor response. The results of these bioassays strongly support the assumption that long-term snuff dipping may also lead to the induction of malignant tumors in man.

Although snuff contains traces of carcinogenic hydrocarbons, ^{210}Po, and possibly other unknown carcinogens, we consider the high concentrations of the tobacco-specific N-nitrosamines to be the major carcinogenic factor in snuff. N'Nitrosonornicotine (NNN) and 4-(methylnitrosamino)-1-(3-pyridyl)-1-butanone (NNK) are highly carcinogenic in mice, rats and hamsters. A single dose of only 1 mg of NNK induces significant numbers of tumors in the respiratory tract of hamsters. In F344 rats, NNK is a more powerful carcinogen than N-nitrosodimethylamine (NDMA) (Hoffmann and Hecht 1985). NNK is metabolically activated to a methylating agent which leads to 7-methylguanine (7-mG) and O^6-methylguanine (O^6-mG) in DNA in vitro and in vivo, an aspect that is discussed by Hecht et al., this volume. To examine the extent of DNA methylation in snuff dippers, we are currently analyzing cells from the oral scrapings of long-term snuff users for O^6-methylguanosine in DNA with a biotin-avidine enzyme-linked immunosorbent assay (BA-ELISA) developed by Foiles et al. (1985).

Betel Quid Chewing and N-Nitrosamines

The risk for cancer of the oral cavity and of the esophagus among chewers of betel quid is increased even more when the quid contains tobacco (Jussawalla and Deshpande 1971). The extract of betel quid is tumorigenic on mouse skin, elicits sarcoma in the connective tissue of mice and rats, and induces hepatoma in mice (Ranadive and Gothoskar 1976; Bhide et al. 1979). However, except for NNN, until recently, not a single carcinogen has been identified in extracts of betel quid (Bhide et al. 1981).

The saliva of betel quid tobacco chewers contains nitrite, thiocyanate, nicotine, and arecoline (Shivapurkar et al. 1980; Nair et al. 1985a). The presence of these agents in the saliva favors the endogenous formation of nitrosamines of both the tobacco alkaloids and the areca-alkaloids in chewers of betel quid. Arecoline makes up about 85-95% of the total alkaloid content of areca (2-4%). Areca alkaloids are arecaidine, guvacoline, and guvacine (Arjungi 1976). In model studies with arecoline, nitrite, and thiocyanate, it was shown that four specific N-nitrosamines can be formed: the areca-specific N-nitrosamines (ASNA), nitrosoguvacoline (NG), nitrosoguvacine (NGC), 3-(methylnitrosamino)propionitrile (MNPN), and 3-(methylnitrosamino)propionaldehyde (MNPA) (Wenke and Hoffmann 1983; Nair et al. 1985a) (Fig. 4). It appears that NG and MNPA are not carcinogenic in rats; NGC has so far not been tested (Lijinsky and Taylor 1976; D. Hoffmann et al., in prep.), but MNPN is a powerful carcinogen in rats (Wenke et al. 1984a).

The analyses of saliva of chewers who use betel quid without tobacco revealed the presence of NG, NGC, and NMPA and, in the case of betel quid with tobacco, NG, NGC, two nitrosamino acids, three tobacco-specific N-nitrosamines and, in a few cases, also volatile N-nitrosamines (Sipahimalani et al. 1984; Wenke et al. 1984b; Nair et al. 1985a,b) (Table 5). Preliminary data indicate that higher levels of ASNA are present in the saliva of chewers of betel quid containing tobacco than in the saliva of those who chew betel quid alone. This may be due to the nitrate content in the tobacco which provides additional nitrosation potential.

Neither MNPN nor MNPA have thus far been identified in saliva. These nitrosamines are probably metabolized too rapidly to be assessed at the time of the saliva analysis. More detailed studies are needed to explain this observation. Although analytical data for ^{210}Po in betel quid and tobacco mixtures are not available, the finding by Harley et al. (1980) of about 0.4 pCi/g in Indian tobacco permits the assumption that traces of this carcinogenic α-emitter are present in the betel quid tobacco mixture.

Genotoxic Agents in Betel Quid

In addition to N-nitrosamines, betel quid contains or may contain agents which are genotoxic in in vitro assays and which are not carcinogenic or have so far not been

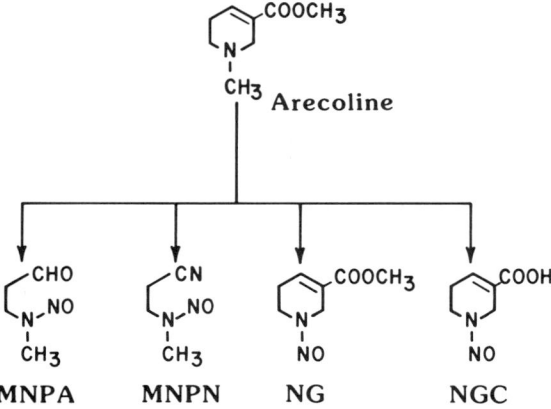

Figure 4
Formation of areca-specific N-nitrosamines

Table 5
Analyses of the Saliva of Chewers of Betel Quid, Chewers of Betel Quid with Tobacco, Cigarette Smokers, and Nontobacco Users

Parameter	BQ	BQT	SM	NT	References
pH	6.3–7.5 (5)	5.9–7.2 (6)	6.9–7.3 (8)	7.3–7.6 (4)	Wenke et al. (1984b)
Thiocyanate	4.6–18.5 (5)	7.5–20.3 (6)	15.7–203 (8)	1.1–21.5 (4)	Wenke et al. (1984b)
$\mu g/ml$					
Nicotine	4.6–31.8 (12)	2.2–15.7 (12)	7.3–102 (15)	16–34.3 (5)	Nair et al. (1985a)
$\mu g/ml$	ND (12)	1.7–311 (12)	0–4.4 (15)	ND (5)	Nair et al. (1985a)
Cotinine	0.005–0.57 (5)	1.6–4.8 (6)	ND–0.26 (8)	ND–0.014 (4)	Wenke et al. (1984b)
$\mu g/ml$	ND (12)	1.0–3.9 (12)	ND–5.2 (15)	ND (5)	Nair et al. (1985a)
Arecoline	0.0–89.9 (12)	2.4–143 (12)	ND	ND	Nair et al. (1985a)
$\mu g/ml$					
NG	3.5–9.5 (5)	4.3–350 (6)	ND–7.6 (8)	ND (4)	Nair et al. (1985a)
ng/ml	0.0–5.9 (12)	0.0–7.1 (12)	ND (15)	ND (5)	Nair et al. (1985a)
NGC	0.0–26.6 (12)	0.0–30.4 (12)	ND (15)	ND (5)	Nair et al. (1985a)
ng/ml					
NMPA	0.0–2.8 (12)	3.7–6.1 (12)	0.0–3.0 (15)	ND (5)	
ng/ml					
NNN	ND (5)	1.2–38 (6)	ND (8)	ND (4)	Wenke et al. (1984b)
ng/ml	ND (12)	1.6–14.7 (12)	ND (15)	ND (5)	Nair et al. (1985a)
		6.4–12.9 (7)			Sipahimalani (1984)
NNK	ND (5)	1.1–2.3 (6)	ND–1.7 (8)	ND (4)	Wenke et al. (1984b)
ng/ml	ND (12)	0.0–2.3 (12)	ND (15)	ND (5)	Nair et al. (1985a)
NAT	ND (5)	3.2–40 (6)	ND (8)	ND (4)	Wenke et al. (1984b)
ng/ml	ND (12)	1.0–10.9 (12)	ND (15)	ND (5)	Wenke et al. (1984b)

Numbers in parentheses are samples analyzed
BQ, betel quid chewers; BQT, chewers of betel quid with tobacco; SM, cigarette smokers; NT, nontobacco users
ND, not detected; NG, nitrosoguvacoline; NGC, nitrosoguvacine; NMPA, 3-(N-nitroso-N-methylamino)propionic acid; NNN, N'nitrisonornicotine; NNK, 4-(methylnitrosamino)-1-(3-pyridyl)-1-butanone; NAT, N'nitrosoanatabine

tested for carcinogenicity in laboratory animals. These are arecoline (Panigrahi and Rao 1982; Shirname et al. 1984), arecaidine (Ashby et al. 1979; Panigrahi and Rao 1984), and eugenol (Stich et al. 1981). Recently, Nair et al. (1985c) identified two synthetic nitro musks in betel quid with tobacco and in perfumed chewing tobaccos such as those used for chewing in India. These are 5-t-butyl-1,3-dinitro-4-methoxy-2-methylbenzene, known as musk ambrette, and 1-t-butyl-3,5-dimethyl-2,4,6-trinitrobenzene, called musk xylene. The concentrations of these synthetic nitro musks in tobacco-containing betel quid samples measured up to 0.2% and in perfumed chewing tobacco up to 2.35% (Table 6). Musk ambrette was mutagenic in TA100 with activation by S9 fraction of liver homogenate of rats pretreated with Aroclor; musk xylene was inactive in the same test.

SUMMARY

Extracts of chewing tobacco and snuff are tumorigenic in laboratory animals. They contain a number of known carcinogens, including volatile and nonvolatile nitrosamines, tobacco-specific nitrosamines, polynuclear aromatic hydrocarbons, and ^{210}Po. The concentration of the carcinogenic TSNA in snuff exceeds by at least two orders of magnitude the concentration of nitrosamines in other consumer products. ^{210}Po measures up to 1.22 pCi in 1 g of snuff. Snuff is also tumorigenic

Table 6
Synthetic Nitro Musks in Samples of Betel Quid with Tobacco and Perfumed Chewing Tobacco

Sample	mg/g wet weight	
	Musk ambrette	Musk xylene
BQT-1	1.10	0.60
BQT-2	1.08	0.45
BQT-3	0.92	0.49
BQT-4	1.44	0.79
BQT-5	0.82	0.47
Z-1	23.5	ND
Z-2	11.2	0.60

Modified from Nair et al. 1985c.
ND, not detected
BQT, betel quid with tobacco; Z, Zarda

in rats and in Syrian golden hamsters. These findings are strongly supportive of epidemiological data which have shown that snuff use significantly increases the risk for cancer of the oral cavity and pharynx. The major reduction of levels of ^{210}Po and of the tobacco-specific nitrosamines in smokeless tobacco, especially in snuff, is strongly indicated, particularly since this is technically feasible.

Chewing of betel quid together with tobacco is strongly correlated with the high incidence of oral cancer in India and other Asian countries. Extracts of the betel quid and tobacco mixture are tumorigenic in experimental animals. In addition to some volatile and nonvolatile nitrosamines and tobacco-specific N-nitrosamines, the saliva of chewers of betel and tobacco mixtures contains at least two nitrosamines which are formed from the major betel nut alkaloid, arecoline. These are N-nitrosoguvacoline and N-nitrosoguvacine. Other areca-specific N-nitrosamines may also be formed during betel quid chewing, but these remain to be identified. Although the presence of ^{210}Po in betel and tobacco mixtures has not been ascertained by analyses, ^{210}Po is likely to be present at levels of 0.1–1 pCi/g tobacco. Recently, two synthetic nitro musk additives have been identified in perfumed chewing tobacco and in betel and tobacco mixtures. One of these two flavor additives, i.e., musk ambrette (5-t-butyl-1,3-dinitro-4-methoxy-2-methylbenzene) is mutagenic. The magnitude of the oral cancer problem in Asia and the extent of the habit of chewing betel and tobacco mixtures there mandates that steps be taken to reduce the levels of carcinogenic N-nitrosamines in these products as soon as possible.

ACKNOWLEDGMENTS

We thank Mrs. I. Hoffmann for editorial assistance. The studies originating from the American Health Foundation are supported by Research Grant PO1-CA-29580 from the National Cancer Institute. J. N. has been awarded a Research Training Fellowship for his studies at the International Agency for Research on Cancer.

REFERENCES

Arjungi, K.N. 1976. Areca nut. A review. *Arzneim. Forsch.* 26: 951.
Ashby, J., J.A. Styles, and E. Boyland. 1979. Betel nuts, arecaidine and oral cancer. *Lancet* i: 112.
Bhide, S.V., N.M. Shivapurkar, S.V. Gothoskar, and K.J. Ranadive. 1979. Carcinogenicity of betel quid ingredients: Feeding mice with aqueous extract and the polyphenol fraction of betel nut. *Br. J. Cancer* 40: 922.
Bhide, S.V., A.I. Pratap, N.M. Shivapurkar, A.T. Sipahimalani, and M.S. Chadha. 1981. Detection of nitrosamines in a commonly used chewing tobacco. *Food Cosmet. Toxicol.* 19: 481.

Brunnemann, K.D. and D. Hoffmann. 1981. Assessment of the carcinogenic N-nitrosodiethanolamine in tobacco products and tobacco smoke. *Carcinogenesis* **2**: 1123.

Brunnemann, K.D., J.C. Scott, and D. Hoffmann. 1982. N-Nitrosomorpholine and other volatile N-nitrosamines in snuff tobacco. *Carcinogenesis* **3**: 693.

———. 1983. N-Nitrosoproline, an indicator for N-nitrosation of amines in processed tobacco. *J. Agric. Food Chem.* **31**: 905.

Brunnemann, K.D., L. Genoble, and D. Hoffmann. 1985. N-Nitrosamines in chewing tobacco: An international comparison. *J. Agric. Food Chem.* **33**: 1178.

Foiles, P.G., N. Trushin, and A. Castonguay. 1985. Measurement of O^6-methyldeoxyguanosine in DNA methylated by the tobacco-specific carcinogen 4-(methylnitrosamino)-1-(3-pyridyl)-1-butanone using a biotin-avidin enzyme-linked immunosorbent assay. *Carcinogenesis* **6**: 989.

Harley, N.H., B. Cohen, and T.C. Tso. 1980. Polonium-210: A questionable risk factor in smoking-related carcinogenesis. *Banbury report 3:* A safe cigarette? (ed. G.B. Gori and F.G. Bock), p. 93. Cold Spring Harbor Laboratory, Cold Spring Harbor, New York.

Hirsch, J.M. and H. Thilander. 1981. Snuff-induced lesions of the oral mucosa—An experimental model in the rat. *J. Oral Pathol.* **10**: 342.

Hirsch, J.M., S.L. Johansson, and A. Vahlne. 1984. Effect of snuff and *herpes simplex* virus-1 on rat oral mucosa: Possible association with the development of squamous cell carcinoma. *J. Oral Pathol.* **13**: 52.

Hoffmann, D. and J.D. Adams. 1981. Carcinogenic tobacco-specific N-nitrosamines in snuff and in the saliva of snuff dippers. *Cancer Res.* **4**: 4305.

Hoffmann, D. and S.S. Hecht. 1985. Nicotine-derived N-nitrosamines and tobacco-related cancer: Current status and future directions. *Cancer Res.* **45**: 935.

Hoffmann, D., K.D. Brunnemann, J.D. Adams, A. Rivenson, and S.S. Hecht. 1982. N-nitrosamines in tobacco carcinogenesis. *Banbury report 12: Nitrosamines and human cancer* (ed. P.N. Magee), p. 211. Cold Spring Harbor Laboratory, Cold Spring Harbor, New York.

Hoffmann, D., N.H. Harley, I. Fisenne, J.D. Adams, and K.D. Brunnemann. 1986. Carcinogenic agents in snuff. *J. Natl. Cancer Inst.* **76**: 435.

IARC. 1985. *Monographs on the evaluation of the carcinogenic risk of chemicals to humans*, vol. 37. International Agency for Research on Cancer, Lyon, France.

Jussawalla, D. and V.A. Deshpande. 1971. Evaluation of cancer risk in tobacco chewers and smokers: An epidemiological assessment. *Cancer* **28**: 244.

Lijinsky, W. and H.W. Taylor. 1976. Carcinogenicity test of two unsaturated derivatives of N-nitrosopiperidine in Sprague-Dawley rats. *J. Natl. Cancer Inst.* **57**: 1315.

Maxwell, J.C. 1985. Smokeless tobacco sales up 2%. *Tob. Rep.* **112**: 62.

Nair, J., H. Ohshima, M. Friesen, A. Croisy, S.V. Bhide, and H. Bartsch. 1985a. Tobacco-specific and betel nut-specific N-nitroso compounds: Occurrence in saliva and urine of betel quid chewers and formation in vitro by nitrosation of betel quid. *Carcinogenesis* **6**: 295.

Nair, J., H. Ohshima, C. Malaveille, M. Friesen, S.V. Bhide, and H. Bartsch. 1985b. N-Nitroso compounds (NOC) in saliva and urine of betel quid chewers:

Studies on the occurrence and formation. *Proc. Am. Assoc. Cancer Res.* **75**: 67.

Nair, J., H. Ohshima, C. Malaveille, M. Friesen, I.K. O'Neill, A.A. Hautefeuille, and H. Bartsch. 1985c. Identification, occurrence and mutagenicity in *S. typhimurium* of two synthetic nitro arenes—Musk ambrette and musk xylene in Indian chewing tobacco and betel quid. *Food Chem. Toxicol.* **24**: 27.

National Research Council. 1981. *The health effects of nitrate, nitrite and N-nitroso compounds*, p. 51. National Academic Press, Washington, D.C.

Ohshima, H., J. Nair, M.-C Burgade, M. Friesen, L. Garven, and H. Bartsch. 1985. Identification and occurrence of two new N-nitrosamino acids in tobacco products: 3-(N-nitroso-N-methylamino)propionic acid and 4(N-nitroso-N-methylamino)butyric acid. *Cancer Lett.* **26**: 153.

Palladino, G., J.D. Adams, K.D. Brunnemann, N.J. Haley, and D. Hoffmann. 1986. Snuff-dipping in college students: A clinical profile. *Military Medicine.* **151**: 342.

Panigrahi, G.B. and A.R. Rao. 1982. Chromosome breaking ability of arecoline, a major betel-nut alkaloid, in mouse bonemarrow cells in vivo. *Mutat. Res.* **103**: 197.

———. 1984. Induction of in vivo sister chromatid exchanges by arecaidine, a betel nut alkaloid, in mouse bone marrow cells. *Cancer Lett.* **23**: 189.

Park, N.H., E.G. Herbosa, and J.P. Sapp. 1985. Oral cancer induced in hamsters with *herpes simplex* infection combined with simulated snuff-dipping. Presented *Tenth international herpes virus workshop*, Ann Arbor, Michigan, August 11–16, 1985, p. 297.

Ranadive, K.J. and S.W. Gothoskar. 1976. Betel quid chewing and oral cancer: Experimental studies: Prevention and detection of cancer. Part I. *Prevention* **2**: 1745.

Rizio, D. 1983. Proliferation of moist snuff use in the U.S. *Tob. Int.* **1**: 17–20.

Shirname, L.P., M.M. Menon, and S.V. Bhide. 1984. Mutagenicity of betel quid and its ingredients using mammalian test systems. *Carcinogenesis* **5**: 501.

Shivapurkar, N.M., A.V. D'Souza, and S.V. Bhide. 1980. Effect of betel quid chewing on nitrite levels in saliva. *Food Cosmet. Toxicol.* **18**: 277.

Sipahimalani, A.T., M.S. Chadha, S.V. Bhide, A.I. Pratap, and J. Nair. 1984. Detection of N-nitrosamines in the saliva of habitual chewers of tobacco. *Food Chem. Toxicol.* **22**: 261.

Stich, H.F., M.P. Rosin, C.H. Wu, and W.D. Parorie. 1981. The action of transition metals on the genotoxicity of simple phenols, phenolic acids and cinnamic acids. *Cancer Lett.* **14**: 251.

Tso, T.C., N.H. Harley, and L.T. Alexander. 1966. Source of lead-210 and polonium-210 in tobacco. *Science* **153**: 880.

Watson, A.P. 1985. Polonium-210 and lead-210 in food and tobacco products: Transfer parameters and normal exposure and dose. *Nucl. Saf.* **26**: 179.

Wenke, G. and D. Hoffmann. 1983. A study of betel quid carcinogenesis. 1. On the in vitro N-nitrosation of arecoline. *Carcinogenesis* **4**: 169.

Wenke, G., A. Rivenson, and D. Hoffmann. 1984a. A study of betel quid carcinogenesis. 3. 3-(Methylnitrosamino)propionitrile, a powerful carcinogen in F344 rats. *Carcinogenesis* **5**: 1137.

Wenke, G., K.D. Brunnemann, D. Hoffmann, and S.V. Bhide. 1984b. A study of betel quid carcinogenesis. 4. Analysis of the saliva of betel chewers: A preliminary report. *J. Cancer Res. Clin. Oncol.* **108**: 110.

Winn, D.M., W.J. Blot, C.M. Shy, L.W. Pickle, A. Toledo, and J.F. Fraumeni, Jr. 1981. Snuff-dipping and oral cancer among women in Southern United States. *New Engl. J. Med.* **304**: 745.

COMMENTS

BELAND: Are there any sites, other than the oral cavity, which are associated with tumor induction by chewing tobacco? In particular, the bladder?

BRUNNEMANN: I'm not aware of any other sites.

BELAND: I am just trying to sort out the relative contribution of nitrosamines as opposed to aromatic amines in bladder tumor induction.

HOFFMANN: There is one study from Schuman in Minnesota and another from Bjelke in Norway which indicate that snuff dippers have a higher risk for pancreas cancer. I am also aware of a study on snuff use and bladder cancer. Recently, Kabat et al. from our institute found three cases of bladder cancer in women who were long-time snuff dippers and who did not smoke or chew tobacco. This finding needs to be confirmed by other studies.

BELAND: I have a question about Eskimo children. Do they also drink? Isn't there a lot of alcohol consumption among Eskimos?

ROSIN: Not so much among the Eskimos we studied. But we've just done a study among the native Indians in Saskatchewan, and they're extremely high consumers of both snuff and alcohol.

TANNENBAUM: The children also?

ROSIN: Yes.

YOAKUM: Klaus [Brunnemann], in the model where you were doing a cocarcinogenesis experiment with tobacco and herpes virus, have you examined the resultant squamous cell carcinomas by restriction fragment length polymorphism mapping or by a secondary transfection analysis to look for active oncogenes that you could target for genetic study?

BRUNNEMANN: Dr. Hoffmann, do you want to answer that?

HOFFMANN: We are just considering studying this aspect with Dr. Vahlne, a virologist from the University of Goeteborg. There are two published studies, one by Hirsch in Goeteborg with rats and the other by Park from U.C.L.A. with hamsters. Both groups demonstrated the formation of invasive carcinoma in the oral cavity as a consequence of the combined effects of herpes simplex virus (HSV) and snuff.

YOAKUM: The question really isn't about the virus, it's about the tumor cells. Have you looked at tumor cell DNA for secondary transfection into recipients such as NIH3T3 to see if you can observe a mutated oncogene from the tumor cells?

HOFFMANN: No, that has not been done.

WINN: Aren't there more snuff dippers in the United States than in Sweden?

HOFFMANN: I am sure you are right. In absolute numbers there are more snuff dippers in the United States. However, per 100,000 men you find more snuff dippers in Sweden.

WINN: It's my understanding that incidence ratios in Sweden for mouth cancer are not high; nevertheless, there has been a case-control study in Sweden by Wynder that showed an association between the use of smokeless tobacco and oral cancer.

STELLMAN: Is there an animal model in carcinogenesis experiments that is analogous to cancer of the buccal mucosa in humans? In other words, some of the nitrosamine carcinogenesis experiments were lung tumors and various other tissues, but were oral cancers researched too?

HOFFMANN: To our knowledge, only one study has bioassayed the carcinogenicity of tobacco-specific nitrosamines in the oral cavity. We found that after we had swabbed the oral cavity of rats for 2 years with a saline solution that contained NNN and NNK, eight out of 30 rats developed benign tumors of the oral cavity.

HARRIS: There has been a great deal of study using the cheek pouch of hamsters—including experiments in which an initiator's been given and then a nonspecific agent, such as just trauma, has led to an increase in the tumors in the cheek pouch.

The Formation of DNA-Protein Cross-links by Aldehydes Present in Tobacco Smoke

HENRY D'A. HECK, MERCEDES CASANOVA, CHIU-WING LAM,* AND
JAMES A. SWENBERG
Department of Biochemical Toxicology and Pathobiology
Chemical Industry Institute of Toxicology
Research Triangle Park, North Carolina 27709

OVERVIEW

Tobacco smoke contains numerous aldehydes, including formaldehyde (methanal: MA) and acetaldehyde (ethanal: EA), both of which have induced nasal cancer in rats, mice, or hamsters during chronic inhalation exposure studies. These aldehydes form DNA-protein cross-links (DPX) in the rat nasal mucosa. The concentration-response curves for DNA-protein cross-linking are nonlinear at low airborne concentrations. In the case of MA, depletion of glutathione (GSH) significantly increased the yield of DPX and caused the concentration-response curve to become more nearly linear, implying that a major saturable defense mechanism is the GSH-dependent oxidation of MA catalyzed by formaldehyde dehydrogenase. In addition to forming DPX, MA reacted covalently with rat nasal mucosal proteins. However, GSH depletion did not increase the amount of MA covalently bound to proteins, indicating that the proteins were primarily extracellular. Acrolein (propenal: PA), another tobacco smoke constituent, was not carcinogenic in hamsters exposed to 4 ppm for 1 year. The formation of DPX in vivo by PA was not demonstrable. However, PA exposure did deplete nasal mucosal GSH, and simultaneous exposure to both PA and MA significantly increased the yield of DPX relative to that obtained in rats exposed to MA alone. These results indicate that saturated aldehydes in tobacco smoke can cross-link DNA to proteins, which appears to be a critical step in the mutagenic activity of these compounds, and that by depletion of GSH unsaturated aldehydes can enhance the toxicity of other smoke components.

INTRODUCTION

Aldehydes, including formaldehyde (MA), acetaldehyde (EA), and acrolein (PA), constitute a class of compounds that are present at high concentrations in tobacco smoke (Table 1). Although the first two of these compounds induced squamous cell carcinomas or adenocarcinomas in the nasal cavity or larynx of rodents during

---

**Present address*: Northrop Services, Inc., Life Sciences Laboratory, P.O. Box 34416, Houston, Texas 77234

Table 1
Aldehyde Concentrations in Cigarette Smoke and Summary of Aldehyde Toxicities

	Formaldehyde $H-CH=O$	Acetaldehyde $CH_3-CH=O$	Acrolein $CH_2=CH-CH=O$
Cigarette smoke (ppm)[a]	84	1120	90
TLV-TWA (ppm)[b]	1	100	0.1
RD_{50} (ppm)[c]	13.1[d]	2991[e]	6.1[f]
Genotoxicity/mutagenicity	+[g]	+[h]	+/−[i]
Carcinogenicity	Rat/mouse[j]	Rat/hamster[k]	?

[a] Newsome et al. (1965)
[b] Threshold limit value expressed as a time-weighted average concentration for a normal 8-hr workday (ACGIH 1984).
[c] Concentration required to elicit a 50% decrease in respiratory rate in F-344 rats.
[d] Barrow et al. (1983)
[e] Babiuk et al. (1985)
[f] W. H. Steinhagen and C. S. Barrow, unpubl.
[g] Ragan and Boreiko (1981); Connor et al. (1983); Goldmacher and Thilly (1983)
[h] Obe and Ristow (1977); Abernethy et al. (1982); Bird et al. (1982)
[i] Beauchamp et al. (1985)
[j] Kerns et al. (1983)
[k] Feron et al. (1982); Woutersen et al. (1984)

long-term inhalation exposure studies (Feron et al. 1982; Kerns et al. 1983; Woutersen et al. 1984), the aldehydes as a group are not considered to be major causative agents of lung cancer in man (Loeb et al. 1984). The volatile phase of tobacco smoke did not induce tumors in animals, although it contains many substances, such as nickel, hydrazine, and vinyl chloride, as well as the aldehydes, that have been shown individually to be carcinogenic (Loeb et al. 1984). In contrast, the particulate phase of tobacco smoke when applied to the skin of mice, the ears of rabbits, or the larynx of hamsters, induced malignant neoplasms (Loeb et al. 1984). This phase contains the polycyclic aromatic hydrocarbons and the tobacco-specific nitrosamines, NNN (N'-nitrosonornicotine) and NNK (4-(N-methyl-N-nitrosamino)-1-(3-pyridyl)-1-butanone), the latter compounds being exceptionally potent carcinogens in rats (Singer and Taylor 1976; Hecht et al. 1980). The particulate phase also contains compounds that appear to act as cocarcinogens and tumor promoters (Loeb et al. 1984).

Since rodents are obligatory nose breathers, the nasal mucosa receives comparatively high doses of inhaled toxicants (Stott and McKenna 1984), which explains, at least in part, the susceptibility of this tissue to the toxic effects of aldehydes. Other factors, which are not fully understood, cause particular regions of the rat nasal passages or particular cells within these regions to be especially sensitive to the toxic effects of specific agents. For example, EA at 400 ppm and PA at 4 ppm induced degenerative changes primarily in the olfactory mucosa (Appelman et al. 1982; Feron et al. 1985), whereas MA primarily affected the respiratory mucosa

(Swenberg et al. 1983). Differences in the capacity of respiratory and olfactory tissues for the bioactivation and detoxication of xenobiotics could at least partially explain the observed intranasal differences in susceptibility to cytotoxicity and carcinogenicity (Brittebo and Tjälve 1982; Hadley and Dahl 1983).

Although nasal cancer is a comparatively rare form of cancer in humans, the induction of squamous cell carcinomas and adenocarcinomas by inhaled aldehydes in the nasal passages of rodents can be utilized to investigate basic mechanisms of carcinogenesis and the factors that influence the susceptibility of tissues to the induction of cancer. The information derived from such mechanistic studies is useful for the assessment of risks due to workplace exposure (Swenberg et al. 1985a). In addition, since several of the most important commercial aldehydes are components of tobacco smoke, such information may also be pertinent to evaluations of the health effects of smoking, which is the subject of this volume.

Recent studies in our laboratory have shown that inhaled MA forms DPX and reacts covalently with proteins in the rat respiratory mucosa (Casanova-Schmitz et al. 1984a). The formation of DPX depends nonlinearly on the inhaled MA concentration between 0 and 6 ppm, whereas the binding of MA to proteins is an apparently linear function of the airborne concentration. The covalent binding of MA to nasal mucosal DNA is a measure of the "delivered dose" to a critical target macromolecule (Starr and Buck 1984) and, hence, is an extremely important parameter for risk assessment. On the other hand, the toxicologic significance of covalent binding to proteins is uncertain since the identity of the proteins as intra- or extracellular was not determined in those studies.

A number of factors, including mucociliary clearance, metabolism (detoxication), DNA repair, and increased cell proliferation could give rise to variabilities in the delivered dose-administered dose relationship. A major goal of the research described in this paper was to examine the role of one of these factors, metabolism of MA, in the observed nonlinear binding of MA to DNA. Conditions were chosen to approximate the exposure conditions used previously (Casanova-Schmitz et al. 1984a), i.e., a single preexposure (3 hours) of male Fischer 344 (F344) rats to unlabeled MA on day 1 followed by a second exposure (3 hours) of the animals on day 2 to [^{3}H]- and [^{14}C]MA. The preexposure stimulates cell turnover in the nasal mucosa (see below), which may enhance the likelihood of covalent binding to DNA, since MA seems to bind only to single-stranded DNA regions (von Hippel and Wong 1971). The use of dual isotopes enables the two mechanisms of labeling of macromolecules, metabolic incorporation and covalent binding, to be differentiated (Casanova-Schmitz et al. 1984a).

After exposure of rats to radioactive MA, the major route of labeling of nasal mucosal nucleic acids is via oxidation of MA to formate and incorporation of the latter into nucleic acid bases by one-carbon metabolic pathways (Casanova-Schmitz et al. 1984a). Formaldehyde dehydrogenase is an important enzyme in the metabolism of MA (Koivusalo et al. 1982; Casanova-Schmitz et al. 1984b), catalyzing the oxidation of the hemithioacetal adduct of MA with glutathione (GSH) to the corresponding S-formyl ester (Uotila and Koivusalo 1974). Since this enzyme requires GSH for activity, depletion of GSH should inhibit the oxidation of MA, resulting in a decrease in the amount of labeled MA that is metabolically incorporated into macromolecules and an increase in the amount that is covalently bound. Evidence that depletion of GSH does, in fact, increase DNA-protein cross-linking by inhaled MA has recently been obtained (Heck et al. 1985).

To investigate the effects of a diminished oxidation rate on the fate of inhaled MA in the nasal mucosa, rats exposed to $[^3H]$- and $[^{14}C]MA$ were injected with phorone (diisopropylidene acetone) (300 mg/kg, i.p.) or with corn oil 2 hours prior to the onset of exposure. At this dose, phorone depletes the concentrations of nonprotein sulfhydryls (NPSH) in the nasal mucosa and liver of rats by approximately 90%, and the NPSH concentrations remain low for about 5 hours before beginning to rebound (Heck et al. 1985). Hence, inhibition of oxidation of MA by formaldehyde dehydrogenase is likely. The rats were killed by decapitation immediately after exposure; DNA and protein were isolated from the nasal respiratory mucosa, and the ^3H and ^{14}C contents of the macromolecules were determined by liquid scintillation counting, as described previously (Casanova-Schmitz et al. 1984a).

Depletion of GSH in the nasal respiratory mucosa can also be achieved by exposure of rats to PA (Lam et al. 1985). Therefore, in a concurrent exposure to both aldehydes, such as occurs in cigarette smoking, PA might potentiate the toxicity of MA by inhibiting the oxidation of the latter. Enhancement of toxicity (as opposed to additivity of toxic effects) could be detected as an increase in the yield of DPX in the nasal respiratory mucosa of rats exposed simultaneously to both compounds relative to the sum of the yields obtained in rats exposed to each compound individually.

The concentration of DPX after MA exposure is highly correlated with the percentage of nasal mucosal DNA that is partitioned into the interface after extraction of solubilized tissue homogenates with phenol/chloroform (Casanova-Schmitz et al. 1984a). Thus, increases in the percent interfacial (IF) DNA can be used to detect the formation of DPX. The possible formation of DPX by PA and the effects of PA exposure on DNA-protein cross-linking by MA were investigated by determining the percent IF DNA from the nasal respiratory mucosa of rats exposed to PA (2 ppm) and MA (6 ppm) singly or together (Lam et al. 1985).

As may be inferred from the preceding remarks, a second major goal of research in our laboratory has been to determine whether DNA-protein cross-linking occurs in the nasal mucosa as a result of exposure to aldehydes other than MA. Inasmuch as the toxicity and chemistry of EA resemble those of MA, it is plausible that these compounds might undergo similar reactions in vivo, including the formation of DPX. Indeed, evidence has been obtained for the formation of cross-links by EA with amino groups in proteins (Mohammad et al. 1949) and in tetrahydrofolate

(LaBaume and Guynn 1985). To determine whether EA can form DPX, rats were exposed to selected concentrations of EA for either 1 day (6 hours) or 5 consecutive days (6 hours/day). The animals were killed immediately after the final exposure, and the percentages of IF DNA in the nasal respiratory and olfactory mucosa were determined. The results of these experiments (Lam et al. 1986) are summarized here.

RESULTS

Formaldehyde

The amounts of MA metabolically incorporated or covalently bound in the DNA of the rat respiratory mucosa were calculated as described previously (Casanova-Schmitz et al. 1984a). As expected, depletion of GSH by i.p. injection with phorone markedly decreased the former and increased the latter in comparison with corn oil-treated controls (Fig. 1), implying that these two pathways of labeling utilize a common MA pool. Covalent binding of $[^{14}C]$MA to DNA in the form of DPX was not detectable at 0.9 ppm in corn oil-treated rats. However, cross-linking did occur at this concentration in GSH-depleted rats.

The ^{14}C-specific activity of the DNA that was due to metabolic incorporation was similar at 0.9 ppm and at 2 ppm in corn oil-treated rats, but the incorporation of $[^{14}C]$formaldehyde into DNA at 4 ppm and at 6 ppm was approximately twice as large as at the two lower concentrations (Figure 1). These results are a function of both the dose of $[^{14}C]$MA delivered to cells and the rate of DNA synthesis. An indication of the proliferative activity of the respiratory mucosa following MA exposures has been obtained by labeling nasal mucosal cells with $[^{3}H]$thymidine 18 hours after exposures to selected concentrations of MA for 1, 3, or 9 days (6 hours/day). The results obtained after 1 day of exposure show that both 0.5 ppm and 2 ppm of MA induce small transient increases in the number of labeled basal cells in the respiratory mucosa, whereas 6 ppm of MA induces a large increase in the number of such cells (Fig. 2). The increase in labeled basal cells of rats exposed to 0.5 ppm or 2 ppm disappears after 3 or 9 days of exposure. Similarly, a lesser response is observed at 6 ppm following repeated exposures to MA.

An increase in cell turnover may predispose the DNA to damage by increasing the number of single-stranded DNA regions. As a result, nonlinear increases in DNA binding might be expected. The yield of DPX in the rat respiratory mucosa was, in fact, a nonlinear function of the $[^{14}C]$MA concentration, both in phorone-treated rats and in controls (Figure 3a). In the latter group, the amount of $[^{14}C]$MA covalently bound to DNA at each of the three lower concentrations (0.9, 2, and 4 ppm) was significantly less than predicted ($P < 0.01$; Newman-Keuls' multiple-range test) by assuming the binding to be proportional to the airborne MA concentration between 0 and 6 ppm. In contrast, in GSH-depleted rats, the

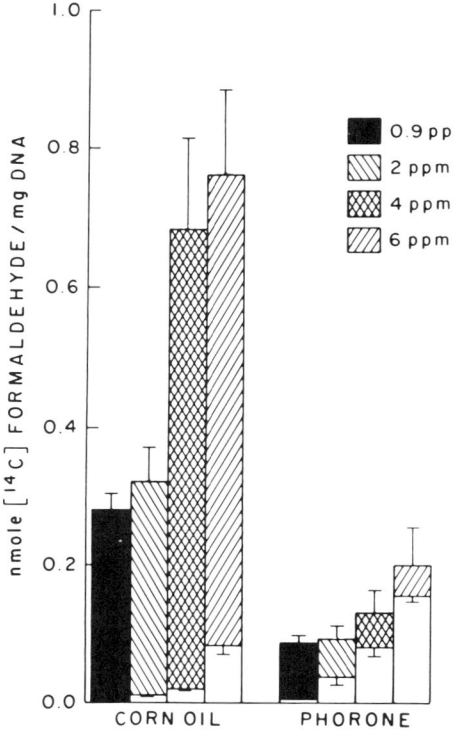

Figure 1
Amounts of MA (nmole/mg) metabolically incorporated or covalently bound in the DNA from the nasal respiratory mucosa of F344 rats after i.p. injection of the animals either with phorone or with corn oil. Exposure to [^{3}H]- and [^{14}C]MA (3 hr) commenced 2 hr after injection, 1 day after a single preexposure (3 hr) to the same concentration of unlabeled MA. Values are mean ± SE. Filled bars, metabolic incorporation; open bars, covalent binding.

binding of [^{14}C]MA to DNA was significantly less ($P < 0.05$) than predicted by this assumption at 0.9 ppm, but not at 2 ppm or at 4 ppm. Thus, in addition to increasing the amount of [^{14}C]MA covalently bound to DNA, depletion of GSH partially linearized the nonlinear concentration-response curve for covalent binding to DNA.

Calculations of the amount of [^{14}C]MA covalently bound to proteins of the nasal respiratory mucosa are shown in Figure 3b. These data are consistent with an approximately linear relationship between protein binding and the inhaled MA concentration, as reported previously (Casanova-Schmitz et al. 1984a). An important result of these measurements is that, unlike the DNA, depletion of GSH had no measurable effect on the quantity of MA covalently bound to proteins. This

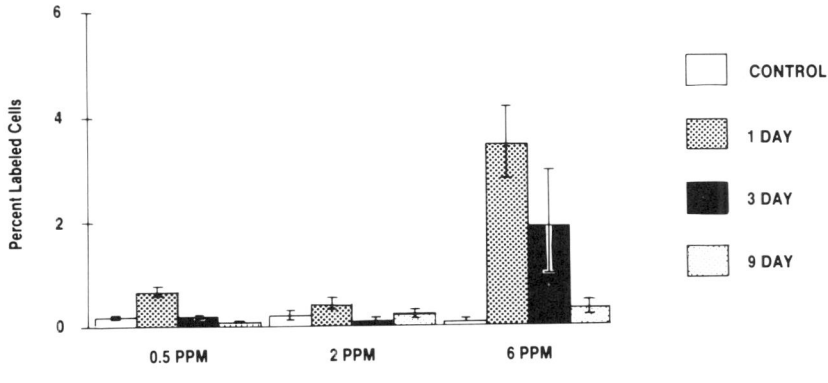

Figure 2
Effect of MA exposure on cell proliferation in the middle portion of the rat nasal respiratory mucosa. All animals were exposed for 6 hr/day. [^{3}H]Thymidine was administered by i.p. injection 18 hr after the last exposure. Data shown are mean ± SE. Reprinted, with permission from Swenberg et al. (1985b).

finding suggests that the proteins to which MA is bound are primarily extracellular since GSH would be expected to exert its protective effects only intracellularly where formaldehyde dehydrogenase is located.

Acrolein

PA exposure at concentrations equal to or greater than 0.5 ppm significantly decreased the concentration of NPSH in the rat nasal respiratory mucosa (Lam et al. 1985). Such depletion could result in an inhibition of MA oxidation, and, thus, might enhance the toxicity of MA in a simultaneous exposure to both compounds. To test this hypothesis, rats were exposed for 6 hours to PA (2 ppm), to MA (6 ppm), or to a mixture of both aldehydes at the concentrations noted. The percent IF DNA in the nasal respiratory mucosa was determined following each of these exposures.

As shown in Table 2, PA exposure did not result in a significant increase in the percent IF DNA relative to air-exposed controls, indicating that few, if any, DPX were induced by PA at 2 ppm, which is 20-fold above the current threshold limit value (TLV) for this compound (ACGIH 1984). In contrast, brief incubation of PA (3 mM) with homogenates of the rat nasal respiratory mucosa (10 min, 0°C, pH 8) resulted in a decreased extractability of the DNA from proteins, indicating that PA can form DPX in vitro (Lam et al.. 1985).

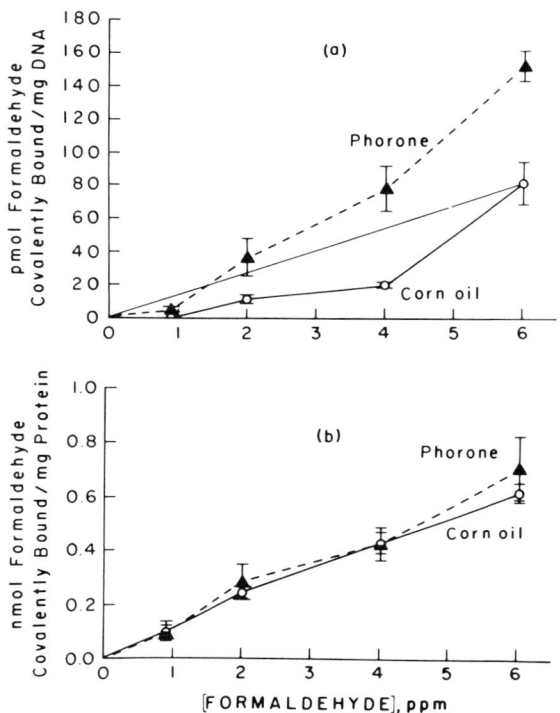

Figure 3
Concentrations of covalently bound MA in DNA (a) and in proteins (b) from the respiratory mucosa of F344 rats injected either with phorone or with corn oil and exposed for 3 hr to 0.9, 2, 4, or 6 ppm of MA. Values are mean ± SE; n = three groups of rats at each concentration (three animals per group [corn oil], five animals per group [phorone]).

As expected, MA exposure at 6 ppm caused detectable DNA-protein cross-linking, as indicated by a significant elevation in the percent IF DNA relative to controls (Table 2). However, when rats were exposed to both PA and MA together, there was a significant further increase in the percent IF DNA from the nasal respiratory mucosa (Table 2). This increase was clearly greater than the sum of the changes caused by the two compounds alone, and, hence, there appears to be a potentiation of toxicity resulting from exposure to both aldehydes.

Acetaldehyde

Exposure of rats to EA (6 hours) causes a concentration-related increase in the percent IF DNA isolated from the nasal respiratory mucosa (Fig. 4), suggesting that EA can form DPX in vivo. Significant increases in the percent IF DNA occurred at

Table 2
Percent Interfacial DNA from the Nasal Respiratory Mucosa of Rats Exposed to Air or to Aldehydes[a]

Exposure	(%) Interfacial DNA[b]
Air	8.1 ± 0.4 (6)
Acrolein (2 ppm)	9.1 ± 0.3 (4)
Formaldehyde (6 ppm)	12.5 ± 1.4 (4)[c]
Formaldehyde (6 ppm) + acrolein (2 ppm)	18.6 ± 1.3 (3)[d]

[a] F-344 rats were exposed to air, acrolein, formaldehyde, or a mixture of acrolein and formaldehyde for 6 hr. Aqueous and interfacial DNA were isolated from the respiratory mucosa as described elsewhere (Lam et al. 1985).
[b] Values are mean ± SE of data obtained from three to six samples. Each sample was the combined respiratory mucosal tissue from three rats.
[c] Significantly greater ($P < 0.05$) than the value obtained using air-exposed rats, following treatment of the data by ANOVA and Scheffé's test (Downie and Heath 1970)
[d] Significantly greater ($P < 0.05$) than the value obtained using rats exposed to formaldehyde alone, following treatment of the data by ANOVA and Scheffé's test. Adapted from Lam et al. (1985).

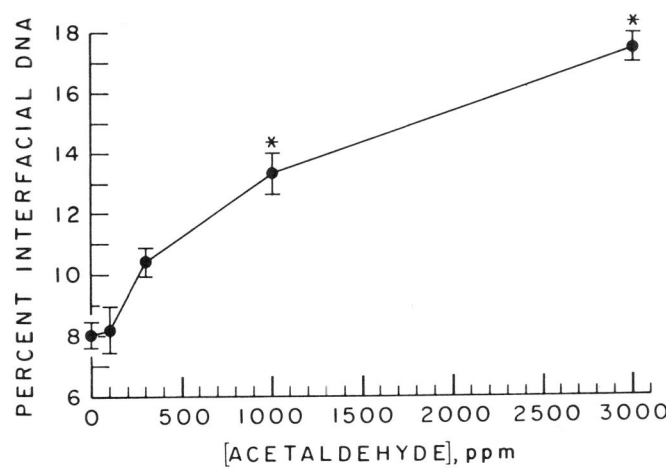

Figure 4
Percent IF DNA from the respiratory mucosa of F344 rats exposed to 0, 100, 303, 1000, or 3016 ppm of EA for 6 hr. Each point represents the mean ± SE of the values from four to six groups of rats (three animals per group). (*) A significant ($P < 0.05$) difference from the value for air-exposed controls. Reprinted, with permission, from Lam et al. 1986.

concentrations equal to or greater than 1000 ppm, which is consistent with the relatively low reactivity of EA as an electrophile in comparison with MA and PA. The results suggest that the formation of the putative cross-links by EA is a nonlinear function of concentration: Cross-linking was undetectable at 100 ppm, increased steeply between 100 ppm and 1000 ppm, and continued to increase, although more slowly, at higher concentrations.

EA did not detectably form DPX in the olfactory mucosa after a single 6-hour exposure to concentrations as high as 3000 ppm. However, an increase in the percent IF DNA from this tissue was observed after 5 consecutive days of exposure (6 hours/day) to 1000 ppm of EA (Lam et al. 1986). The apparent formation of cross-links after repeated exposures could have resulted from an increase in cell turnover due to cytotoxicity (Appelman et al. 1982; Feron et al. 1982), which might cause an increase in the amount of EA bound to DNA if EA, like MA, binds preferentially to single-stranded DNA regions. Investigations of cell proliferation in the olfactory mucosa are needed to understand more clearly the toxic effects of EA in this region of the nasal passages.

DISCUSSION

Research on the mechanisms of toxicity of the aldehydes has shown the potential of compounds in this class to react with DNA and to form DPX in vivo. The relevance of DNA-protein cross-linking to carcinogenesis has not yet been established, but evidence is accumulating that cross-links formed by MA can result in certain types of DNA damage. Thus, MA caused various small deletions (rather than single-base substitutions) to occur in a sequenced *Drosophila* gene, which can be explained by a slipped mispairing mechanism during replication that could be due to the formation of DPX (Benyajati et al. 1983). In addition, cytogenetic evidence indicates that MA induces chromosomal aberrations (gaps, breaks, and exchanges) and SCEs in Chinese hamster ovary cells during DNA replication, a result which is typical of cross-linking agents (Natarajan et al. 1983). These findings suggest that the occurrence of cross-links during the replication stage of the DNA may be a critical event leading to a heritable mutation.

The evidence presented in this article and elsewhere (Lam et al. 1986) indicates that not only MA but also EA can form DPX, and, therefore, that the carcinogenicity of these compounds may be caused by a similar mechanism. In both cases, the formation of cross-links was a nonlinear function of the inhaled concentration of the aldehyde. Mechanistic research has identified several factors that could contribute to a nonlinear response in the binding of MA to DNA and in the induction of nasal squamous cell carcinomas (Starr et al. 1985). It is clear that one of the most important factors is the GSH-dependent oxidation of MA occurring in the target cells.

Metabolism is a saturable process, the efficiency of which decreases with increasing concentrations of the toxicant. Strong support for the conclusion that detoxication is a key mechanism of nonlinearity is provided by the observation that when detoxication was inhibited, the nonlinear concentration-response curve for covalent binding of MA to DNA became more nearly linear. However, even in animals whose metabolic capacity with respect to MA oxidation was severely compromised by injection with phorone, the yield of DPX at 0.9 ppm was significantly less than predicted by assuming a linear response between 0 and 6 ppm. This result suggests the existence of other defense mechanisms in the rat nasal mucosa that are not dependent on GSH and are effective at low MA concentrations. Such mechanisms may include alternative pathways for metabolism of MA or saturable pathways for its removal, such as the mucociliary clearance apparatus (Morgan et al. 1986).

Extensive evidence indicates that cell proliferation is an essential step in the pathogenesis of neoplasms (Farber 1982). Exposures to high concentrations of MA and EA result in marked increases in the rate of cell turnover, which can increase the rate of both initiating and promoting events (Swenberg et al. 1985b). The cell populations that result are altered both morphologically and biochemically from normal populations. The layers of replacement cells are thicker and more keratinous than those found in the normal rat nose. Consequently, penetration of inhaled MA to basal (proliferating) cells is likely to be decreased in such populations. Such changes in nasal morphology constitute another defense mechanism by which nasal tissues can adapt to toxic insult in a manner that is disproportionate to the inhaled concentration of the toxicant.

The inhalation of tobacco smoke involves exposure to a multiplicity of carcinogens. The effects of these compounds on respiratory tract tissues can be additive, synergistic, or antagonistic. Compounds such as PA, which are either noncarcinogenic or only weakly carcinogenic in themselves, can potentiate the toxicity of other materials by depleting GSH and, thereby, decreasing the rate of detoxication of more potent carcinogens. Thus, although the carcinogenic potency of the aldehydes is slight in comparison with compounds such as NNN, NNK, and the polycyclic aromatic hydrocarbons, their role in tobacco-associated respiratory tract cancer may not be insignificant.

REFERENCES

Abernethy, D. J., J. H. Frazelle, and C. J. Boreiko. 1982. Effects of ethanol, acetaldehyde and acetic acid in the C3H/10T1/2 Cl 8 cell transformation system. *Environ. Mutagen.* **4**: 331.

American Conference of Governmental Industrial Hygienists (ACGIH). 1984. *Documentation of the threshold limit values*, 4th ed. Cincinnati, Ohio.

Appelman, L. M., R. A. Woutersen, and V. J. Feron. 1982. Inhalation toxicity of acetaldehyde in rats. I. Acute and subacute studies. *Toxicology* **23**: 293.

Babiuk, C., W. H. Steinhagen, and C. S. Barrow. 1985. Sensory irritation response to inhaled aldehydes after formaldehyde pretreatment. *Toxicol. Appl. Pharmacol.* **79**: 143.

Barrow, C. S., W. H. Steinhagen, and J. C. F. Chang. 1983. Formaldehyde sensory irritation. In *Formaldehyde toxicity* (ed. J. E. Gibson), p. 16. Hemisphere, Washington, D. C.

Beauchamp, R. O., Jr., D. A. Andjelkovich, A. D. Kligerman, K. T. Morgan, and H. d'A. Heck. 1985. A critical review of the literature on acrolein toxicity. *CRC Crit. Rev. Toxicol.* **14**: 309.

Benyajati, C., A. R. Place, and W. Sofer. 1983. Formaldehyde mutagenesis in *Drosophila*: Molecular analysis of ADH-negative mutants. *Mutat. Res.* **111**: 1.

Bird, R. P., H. H. Draper, and P. K. Basrur. 1982. Effect of malonaldehyde and acetaldehyde on cultured mammalian cells: Production of micronuclei and chromosomal aberrations. *Mutat. Res.* **101**: 237.

Brittebo, E. B. and H. Tjälve. 1982. Tissue-specificity of N-nitrosodibutylamine metabolism in Sprague-Dawley rats. *Chem.-Biol. Interact.* **38**: 231.

Casanova-Schmitz, M., T. B. Starr, and H. d'A. Heck. 1984a. Differentiation between metabolic incorporation and covalent binding in the labeling of macromolecules in the rat nasal mucosa and bone marrow by inhaled [^{14}C]- and [^{3}H]formaldehyde. *Toxicol. Appl. Pharmacol.* **76**: 26.

Casanova-Schmitz, M., R. M. David, and H. d'A. Heck. 1984b. Oxidation of formaldehyde and acetaldehyde by NAD^+-dependent dehydrogenases in rat nasal mucosal homogenates. *Biochem. Pharmacol.* **33**: 1137.

Connor, T. H., M. D. Barrie, J. C. Theiss, T. S. Matney, and J. B. Ward, Jr. 1983. Mutagenicity of formalin in the Ames assay. *Mutat. Res.* **119**: 145.

Downie, N. M. and R. W. Heath. 1970. *Basic statistical methods*, 3rd ed., p. 221. Harper & Row, New York.

Farber, E. 1982. Chemical carcinogenesis: A biologic perspective. *Am. J. Pathol.* **106**: 272.

Feron, V. J., A. Kruysse, and R. A. Woutersen. 1982. Respiratory tract tumours in hamsters exposed to acetaldehyde vapor alone or simultaneously to benzo(*a*)pyrene or diethylnitrosamine. *Eur. J. Cancer Clin. Oncol.* **18**: 13.

Feron, V. J., R. A. Woutersen, and B. J. Spit. 1985. Pathology of chronic nasal toxic responses including cancer. In *Toxicology of the nasal passages* (ed. C.S. Barrow), p. 67. Hemisphere, Washington, D.C.

Goldmacher, V. S. and W. G. Thilly. 1983. Formaldehyde is mutagenic for cultured human cells. *Mutat. Res.* **116**: 417.

Hadley, W. M. and A. R. Dahl. 1983. Cytochrome P-450-dependent monooxygenase activity in nasal membranes of six species. *Drug. Metab. Dispos.* **11**: 275.

Hecht, S. S., C. B. Chen, T. Ohmori, and D. Hoffmann. 1980. Comparative carcinogenicity in F344 rats of the tobacco-specific nitrosamines, N-nitrosonornicotine and 4-(N-methyl-N-nitrosamino)-1-(3-pyridyl)-1-butanone. *Cancer Res.* **40**: 298.

Heck, H. d'A., M. Casanova, M. J. McNulty, and C.-W. Lam. 1985. Mechanisms of nasal toxicity induced by formaldehyde and acrolein. In *Toxicology of the nasal passages* (ed. C.S. Barrow), p.235. Hemisphere, Washington, D.C.

Kerns, W. D., K. L. Pavkov, D. J. Donofrio, E. J. Gralla, and J. A. Swenberg. 1983. Carcinogenicity of formaldehyde in rats and mice after long-term inhalation exposure. *Cancer Res.* **43**: 4382.

Koivusalo, M., T. Koivula, and L. Uotila. 1982. Oxidation of formaldehyde by nicotinamide nucleotide dependent dehydrogenases. In *Enzymology of carbonyl metabolism: Aldehyde dehydrogenase and aldo/keto reductase* (ed. H. Weiner and B. Wermuth), p. 155. Alan R. Liss, New York.

LaBaume, L. B. and R. W. Guynn. 1985. Investigation into the substrate capacity of the acetaldehyde-tetrahydrofolate condensation product. In *Aldehyde adducts in alcoholism* (ed. M. A. Collins), p. 189. Alan R. Liss, New York.

Lam, C.-W., M. Casanova, and H. d'A. Heck. 1985. Depletion of nasal mucosal glutathione by acrolein and enhancement of formaldehyde-induced DNA-protein cross-linking by simultaneous exposure to acrolein. *Arch. Toxicol.* **58**: 67.

Lam, C.-W., M. Casanova, and H. d'A. Heck. 1986. Decreased extractability of DNA from proteins in the rat nasal mucosa after acetaldehyde exposure. *Fundam. Appl. Toxicol.* **6**: 541.

Loeb, L. A., V. L. Ernster, K. E. Warner, J. Abbotts, and J. Laszlo. 1984. Smoking and lung cancer: An overview. *Cancer Res.* **44**: 5940.

Mohammad, A., H. S. Olcott, and H. Fraenkel-Conrat. 1949. The reaction of proteins with acetaldehyde. *Arch. Biochem.* **24**: 270.

Morgan, K. T., D. L. Patterson, and E. A. Gross. 1986. Responses of the nasal mucociliary apparatus of F-344 rats to formaldehyde gas. *Toxicol. Appl. Pharmacol.* **82**: 1.

Natarajan, A. T., F. Darroudi, C. J. M. Bussman, and A. C. van Kesteren-van Leeuwen. 1983. Evaluation of the mutagenicity of formaldehyde in mammalian cytogenetic assays in vivo and vitro. *Mutat. Res.* **122**: 355.

Newsome, J. R., V. Norman, and C. H. Keith. 1965. Vapor phase analysis of tobacco smoke. *Tob. Sci.* **9**: 102.

Obe, G. and H. Ristow. 1977. Acetaldehyde, but not ethanol, induces sister chromatid exchanges in Chinese hamster cells in vitro. *Mutat. Res.* **56**: 211.

Ragan, D. L. and C. J. Boreiko. 1981. Initiation of C3H/10T1/2 cell transformation by formaldehyde. *Cancer Lett.* **13**: 325.

Singer, G. M. and H. W. Taylor. 1976. Carcinogenicity of N'-nitrosonornicotine in Sprague-Dawley rats. *J. Natl. Cancer Inst.* **57**: 1275.

Starr, T. B. and R. D. Buck. 1984. The importance of delivered dose in estimating low-dose cancer risk from inhalation exposure to formaldehyde. *Fundam. Appl. Toxicol.* **4**: 740.

Starr, T. B., J. E. Gibson, C. S. Barrow, C. J. Boreiko, H. d'A. Heck, R. J. Levine, K. T. Morgan, and J. A. Swenberg. 1985. Estimating human cancer risk from formaldehyde: Critical issues. In *Formaldehyde: analytical chemistry and toxicology* (ed. V. Turoski), p. 299. American Chemical Society, Washington, D. C.

Stott, W. T. and M. J. McKenna. 1984. The comparative absorption and excretion of chemical vapors by the upper, lower, and intact respiratory tract of rats. *Fundam. Appl. Toxicol.* **4**: 594.

Swenberg, J. A., E. A. Gross, J. Martin, and J. A. Popp. 1983. Mechanisms of formaldehyde toxicity. In *Formaldehyde toxicity* (ed. J. E. Gibson), p. 132. Hemisphere, Washington, D. C.

Swenberg, J. A., H. d'A. Heck, K. T. Morgan, and T. B. Starr. 1985a. A scientific approach to formaldehyde risk assessment. In *Banbury report 19: Risk quantitation and regulatory policy* (ed. D. G. Hoel, R. A. Merrill, and F. P. Perera), p. 255. Cold Spring Harbor Laboratory, Cold Spring Harbor, New York.

Swenberg, J. A., E. A. Gross, and H. W. Randall. 1985b. Localization and quantitation of cell proliferation following exposure to nasal irritants. In *Toxicology of the nasal passages* (ed. C.S. Barrow), p. 291. Hemisphere, Washington, D.C.

Uotila, L. and M. Koivusalo. 1974. Formaldehyde dehydrogenase from human liver: Purification, properties and evidence for the formation of glutathione thiol esters by the enzyme. *J. Biol. Chem.* **249**: 7653.

von Hippel, P. H. and K.-Y. Wong. 1971. Dynamic aspects of native DNA structure: Kinetics of the formaldehyde reaction with calf thymus DNA. *J. Mol. Biol.* **61**: 587.

Woutersen, R. A., L. M. Appelman, V. J. Feron, and C. A. van der Heijden. 1984. Inhalation toxicity of acetaldehyde in rats. II. Carcinogenicity study: Interim results after 15 months. *Toxicology* **31**: 123.

COMMENTS

MAGEE: Would you expand on your methods?

HECK: We published that in volume 76 of *Toxicology and Applied Pharmacology*. Basically, you separate the DNA into aqueous and interfacial portions which are labeled with tritium and carbon-14. The aqueous portion of DNA is not cross-linked to proteins, and the isotope ratio of that portion is independent of the airborne concentration. The isotope ratio of the interfacial DNA increases with the airborne concentration, due presumably to the formation of cross links. By knowing the isotope ratios of the two DNA fractions and the amounts of the DNA in the two fractions, we can calculate how much of the labeling is due to binding and how much is due to metabolism.

PEGG: Just for me to get this clear, is what you're calling "binding" formaldehyde adducts? Would it include things in which formaldehyde was involved in a cross link to a protein?

HECK: Yes.

PEGG: So you would have two separate components then. There may be adducts that don't involve cross-linking.

HECK: There may be adducts that don't involve cross links. We haven't seen evidence of those in vivo although they may be there at a lower level than the cross links.

GRAFSTROM: Could you speculate why thiol depletion causes increased DNA protein cross-linking?

HECK: Well, glutathione is required for oxidation of formaldehyde; and I suppose what happens is that when you deplete glutathione, you effectively increase the concentration of formaldehyde in the target tissue.

GRAFSTRÖM: I am asking because formaldehyde is only temporarily bound to glutathione and not consumed in the enzyme catalyzed oxidation reactions.

HECK: Right. In the normal rat.

BELAND: What are the tissue concentrations of glutathione because even if you are decreasing it by 90%, isn't it still far in excess of the formaldehyde concentration you are administering? An alternate interpretation of your results is that the compound you are using to deplete glutathione is reacting with the DNA, thus exposing additional sites for reaction with formaldehyde.

HECK: In regard to your first question, the level of glutathione in the rat respiratory mucosa is about 2.8 $\mu M/g$. It is about one-third or one-half what you find in the liver. The reaction with formaldehyde is reversible, and at the low concentrations of glutathione that occur following phorone treatment, probably very little formaldehyde is bound to glutathione. Now as far as what phorone may be doing, reacting with DNA, all I can say on that is that when we treat the animals with phorone only, we do not see any increase in the interfacial DNA as compared with untreated animals. You require formaldehyde exposure in addition to phorone treatment to cause the cross-linking to occur. You also have to have external formaldehyde coming in to get the cross link. In any case, phorone clearly inhibits formaldehyde metabolism, so we think that is the most likely mechanism of its action.

TANNENBAUM: Could you give a hypothetical structure for an acetaldehyde cross link?

HECK: Acetaldehyde is known to cross link with quite a few compounds. You may have a structure similar to that which occurs with tetrahydrofolate, for example.

HARRIS: I think that it is worth remembering that not only are aldehydes formed when you burn tobacco, but N-nitrosamines give rise to equal molar concentrations of aldehydes when they're metabolized. In this case, the aldehyde is intracellular and is probably produced in the same instant as the alkyldiazonium ions, the operating species.

HECK: Yes. Dr. Enzell's work showed quite a few other aldehydes that can be in tobacco smoke.

HECHT: What is the acrolein toxicity due to?

HECK: Acrolein is a very toxic chemical. For example, you may end up with lipid peroxidation. It's a very, very toxic material.

HECHT: Is the mechanism of the toxicity really established?

HECK: No one has studied it.

GRAFSTRÖM: With isolated hepatocytes many studies show that depletion of thiols precede the cytotoxicity. Similarly, in cultured human cells, we also see a depletion of thiols from exposure to acrolein. However, thiol depletion does not seem to be a prerequisite to inhibit proliferation of cells.

Session 3: Biochemical, Cellular, and Molecular Studies on Human Tissues and Cells

Differences in Metabolism and Biological Effects of NNK in Human Target Cells

ISMAIL PARSA,* CLARENCE A. FOYE,* CATHLEEN M. CLEARY,* AND DIETRICH HOFFMANN†
*State University of New York
Downstate Medical Center
Brooklyn, New York 11203
†Naylor Dana Institute for Disease Prevention
American Health Foundation
Valhalla, New York 10595

INTRODUCTION

Smoking, exposure to tobacco smoke, and environmental pollutants are considered major contributors to human cancers. The polycyclic aromatic hydrocarbons (PAH) and nitrosamines in tobacco smoke are regarded as factors in the development of human lung and pancreas carcinoma. The tobacco-specific N-nitrosamine 4-(methylnitrosamino)-1-(3-pyridyl)-1-butanone (NNK) is shown to be present at a significant concentration per cigarette in both mainstream and sidestream smoke (Hoffmann et al. 1979). Its presence was also demonstrated in chewing tobacco and was detected in the saliva of snuff-dipping women (Hoffmann and Adams 1981). The carcinogenicity and metabolic activation of NNK in rodents have been extensively described (Hecht et al. 1984). It is considered that the carcinogenicity of NNK for a given tissue depends to a great extent on its α-hydroxylation by the tissue to form α-hydroxylnitrosamine and subsequent DNA methylation. This is supported in part by the demonstration of O^6-methylguanine (O^6-mG) in target tissues exposed to NNK (Castonguay et al. 1983; Foiles et al. 1985). The DNA-damaging potential of oxobutyldiazohydroxide, resulting from methyl hydroxylation of NNK, is also suggested to contribute to the NNK carcinogenicity.

A human model of carcinogenesis has been reported from this laboratory describing several morphologically recognizable steps in this process. In this model repeated treatments with methylnitrosourea of pancreas explants for several weeks results in ductal metaplasia, ductal hyperplasia, focal atypia, and the development of transplantable carcinoma (Parsa et al. 1984). Induction of squamous metaplasia, hyperplasia, atypia, and carcinoma of the respiratory epithelium in this model using fetal human tracheobronchial explants has been achieved by repeated exposure to N-methyl-N-nitrosoguanidine (MNNG) (Parsa and Belich 1984). Clonal growth derived from the altered epithelium allowed the correlation of the morphological alterations: metaplasia, hyperplasia, dysplasia, atypia, and anaplasia; with growth enhancement, immortality, and tumorigenicity.

A monoclonal IgG_{2b} with a high affinity for O^6-mG was developed in this laboratory allowing immunohistochemical localization of this adduct in routine histologic sections. It has been possible to demonstrate the selective persistence of O^6-mG in target cell nuclei of human pancreas explants exposed to dimethylnitrosamine by indirect immunofluorescence using this antibody (I. Parsa et al., in prep.).

This paper compares the effect of MNNG and NNK on organ-cultured human fetal tracheobronchial and pancreas explants. Morphological alteration, tumorigenicity, and the presence and/or persistence of O^6-mG in the respiratory and pancreatic epithelium were studied.

RESULTS

Respiratory Epithelium

Explants, 1 mm in thickness, prepared from trachea and main bronchi of prostaglandin-induced 12-14-week-old fetuses were cultured in a chemically defined medium (Parsa et al. 1984) for up to 12 months. The respiratory epithelium of untreated or acetone (1 µl/ml)-treated cultures appeared ciliated, remained unremarkable except for focal squamous metaplasia, and by the end of the fourth month became atrophic, 1-2 layers thick. Clonal growths of cells derived from these explants were limited and senesced after the second subculturing, some with terminal differentiation.

MNNG treatment of explants, 0.4 µg/ml for 2 hours, twice a week, resulted in an increase of necrosis to 13%. The remaining explants showed squamous metaplasia by the second month of culture with minimal keratinization. Focal hyperplasia were common by the third month of culture. Dysplasia and atypia developed after 3 months of culture and were associated with a lack of cell-to-cell adhesiveness. Carcinoma in situ developed as early as the fifth month of culture and was seen in 82% of explants examined 6 months after treatment (Fig. 1). Due to epithelial shedding the anaplastic foci seen after 6 months were small and were composed of few cells (Fig. 2). Cells derived from explants treated for 6 months produced multiple tumor nodules in nude mice 8 weeks after inoculation, histologically consistent with squamous cell carcinoma. Clonal growths of cells derived from explants exposed to MNNG for more than 3 months led to the development of cell lines five of which were tumorigenic in nude mice.

Explants cultured in the presence of NNK, 20 µg/ml, freshly added to the medium twice a week, developed extensive basal cell hyperplasia with foci of squamous metaplasia by the third month of treatment. In contrast with MNNG-induced lesions, the ciliated surface epithelium was essentially preserved (Fig. 3).

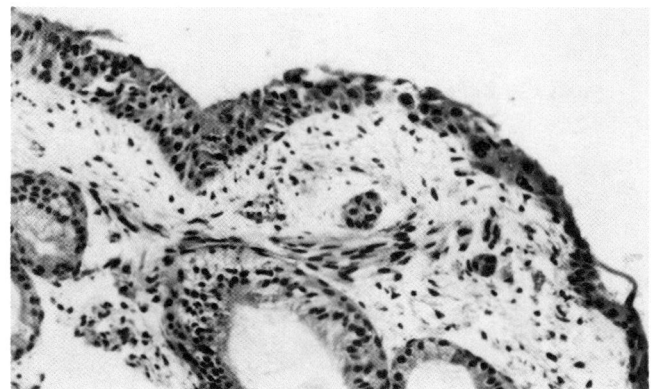

Figure 1
Section from tracheobronchial explant treated with MNNG for 5 months showing in situ carcinoma (×400)

Foci of dysplasia and atypia developed by the end of 7 culture months (Fig. 4). Carcinoma in situ was present in 17% of the explants examined after 8 months. Cells derived from explants treated for 12 months produced subcutaneous tumors in two out of 20 nude mice 8 weeks after inoculation, histologically consistent with undifferentiated carcinoma (Fig. 5).

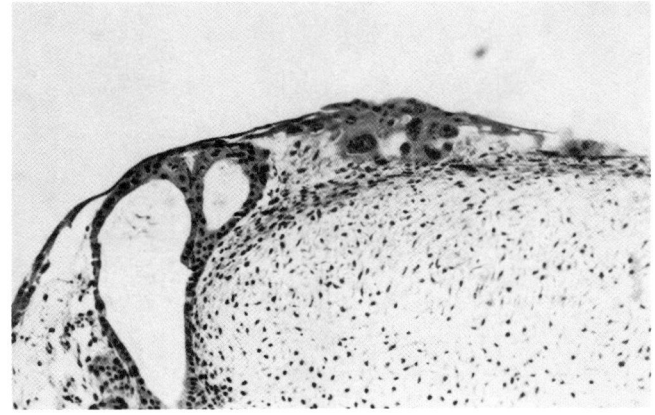

Figure 2
Section from tracheobronchial explant treated with MNNG for 8 months showing anaplastic cells with large nuclei and loss of cell-to-cell adhesion (×400)

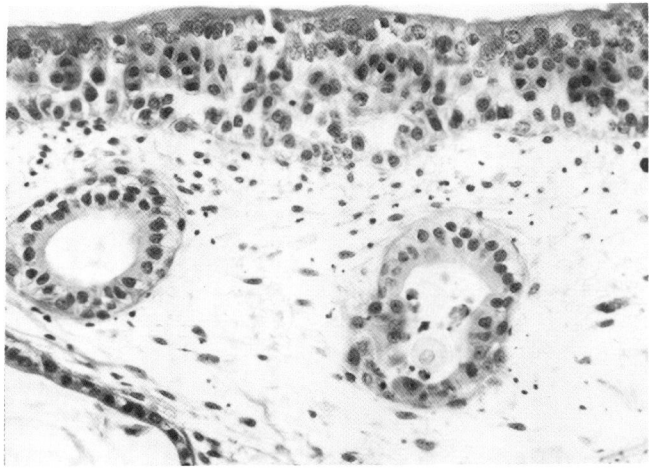

Figure 3
Section from tracheobronchial explant exposed to NNK for 3 months showing basal hyperplasia (×400)

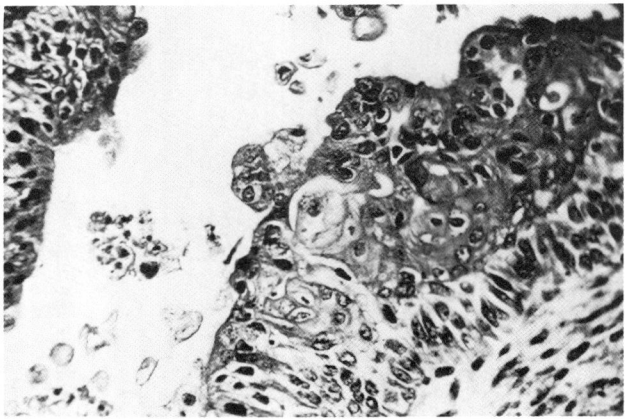

Figure 4
Section from tracheobronchial explant exposed to NNK for 7 months showing foci of dysplasia and atypia (×400)

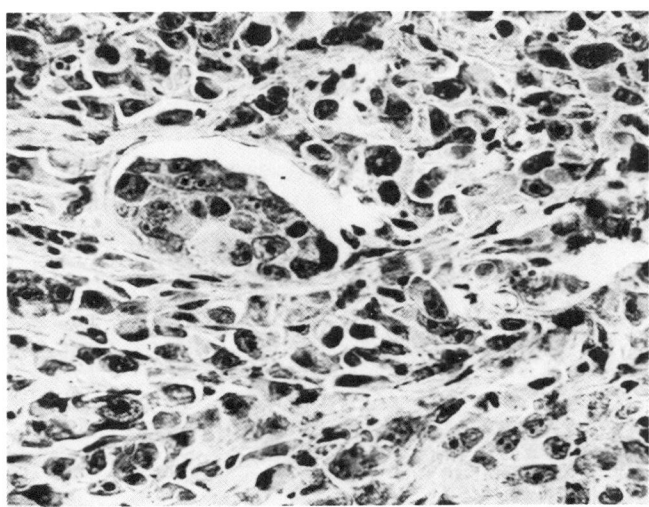

Figure 5
Section from subcutaneous tumor of nude mice 8 weeks after inoculation with cells from tracheobronchial explants treated with NNK for 12 months showing undifferentiated carcinoma (×400)

Pancreatic Epithelium

Explants, 1 mm in thickness, prepared from pancreases of prostaglandin-induced fetuses were cultured under the same conditions and carcinogen treatments as those of the tracheobronchial explants. Differentiation of exocrine pancreas occurred in culture, and explants cultured for 4 weeks or longer revealed normal acinar structures with zymogen granules. Similarly, ducts and ductules developed normally.

Explants exposed to MNNG (2 hours, twice a week) showed minimal necrosis and degeneration, ductal metaplasia, proliferation of ductular epithelium, and numerous foci of ductal hyperplasia. In explants cultured for more than 3 months, foci of carcinoma were present. Cells derived from these explants formed adenocarcinoma in six out of six nude mice when xenografted subcutaneously.

Explants cultured in the presence of NNK (20 μg/ml) differentiated fully and developed ductal metaplasia and multiple foci of ductal hyperplasia within 3 months of treatment (Fig. 6). Sections from explants cultured for up to 12 months in the presence of NNK revealed hyperplasia but no atypia. Sheets of cells with regular nuclei and frequent mitotic figures were often present after 6 months of culture.

Explants exposed alternately to 1 week of NNK (20 μg/ml, twice a week) and 1 week of 12-O-tetradecanoyl-phorbole-13-acetate (TPA), 0.1 μg/ml, (once a week),

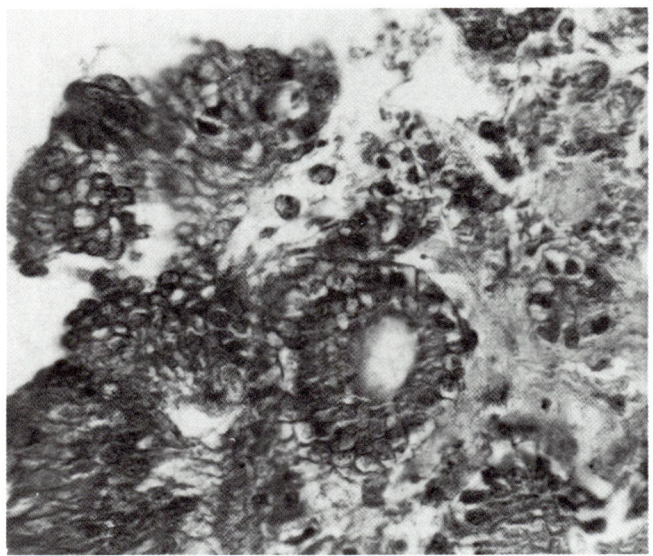

Figure 6
Section from pancreas explant treated with NNK for 12 months showing ductal hyperplasia (×400)

developed ductal metaplasia and ductal hyperplasia within 3 months. Cellular atypia appeared during the fifth month of treatment. Explants examined after 8 months of NNK-TPA treatment showed extensive necrosis in 61%, hyperplasia and atypia in 32%, and foci of anaplastic growth consistent with carcinoma in 7% of the explants (Fig. 7). Explants exposed to TPA (0.1 µg/ml, once a week) and cultured for up to 8 months showed no hyperplasia, atypia, or carcinoma.

O^6-Methylguanine

Sections from untreated, MNNG-, and NNK-treated explants were incubated at 70°C for 30 minutes, then deparafinnized in xylene, hydrated in gradients of ethanol in water and placed in PBS. Sections were stained with fluorescein- or peroxidase-conjugated anti-mouse IgG after a 30-minute incubation in monoclonal antibody to O^6-mG. There was no staining in sections from untreated explants.

The nuclear chromatin in sections from MNNG-treated pancreas or tracheobronchial explants at 1 day after treatment were stained with variable intensity (Fig. 8). Sections from MNNG-treated explants at 7 and 14 days after a single exposure revealed only few nuclei with intense staining; the remaining nuclei were negative.

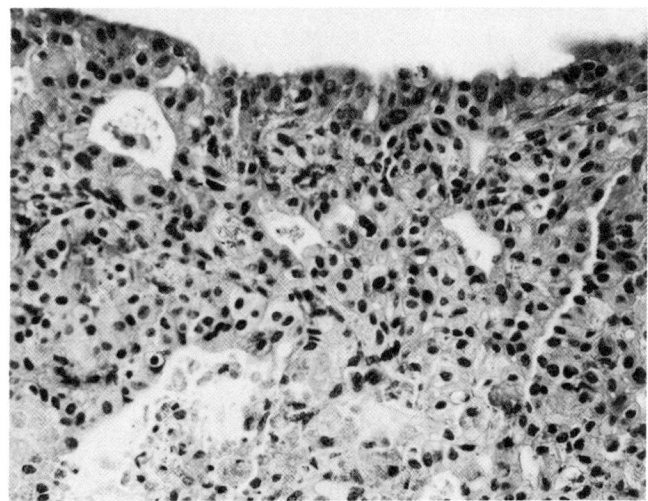

Figure 7
Section from pancreas explant treated alternately with NNK and TPA for 8 months showing anaplastic growth compatible with carcinoma (×250)

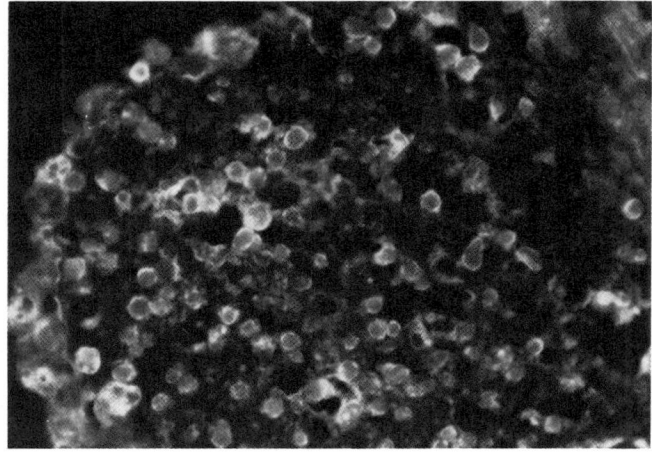

Figure 8
Section from tracheobronchial explant treated with MNNG and stained for O^6-mG showing nuclear staining (×400)

240 / I. Parsa et al.

The nuclear chromatin in NNK-treated tracheobronchial explants were faintly stained 1 day after treatment. The intensity of stain in a few nuclei was increased within 7 days after continuous exposure while the other nuclei revealed faint or negative staining (Fig. 9). In sections from explants exposed to NNK for 1 day and cultured further for 7 days, the nuclear staining was slight and limited to only a few nuclei.

Pancreas explants cultured in the presence of NNK or treated with a NNK-TPA regimen for up to 4 weeks revealed neither nuclear nor cytoplasmic staining.

DISCUSSION

To date no causative agent for human pancreatic carcinoma has been identified. Extrapolation from experimental animal models of pancreas carcinogenesis suggests that nitroso compounds are probably the initiators of human pancreas carcinoma. Human cells are found to be more resistant than those of rodents to tumorigenesis by chemical carcinogens. The success in the development of an in vitro model system of adult human pancreas carcinogenesis in this laboratory using nitroso compounds (Parsa et al. 1981), induction of transplantable carcinoma in organ-cultured fetal human pancreas by methylnitrosourea (Parsa et al. 1984), and the development of transplantable carcinoma in the model described here tend to support such

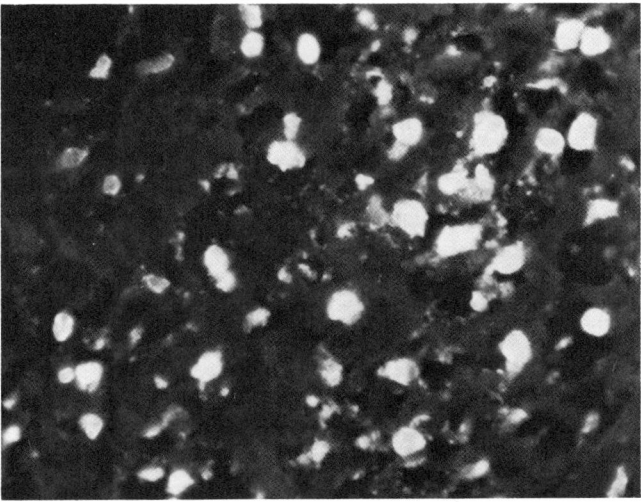

Figure 9
Section from tracheobronchial explant treated with NNK and stained for O^6-mG showing intense staining of a few nuclei ($\times 400$)

an extrapolation. Furthermore, in this model it has been possible to demonstrate the stepwise development of metaplasia, hyperplasia, and atypia leading to transplantable carcinoma.

The epidemiological data consider tobacco to be an important contributor to the development of pancreas carcinoma in man, and since NNK has been shown to be the most potent tobacco nitrosamine for initiation of tumors in rodents, it was natural to examine the role of NNK in the induction of human pancreatic cancer. The present data indicate that NNK is responsible for the induction of early morphological events—metaplasia and hyperplasia—in human pancreas explants but does not produce atypia or carcinoma in this system. The combined use of NNK and TPA, however, result in atypia leading to the development of anaplastic carcinoma. Ductal metaplasia has also been described in the noncancerous portion of the human pancreas of an individual with pancreatic carcinoma (Parsa et al. 1985) and may represent a noncarcinogenic response to the toxicity of carcinogens. Ductal hyperplasia, on the other hand, is considered to be a step in carcinogenesis from which the progenitor cells of cancer emerge. The molecular events leading to the initiation of human pancreas cells by NNK are yet to be examined.

Cigarette smoking is considered the major cause of lung cancer, and both classes of compounds, the polynuclear aromatic hydrocarbons and the tobacco-specific nitrosamines, have been the subjects of intensive study in the past decade. Our knowledge of the effects of these compounds on human respiratory epithelium is limited to short-term studies dealing with their metabolism (Harris et al. 1976,1977,1982). The development of an in vitro model of human lung carcinogenesis offers the potential for a quantitative study of this process in respiratory epithelium by other compounds.

The successful induction of bronchogenic carcinoma in this model by NNK supports the in vivo carcinogenic role of this compound for the human respiratory tract. In this model NNK produced fewer tumors and had a much longer latency period than MNNG. Factors affecting its rate of activation and its potency in this model are yet to be established.

A number of nitroso compounds-adducts are reported in the literature. Of these, mainly O-alkyl-guanine and O-alkyl-thymidine are thought to produce misreadings. The only one with substantial documentation, though controversial, is O^6-alkyl-guanine. It is now established that there is no correlation between the persistence of this adduct in total DNA of tissue or organ and tumorigenicity of nitroso compounds. Correlation of the persistence of the adducts by immunohistochemical techniques in those cells which are or which become repair-deficient with cell initiation and tumor induction by nitroso compounds, however, may be more significant than measurement of modified base in total DNA. The present study demonstrates the formation of O^6-mG in nuclear chromatin of pancreatic and respiratory epithelium exposed to MNNG and its persistence in some nuclei 2 weeks after exposure. This and the formation and persistence of O^6-mG in the nuclei of some NNK-treated bronchial cells correlate well with the development of transplantable carcinomas in these tissues. In contrast with the NNK-treated respiratory epithelium, the pancreas cells treated with NNK failed to form demonstrable O^6-mG, indicating possible differences in the metabolism of NNK in these tissues.

REFERENCES

Castonguay, A., G.D. Stoner, P. Radok, K. Furuya, S.S. Hecht, and H.A.J. Schut. 1983. Metabolism of tobacco-specific N-nitrosamines by cultured human tissues. *Proc. Natl. Acad. Sci. U.S.A.* **80**: 6694.

Foiles, P.G., N. Trushin, and A. Castonguay. 1985. Measurement of O^6-methyldeoxyguanosine in DNA methylated by the tobacco-specific carcinogen 4-(methylnitrosamine)-1-(3-pyridyl)-1-butanone using a biotin-avidin enzyme-linked immunosorbent assay. *Carcinogenesis.* **6**: 989.

Harris, C.C., B.F. Trump, R.C. Grafstrom, and H. Autrup. 1982. Differences in metabolism of chemical carcinogens in cultured human epithelial tissues and cells. In *Mechanisms of chemical carcinogenesis* (ed. C.C. Harris and P. Cerutti). Alan R. Liss, New York.

Harris, C.C., H. Autrup, G. Stoner, E. McDowell, B.F. Trump, and P. Schafer. 1977. Metabolism of acyclic and cyclic N-nitrosamines in cultured human bronchi. *J. Natl. Cancer Inst.* **59**: 1401.

Harris, C.C., A. Frank, C. Van Haaften, D. Kaufman, R. Connor, F. Jackson, L. Barret, E. McDowell, and B.F. Trump. 1976. Binding of (^{3}H)benzo(a)pyrene to DNA in cultured human bronchus. *Cancer Res.* **36**: 1011.

Harris, C.C., H. Autrup, G. Stoner, S.K. Young, J.C. Lentz, H.V. Gelobin, J.K. Selkirk, R.J. Conner, L.A. Barrett, R.T. Jones, E. McDowell, and B.F. Trump. 1977. Metabolism of benzo(a)pyrene and 7,12 dimethylbenz(a)anthracene in cultured human bronchus and pancreatic duct. *Cancer Res.* **37**: 3349.

Hecht, S.S., A. Castonguay, F.-L. Chung, and D. Hoffmann. 1984. Carcinogenic and metabolic activation of tobacco-specific nitrosamines: Current status and future prospects. In *N-nitroso compounds: Occurrence, biological effects and relevance to human cancer* (ed. I.K. O'Neill, R.C. Von Borstel, C.T. Miller, J. Long, and H. Bartsch), p. 763. IARC Scientific Publication No. 57, International Agency for Cancer, Lyon, France.

Hoffmann, D. and J.D. Adams. 1981. Carcinogenic tobacco-specific N-nitrosamines in snuff and in the saliva of snuff dippers. *Cancer Res.* **41**: 4305.

Hoffmann, D., J.D. Adams, and S.S. Hecht. 1979. Assessment of tobacco-specific N-nitrosamines in tobacco products. *Cancer Res.* **39**: 2505.

Parsa, I., W.H. Marsh, A.L. Sutton, and K.M.H. Butt. 1981. Effects of dimethylnitrosamine on organ-cultured adult human pancreas. *Am. J. Pathol.* **102**: 403.

Parsa, I. and J.M. Belich. 1984. An *in vitro* model of human lung carcinogenesis. *Fed. Proc.* **43**: 662.

Parsa, I., R.D. Bloomfield, A.C. Foye, and A.L. Sutton. 1984. Methylnitrosourea-induced carcinoma in organ-cultured fetal human pancreas. *Cancer Res.* **44**: 3530.

Parsa, I., D.S. Longnecker, D.G. Scarpelli, P. Pour, J.K. Reddy, and M. Lefkowitz. 1985. Ductal metaplasia of human exocrine pancreas and its association with carcinoma. *Cancer Res.* **45**: 1265.

COMMENTS

POIRIER: Have you done quantitative studies to determine what the DNA modification levels are at the lower end of your sensitivity range? What is the lowest finding level you are able to see?

PARSA: Well, that depends on whether a bivalent antibody is used with indirect fluorescence technique or direct fluorescent technique. The indirect fluorescent matches the measurement using anti-O^6-methyl and then labeled antimouse IgG to precipitate it, and counting the labeling in the pellet.

POIRIER: I was just wondering if maybe your binding levels in the pancreas were so low that even though you may have adducts there, you cannot detect them.

PARSA: In the case of MNNG it is quite high. It is low with DMN and absent or not measurable with NNK.

MAGEE: Were the autoradiographic grains on the same nuclei as the antibodies for the O^6-methylguanine?

PARSA: That's right.

MAGEE: And the cells are not dividing at all? Could there be any incorporation of isotope, metabolically, from the one carbon produced, or must it all be metabolized?

PARSA: No, we are speaking about the DMN in adult pancreas, 7 days, is that right?

MAGEE: That's right.

PARSA: There is not much mitosis at that time.

YOAKUM: I assume you can grow your tumors as transferable cell lines in the mice?

PARSA: Some of them.

YOAKUM: Have you tested any of these for activated oncogenes?

PARSA: No, not as yet.

PEGG: Does your antibody only react with O^6-methylguanine in DNA and not RNA. Otherwise, why doesn't the RNA show up?

PARSA: We did try and it reacts with O^6-methyl-RNA; and we did remove the RNA, but 7 days after one exposure to DMN there's not much of a label in the total RNA. In other words, there was no difference in labeling between the RNA-extracted tissue and the tissue that has RNA. In the particular sets of experiments I showed you, there was not much labeling in RNA, except when treated with MNNG and only at the very beginning.

PEGG: So, that's due to just RNA turnover, is it?

PARSA: RNA was removed in order to measure the O^6-methyl DNA. In other words, RNA has to be removed either by NaOH or RNAse before measurement of O^6-methylguanine. That's the procedure used.

HOFFMANN: It may be of interest that we have looked very carefully for lesions in the pancreas of rats and hamsters treated with NNN and NNK. We have never detected tumors in the pancreas; but with NNN, we have detected tumors of the nasal cavity, esophagus, and lung and with NNK, tumors of the nasal cavity, lung, and liver. These tobacco-specific N-nitrosamines are procarcinogens whereas NMNG is a direct alkylating agent which does not require metabolic activation. Thus, the human pancreas explant may not be an ideal system for the in vitro assay of NNN or NNK.

CONNEY: Would it be worthwhile to add a metabolic activating system to the pancreas culture?

PARSA: I'm sure it's possible.

CONNEY: Is the pancreas intrinsically resistant or does it have something to do with the xenobiotic metabolizing system?

HECHT: It would be interesting to do a comparative study of metabolism in the bronchus and the pancreas.

Recent Studies on the Metabolic Activation of Tobacco-specific Nitrosamines: Prospects for Dosimetry in Humans

STEPHEN S. HECHT, PETER G. FOILES, STEVEN G. CARMELLA, NEIL TRUSHIN, ABRAHAM RIVENSON, AND DIETRICH HOFFMANN
Naylor Dana Institute for Disease Prevention
American Health Foundation
Valhalla, New York 10595

OVERVIEW

The tobacco-specific nitrosamines N'-nitrosonornicotine (NNN) and 4-(methylnitrosamino)-1-(3-pyridyl)-1-butanone (NNK) are present in relatively high quantities in tobacco and tobacco smoke. Recent studies on the metabolic activation of NNK and NNN, and possible applications of these studies to human dosimetry, are discussed. NNK was found to be a more potent carcinogen in the F344 rat than the related methylating nitrosamine, N-nitrosodimethylamine (NDMA). However, NDMA was a more efficient DNA methylating agent than was NNK, indicating that factors other than DNA methylation are important in NNK carcinogenesis. One such factor might be DNA pyridyloxobutylation by NNK; studies on the structures of putative adducts resulting from this pathway were carried out. Sensitive immunochemical methods for the detection of methylated DNA in exfoliated cells and related methods for detecting pyridyloxobutylation of DNA and hemoglobin are being developed. Such approaches may be important in identifying individuals susceptible to tobacco carcinogenesis.

INTRODUCTION

Among the many compounds in tobacco and tobacco smoke, nicotine is perhaps the most important. Its habituating properties are one of the main reasons that millions of people use tobacco despite widespread knowledge of its harmful effects. Nicotine and the related compounds, nornicotine, anabasine, and anatabine, are not known to be carcinogenic, but these tobacco alkaloids are the precursors to a group of carcinogens called the tobacco-specific nitrosamines (Hoffmann and Hecht 1985). Two of these nitrosamines, N'-nitrosonornicotine (NNN) and 4-(methylnitrosamino)-1-(3-pyridyl)-1-butanone (NNK), have wide ranging carcinogenic effects. Since they are present in both tobacco and tobacco smoke in significant quantities, they have been a focus of our recent studies. We believe that research on the metabolic activation of these nitrosamines will lead to new insights on the prevention of tobacco-related cancer. In particular, it is probable that methods for assessing human uptake and metabolic activation of these nitrosamines can be developed. Since NNK and NNN are found only in tobacco and tobacco smoke, in contrast to other carcinogens such as the polynuclear aromatic hydrocarbons, they appear to be uniquely suited as potential dosimeters for tobacco carcinogenesis. In this paper, we summarize some of our recent results on the metabolic activation of NNK and NNN in rats and discuss their possible applications in human dosimetry.

NNK is an *N*-methyl nitrosamine and as such is structurally related to *N*-nitrosodimethylamine (NDMA) (Fig. 1). The carcinogenic properties and metabolic activation pathways of NDMA are well characterized (Preussmann and Stewart 1984). Therefore, to learn more about the mechanism of tumor induction by NNK, we have compared the carcinogenicity and DNA methylating properties of NDMA and NNK in the rat. In parallel studies, we have developed immunoassays for measuring DNA methylation by NNK. Since methylation alone does not seem to account for the ability of NNK to induce tumors in various rat tissues, we have carried out model studies on the potential DNA interactions of 4-(3-pyridyl)-4-oxobutyldiazohydroxide, which should also be formed in the metabolism of NNK (Fig. 1). The same intermediate is thought to be involved in the metabolic activation of NNN (Hoffmann and Hecht 1985). Methods for assaying the potential interaction of such intermediates with DNA and with proteins such as hemoglobin have been investigated.

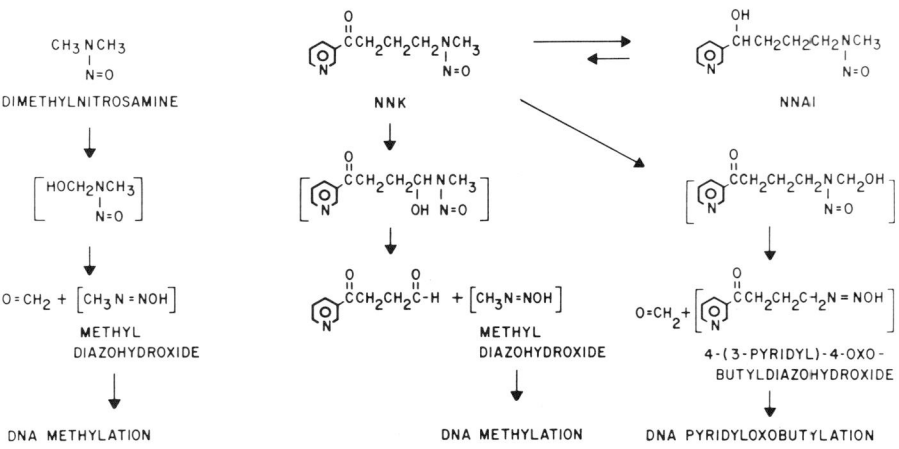

Figure 1
Pathways of metabolism of NDMA or NNK leading to DNA methylation or DNA pyridyloxobutylation

RESULTS

Comparative Carcinogenicity of NNK and NDMA

Groups of male F344 rats were given subcutaneous injections of either NNK or NDMA, three times weekly for 20 weeks. The total doses were 0.33 mmole/kg of each nitrosamine. The experiment was terminated after 104 weeks. The results are summarized in Table 1. Both compounds induced a low incidence of liver tumors. However, NNK also induced a significant incidence of lung and nasal cavity tumors; only one nasal cavity tumor was observed in the animals treated with NDMA. Thus, NNK was significantly more tumorigenic than was NDMA toward the rat lung and nasal cavity (Hecht et al. 1986a).

Comparative DNA Methylation by NNK and NDMA

Groups of male F344 rats were given a single subcutaneous injection of 0.39 mmole/kg of either NNK or NDMA in trioctanoin. They were sacrificed at intervals after treatment and the levels of 7-methylguanine (7-mG) and O^6-methylguanine (O^6-mG) were measured in DNA of liver, lung, and nasal mucosa. The results are summarized in Table 2 and Figures 2 and 3. In liver and lung, NDMA methylation was significantly greater ($P < 0.001$) than NNK methylation at all intervals; NDMA methylation also exceeded NNK methylation in the nasal mucosa. After a single subcutaneous dose of 0.055 mmole/kg, NDMA methylation 4 hours or 24 hours after treatment exceeded NNK methylation in liver; but the levels of DNA methylation in nasal mucosa were similar for the two nitrosamines (Hecht et al. 1986a).

Immunochemical Measurement of DNA Methylation by NNK

Anti-O^6-methyldeoxyguanosine antibody was raised in rabbits, using an O^6-methylguanosine conjugate. The purified antibody was used to develop a biotin-avidin enzyme-linked immunosorbent assay (BA-ELISA). The specificity and sensitivity of the antibody used in the BA-ELISA is illustrated in Figure 4. With this specificity, the lower limit of DNA added to each well was about 5 µg. By coupling high-performance liquid chromatography (HPLC) to the BA-ELISA, this limitation was overcome and the amount of DNA analyzed could be increased to 1 mg or more. The detection limit was approximately 1 µmole of O^6-methyldeoxyguanosine per mole deoxyguanosine. Figure 5 shows the results of an analysis, by HPLC-BA-ELISA, of nasal mucosa DNA from a rat treated with NNK (Foiles et al. 1985).

The sensitivity of the assay was further improved by a modification of the immuno-blotting technique described by Nehls et al. 1984. Samples of DNA ($\simeq 5$ µg) were absorbed on nitrocellulose membranes. Individual blots were then placed in test tubes and incubated with the anti-O^6-methyldeoxyguanosine antibody. Binding was detected by the biotin-avidin-horse radish peroxidase method used above. The applicability of this direct binding assay to small samples of DNA

Table 1
Induction of Tumors by NNK and NDMA in F344 rats[a]

Group	Effective no. of rats[b]	No. of rats with tumors[c]					
		Liver		Lung[d]		Nasal cavity[e]	
		Hepatoma	Adenoma	Adenocarcinoma	Adenoma	Squamous cell carcinoma	papilloma
NNK	27	2	8	4	9	1	5
NDMA	27	2	4	0	0	0	1
Vehicle	26	0	0	0	1	0	0

[a]Rats were given s.c. injections of NDMA or NNK in trioctanoin, three times weekly for 20 weeks; total doses were 0.33 mmole/kg of each nitrosamine. The experiment was terminated after 104 weeks.
[b]No. of rats autopsied
[c]Other tumors: Leydig tumors, NDMA group, 21; NNK group, 22; vehicle control group 20; abdominal mesothelioma, NDMA group, 2; NNK group, 2; vehicle control, 0; subcutaneous sarcoma, NDMA group, 5; NNK group, 2; vehicle control group, 2; prostate in situ carcinoma, NDMA group, 4; NNK group, 3; vehicle control group, 1; leukemia/lymphoma, NDMA group, 4; NNK group, 3; vehicle control group, 4
[d]Tumor incidence in NNK group > NDMA group, $P < 0.01$
[e]Tumor incidence in NNK group > NDMA group, $P < 0.05$

Table 2
Levels of 7 mG and O^6-mG in F344 Rat Tissues at Intervals after S.C. Injection of 0.39 mmole/kg NNK or NDMA[a]

Treatment	Survival interval (hrs)	Liver		Guanine (μmole/mole) Lung		Nasal mucosa	
		7-mG	O^6-mG	7-mG	O^6-mG	7-mG	O^6-mG
NNK	1	367 ± 27	26 ± 3.5	ND	ND	1520	170
NDMA	1	1850 ± 230	230 ± 35	203 ± 29	15 ± 3	1580	168
NNK	4	817 ± 31	74 ± 5.2	ND	3 ± 3	1960	230
NDMA	4	7110 ± 300	980 ± 12	580 ± 62	71 ± 7	3470	380
NNK	12	935 ± 22	108 ± 5	ND	6.7 ± 0.1	2060	251
NDMA	12	7650 ± 340	1230 ± 47	635 ± 7	70 ± 6	3300	441
NNK	24	1107 ± 96	87 ± 7	62 ± 4.3	7.9 ± 1.2	1400	210
NDMA	24	6270 ± 150	1240 ± 20	523 ± 76	65 ± 15	2910	490
NNK	36	853 ± 96	51 ± 21	87 ± 24	8.9 ± 0.2	1220	190
NDMA	36	3450 ± 500	750 ± 90	400 ± 26	60 ± 11	2050	400
NNK	48	559 ± 14	18 ± 3	ND	5.7 ± 0.7	589	142
NDMA	48	2020 ± 143	400 ± 21	318 ± 20	62 ± 4	1620	311

[a] Groups of three male F344 rats were given an s.c. injection of NNK or NDMA in trioctanoin (0.39 mg/kg) and sacrificed at the intervals noted. Values are mean ± SD of duplicate determinations on DNA from liver and lung of each of three rats and mean ± SD of duplicate determinations on DNA pooled from the nasal mucosa of three rats.
[b] ND = not detected

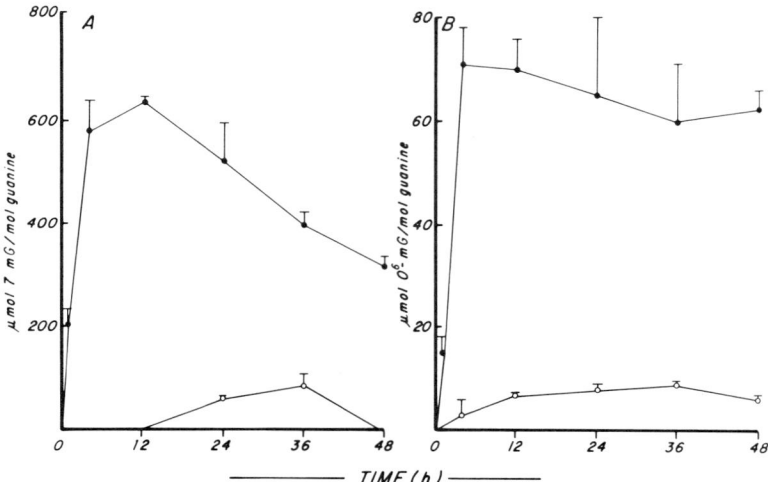

Figure 2
Comparative levels of (A) 7-mG and (B) O^6-mG in lung DNA at intervals after treatment with NDMA (●) or NNK (○)

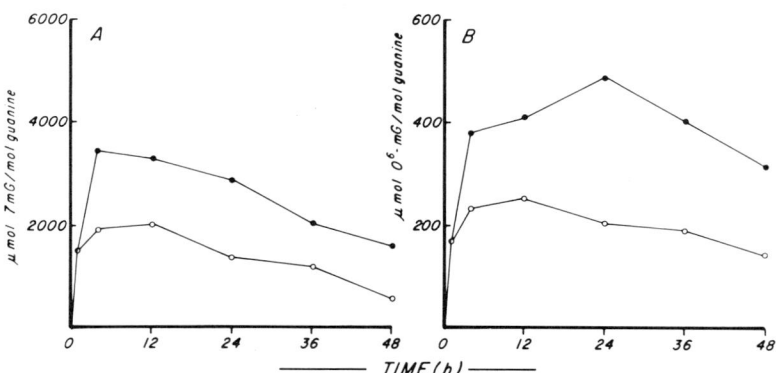

Figure 3
Comparative levels of (A) 7-mG and (B) O^6-mG in nasal mucosa DNA at intervals after treatment with NDMA (●) or NNK (○)

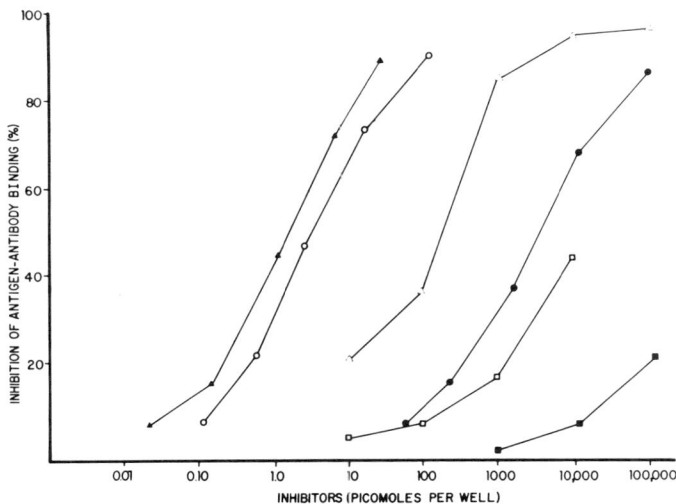

Figure 4
Inhibition of anti-O^6-methyldeoxyguanosine antibody binding to immobilized O^6-methylguanosine-bovine serum albumin by O^6-methyldeoxyguanosine (▲); O^6-methylguanosine (○); O^6-mG (△); N^6-methyldeoxyadenosine (●); 7-methyldeoxyguanosine (□); and 2'-deoxyguanosine (■)

should allow its use in analyzing O^6-methyldeoxyguanosine in DNA extracted from exfoliated oral cells.

Reactions with Deoxyguanosine of 4-(Carbethoxynitrosamino)-1-(3-pyridyl)-1-butanone

The title compound is a stable precursor to 4-(3-pyridyl)-4-oxobutyldiazohydroxide (Fig. 1). Its reactions with deoxyguanosine were investigated to provide information on the potential DNA interactions of NNK and NNN. The principle deoxyguanosine adduct was the rearranged, branched chain N^2-adduct illustrated in Fig. 6. Its structure was established by its spectral properties and by independent synthesis from the α,β-unsaturated ketone, 1-(3-pyridyl)-2-buten-1-one. In the reaction of deoxyguanosine with 4-(carbethoxynitrosamino)-1-(3-pyridyl)-1-butanone, the rearranged N^2-adduct could be formed either through the small amount of α,β-unsaturated ketone produced in this reaction or through carbonium ion rearrangement as illustrated in Figure 6 (Hecht et al. 1986b). This adduct has been coupled to keyhole limpet hemocyanin, and mice have been treated with the conjugate. We will attempt to isolate monoclonal antibodies for use in developing immunoassays for the adduct in tissue DNA of rats treated with NNK, and in exfoliated cells from tobacco smokers and chewers.

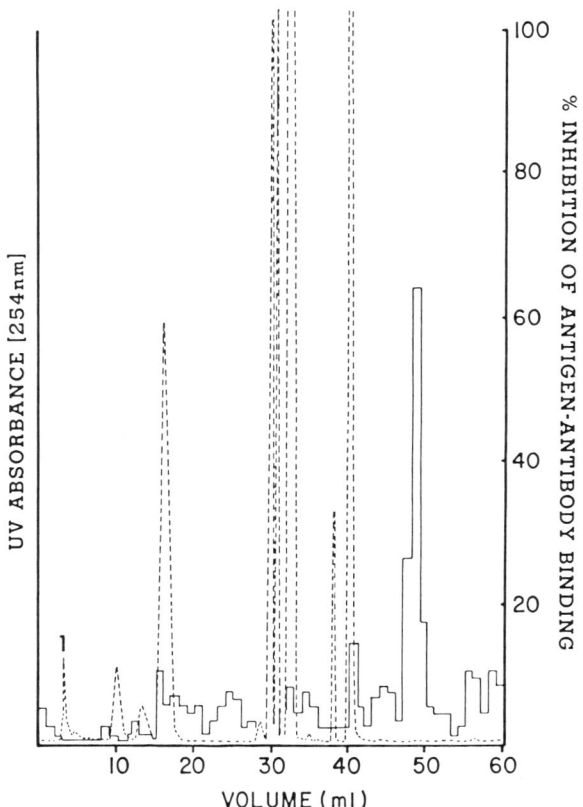

Figure 5
HPLC-BA-ELISA analysis of DNA from nasal mucosa of a rat treated with NNK. UV (– – –); inhibition of antigen antibody binding (———). The peak at 49 ml corresponds to 5.2 pmole of O^6-methyldeoxyguanosine.

Reactions with N-Acetylcysteine of 4-(Carbethoxynitrosamino)-1-(3-pyridyl)-1-butanone

Groups of two rats were given single intraperitoneal injections of either [5-^{3}H]NNK or [5-^{3}H]NNN, 0.1 mCi/0.1 μmole. After 24-48 hours, blood was obtained by cardiac puncture. Globin was isolated from the erythrocytes as described (Green et al. 1984) and analyzed for radioactivity by combustion. The results demonstrated that approximately 0.01% of the dose was bound to globin. Since this level of binding is potentially great enough to allow detection of adducts in smokers, studies aimed at characterization of adducts were carried out. The model compound, 4-(carbethoxynitrosamino)-1-(3-pyridyl)-1-butanone, was

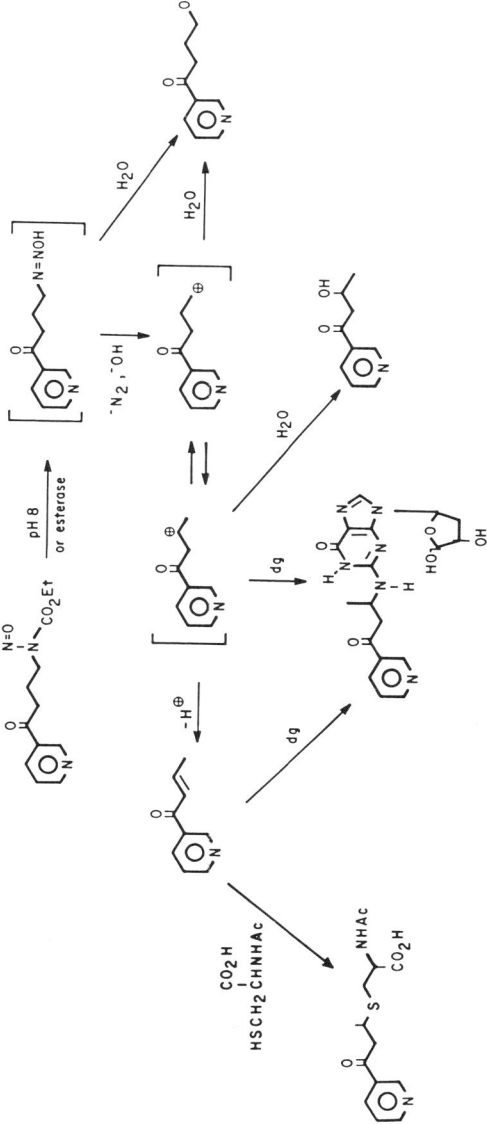

Figure 6
Reactions of 4-(carbethoxynitrosamino)-1-(3-pyridyl)-1-butanone with deoxyguanosine (dG), H_2O, and N-acetylcysteine

allowed to react with N-acetylcysteine at 37°C, pH 8. A major product was identified as the adduct illustrated in Figure 6. The adduct diastereomers are apparently formed by reaction of N-acetylcysteine with 1-(3-pyridyl)-2-buten-1-one.

DISCUSSION

The results of the comparative carcinogenicity assay of NNK and NDMA demonstrate that NNK is more carcinogenic than NDMA, at least under the conditions of this protocol in the F344 rat. This is important because of the relatively high exposure of smokers, chewers, and snuff dippers to NNK. Extensive dose-response studies of NDMA have shown that its hepatocarcinogenicity was clearly observable at a daily dose of 0.02 mg/kg body weight, corresponding to a total dose of approximately 0.3 mmole/kg, as in our study (Peto et al. 1984). This dose is only ten times higher than the estimated lifetime NNK dose of a snuff dipper (Hecht et al. 1986a). The higher carcinogenicity of NNK than of NDMA suggests that this dose might be sufficient to induce cancer.

The tumorigenic properties of NNK are probably mediated at least in part by the miscoding lesion, O^6-mG, which was detected in target tissues by HPLC, with detection either by fluorescence or BA-ELISA. Nevertheless, the comparative DNA methylation studies of NDMA and NNK suggest that factors in addition to O^6-mG must be involved in the induction of tumors by NNK. Whereas NNK was more tumorigenic than NDMA in the lung, levels of O^6-mG in lung DNA upon treatment with NDMA were 7-22 times greater than those caused by NNK. NNK was also more tumorigenic than NDMA in the nasal mucosa, but the levels of O^6-mG caused by the two compounds were similar. In liver, NNK and NDMA had similar tumorigenic activities, but levels of O^6-mG upon treatment with NDMA were 9-22 times greater than upon treatment with NNK.

To obtain meaningful information on the uptake and metabolic activation of NNK by tobacco users, it will probably be necessary to measure levels of methylation, as well as levels of other adducts. Methylation alone does not seem to be sufficient for cancer induction by NNK and, of course, can result from exposures to methylating agents other than NNK. However, the biochemistry of DNA methylation is presently fairly well understood (Pegg 1983; Singer and Grunberger 1983), and our results with the immunoassays suggest that it should be measurable in exfoliated cells. Measurements of O^6-methyldeoxyguanosine in surgical specimens of human esophagus and stomach have recently been reported (Umbenhauer et al. 1985). Immunoassays for the pyridyloxobutyl adducts of NNK and NNN will presumably be more valuable than those for methylation because such adducts, if formed, are likely to be unique to tobacco-specific nitrosamines. The results of the comparative DNA methylation study also suggest that they are probably important in NNK carcinogenesis.

Hemoglobin adducts may provide an alternate method for NNK and NNN dosimetry in tobacco users. A smoker may inhale about 100 ng of NNK per cigarette, according to machine smoking measurements (Hoffmann and Hecht 1985). This is about 4 µg/day in a smoker of two packs per day. According to the results in rats, about 0.4 ng/day may become bound to hemoglobin. Since the lifetime of the human red blood cell is about 120 days, this dose will accumulate. In 60 days, about 24 ng may be bound. This amount will be diluted in approximately 5 liters of blood, giving about 5 pg/ml. Such levels may be detectable, depending, of course, on the nature of the adduct. Although such protein adducts may not be as biologically important as DNA adducts, they may be easier to measure because they may accumulate whereas DNA adducts may be repaired. Their levels should reflect the capacity of the individual to metabolically convert NNK or NNN to an electrophile. This capacity may be related to the individual's susceptibility to cancer induction by these nitrosamines.

SUMMARY

The nicotine-derived nitrosamine, 4-(methylnitrosamino)-1-(3-pyridyl)-1-butanone (NNK) is more carcinogenic in the F344 rat than the related methylating nitrosamine N-nitrosodimethylamine (NDMA). A comparative study of DNA methylation by NNK and NDMA showed that NDMA was a stronger methylating agent than was NNK in rat liver, lung, and nasal mucosa. Since the latter two tissues develop tumors upon treatment with NNK, but not with NDMA, the results indicate that factors in addition to DNA methylation are involved in NNK tumorigenesis. Such factors may include DNA pyridyloxobutylation. According to model studies, pyridyloxobutyl diazohydroxide intermediates generated metabolically from NNK, as well as N'-nitrosonornicotine (NNN), can form N^2-adducts with deoxyguanosine. Such adducts, as well as methyl adducts in DNA, may provide indicators of human exposure to, and activation of, tobacco-specific nitrosamines. Immunochemical methods for detection of O^6-methyldeoxyguanosine in DNA of exfoliated cells, and assays for detection of pyridyloxobutyl adducts are being developed. Adducts of NNK or NNN with hemoglobin are also formed and seem to represent a promising alternate approach to assessing uptake and activation of tobacco-specific nitrosamines in humans.

ACKNOWLEDGMENTS

This study was supported by NCI grants 21393, 29580, and 32391.

REFERENCES

Foiles, P.G., N. Trushin, and A. Castonguay. 1985. Measurement of O^6-methyldeoxyguanosine in DNA methylated by the tobacco-specific carcinogen

4-(methylnitrosamino)-1-(3-pyridyl)-1-butanone using a biotin-avidin enzyme-linked immunosorbent assay. *Carcinogenesis* **6**: 989.

Green, L.C., P.L. Skipper, R.J. Turesky, M.S. Bryant, and S.R. Tannenbaum. 1984. In vivo dosimetry of 4-aminobiphenyl in rats via a cysteine adduct in hemoglobin. *Cancer Res.* **44**: 4245.

Hecht, S.S., N. Trushin, A. Castonguay, and A. Rivenson. 1986a. Comparative carcinogenicity and DNA methylation in F344 rats by 4-(methylnitroso)-1-(3-pyridyl)-1-butanone and N-nitrosodimethylamine. *Cancer Res.* **46**: 498.

Hecht, S.S., D. Lin, J. Chang, and A. Castonguay. 1986b. Reactions with deoxyguanosine of 4-(carbethoxynitrosamino)-1-(3-pyridyl)-1-butanone, a model compound for α-hydroxylation of tobacco-specific nitrosamines. *J. Am. Chem. Soc.* **108**: 1292.

Hoffmann, D. and S.S. Hecht. 1985. Nicotine-derived N-nitrosamines and tobacco related cancer: Current status and future directions. *Cancer Res.* **45**: 935.

Nehls, P., J. Adamkiewicz, and M.F. Rajewsky. 1984. Immuno-slot-blot: A highly sensitive immunoassay for the quantitation of carcinogen-modified nucleosides in DNA. *J. Cancer Res. Clin. Oncol.* **108**: 23.

Pegg, A.E. 1983. Alhylation and subsequent repair of DNA after exposure to dimethylnitrosamine and related carcinogens. *Rev. Biochem. Toxicol.* **5**: 83.

Peto, R., R. Gray, P. Brantom, and P. Grasso. 1984. Nitrosamine carcinogenesis in 5120 rodents: Chronic administration of sixteen different concentrations of NDEA, NDMA, NPYR, and NPIP in the water of 1440 inbred rats, with parallel studies on NDEA alone of the effect of age of starting (3, 6, or 20 weeks) and of species (rats, mice or hamsters). In *N-nitroso compounds: Occurrence, biological effects and relevance to human cancer* (ed. I.K. O'Neill, R.C. VonBorstel, C.T. Miller, J. Long, and H. Bartsch). Pub. no. 57, p. 627. International Agency for Research on Cancer, Lyon, France.

Preussman, R. and B.W. Stewart. 1984. N-nitroso carcinogens. In *Chemical carcinogens*, second ed. (ed. C.E. Searle), p. 643. American Chemical Society, Washington, D.C.

Singer, B. and D. Grunberger. 1983. *Molecular biology of mutagens and carcinogens*, p. 221. Plenum Publishing, New York.

Umbenhauer, D., C.P. Wild, R. Montesano, R. Saffhill, J.M. Boyle, N. Huh, U. Kirstein, J. Thomaele, M.F. Rajewsky, and S.H. Lu. 1985. Detection of alkylated bases in DNA and of alkyltransferase activity in human tissues. *Proc. Am. Assoc. Cancer Res.* **26**: 82.

COMMENTS

BELAND: Based upon your work, do you have any idea how much hydroxylation is occurring on each side of the nitrogen? Do you get more methylation or more of the other type of adduct?

HECHT: It seems from the work that we have done so far that the pyridyloxobutyl adducts are about one-tenth to one-hundredth of what we get of O^6-methylguanine. However, from our in vitro work, the hydroxylations on each side are similar.

HARRIS: I would like to encourage you, Steve [Hecht], to investigate human buccal mucosa. Both Dr. Grafstrom and Dr. Autrup have developed methods for culturing those cells. Therefore, you can go directly to your target, the target tissue for humans.

HECHT: We have done a collaborative study with Gary Stoner, which was published a couple of years ago, in which we used various cultured tissues obtained from immediate autopsy. One of them was buccal mucosa. All these tissues metabolize both NNK and NNN in ways that you would expect to lead to DNA methylation and pyridyloxobutylation although that was not measured in that study.

CONNEY: There are a large number of adducts from NNK. Are you trying to relate some of these adducts to the biological activity of NNK?

HECHT: Naturally.

MAGEE: The urethane analog of NNK was highly mutagenic. Did you also test for carcinogenicity?

HECHT: No, mainly because there are many studies that have shown that direct-acting model compounds, such as nitrosourethanes and alpha-acetoxy-*N*-nitrosamines, are contact carcinogens in animals. I feel certain that our nitrosourethane model compound would cause tumors, but perhaps it's worth doing the experiment.

Metabolism of Polycyclic Aromatic Hydrocarbons in Human Target Tissues

HERMAN AUTRUP
Laboratory of Environmental Carcinogenesis
Fibinger Institute
Copenhagen, Denmark

OVERVIEW

Polycyclic aromatic hydrocarbons (PAH), e.g., benzo[a]pyrene (B[a]P), are among the major carcinogenic fractions in the particulate phase of cigarette smoke. The compounds require metabolic activation to exert their harmful biological effects. The oral cavity, lung, and bladder are some of the organs associated with increased risk of cancer as a consequence of smoking. The metabolism of B[a]P has been investigated in either cell or explant cultures from these human tissues and was quite similar in these organs, as measured by binding of the ultimate carcinogenic form of B[a]P to DNA, by the metabolic profile, and by the relative distribution of the B[a]P-DNA adducts. These tissues had a slightly higher activity as measured by binding of B[a]P to DNA, and they converted the primary B[a]P metabolites into nontoxic, water excretable metabolites less efficiently than nontarget organs, e.g., the liver and colon.

INTRODUCTION

Polycyclic aromatic hydrocarbons (PAH) constitute by far the largest group of carcinogens in tobacco smoke (Hoffmann et al. 1978). Many of these compounds are highly carcinogenic in experimental animals and mutagenic in both bacterial and mammalian mutation assays. The compounds are procarcinogens that require metabolic activation before they can exert their cytotoxic, mutagenic, and carcinogenic effects. The metabolism requires several enzymatic steps involving the cytochrome P-450-associated mixed-function oxidase, epoxide hydratases, and cytoplasmic and microsomal transferases. The principal carcinogenic metabolites have been identified as bay-region dihydrodiol epoxides that mainly react with the exocyclic 2-amino group of deoxyguanosine in DNA. However, the other bases may also be target but to a lesser extent. The enzyme systems responsible for the activation of PAH to their carcinogenic metabolites are also involved in the detoxification of the PAH to less harmful compounds. Therefore, the ratio between activation and deactivation of the PAH may be an important determinant in organ, species, and individual susceptibility to the carcinogenic action.

Formation of a covalent carcinogen-DNA adduct is currently considered a significant event in the initiation of the carcinogenic process although the reaction with other macromolecules may also be important (Miller 1978). The principal benzo[a]pyrene-DNA adducts have been identified as N^2-(10[7b,8a,9a-trihydroxy-7,8,9,10-tetrahydrobenzo(a)pyrene]yl)deoxyguanosine. The amount of these specific B[a]P-DNA adducts has been associated with induction of skin tumors in mice (Nakayama et al. 1984), transformation frequency in C3H 10T1/2 cl 8, and mutation frequency in *Salmonella* T100 (Theall et al. 1982). Although the liver is generally considered the major site for biotransformation of xenobiotics, in situ metabolism in extrahepatic tissues may be an important determinant in organ toxicity (Boyd et al. 1983) and in initiation of carcinogenesis of these sites.

The metabolism of B[a]P has been extensively investigated in both intact human and animal tissues and in subcellular fractions. The metabolism of B[a]P is qualitatively similar in tracheobronchial tissues from both humans and animal species in which B[a]P has been experimentally shown to be carcinogenic (Autrup et al. 1980). However, a wide interindividual variation in the activation of B[a]P-to DNA-binding metabolites has been observed in all organs investigated (Harris et al. 1984). When the metabolism of B[a]P was studied in fibroblast and epithelial cells derived from the same individual, a higher activity was observed in the epithelial cells (Lechner et al. 1981; Stampfer et al. 1981; Kuroki et al. 1982). These epithelial cells may be considered the target cells, as most human tumors are of epithelial origin.

Several studies have demonstrated the importance of using an intact cellular system to correlate experimental data to the in vivo situation instead of a cell-free system. The metabolism of B[a]P by intact bronchial cells, in which the entire cellular biochemistry is present, gives both a different metabolic profile and B[a]P-DNA adduct profile when compared to a cell-free system (Autrup et al. 1983; Mass and Kaufman 1983).

The metabolism of other carcinogenic PAH present in tobacco smoke has not been investigated in human tissues. The metabolism of chrysene has been studied in hamster embryo cells (Vigny et al. 1982) and 5-methylchrysene in mouse epidermis in vivo (Melikian et al. 1983). The metabolism of a series of benzfluoranthenes in cell-free systems has been studied by identification of mutagenic metabolites (Hecht et al. 1980; LaVoie et al. 1982) or by binding to DNA (Perin-Roussel et al. 1983). The metabolism of benz[a]anthracene (van Bladeren et al. 1982), chrysene (Hodgson et al. 1982; Vyas et al. 1982), and benzo(c)phenanthrene (Ittah et al. 1983) have been studied using reconstituted P-450 systems.

The development of appropriate culture conditions for human target tissues has made it possible to study the metabolism of carcinogens found in tobacco in the tissues that exhibit a higher cancer incidence in smokers than in nonsmokers.

RESULTS

The metabolism of B[a]P has been studied in explant cultures or cell cultures derived from surgical biopsies. The explants and the cells were grown under controlled conditions as previously described (Harris et al. 1982; Autrup et al. 1984,1985). The cells were incubated with radiolabeled B[a]P for 24 hours, and the binding of B[a]P to cellular DNA was determined. At least 90% of the total radioactivity associated with cellular DNA is adducts formed between the ultimate carcinogenic form of B[a]P and bases in DNA (Autrup and Harris 1983). The highest mean activity was found in explants from the peripheral lung and bladder (Table 1) and the lowest, in liver and colon explants, organs that do not have an excessive cancer risk in smokers. The highest level of binding corresponded to one B[a]P moiety per 160,000 bases. A wide interindividual variation in the binding level was observed in explants from all organs, but significantly less variation was seen in primary cell cultures derived from the same organs (Table 2). Potential target cells for B[a]P carcinogenesis were less efficient in converting primary B[a]P metabolites to detoxified, water soluble metabolites (Table 3). The metabolites extractable with acetone/ethylacetate (1/1) accounted for 65-80% of all the metabolites excreted into the tissue culture media from the explant cultures of target organs. High-pressure liquid chromatographic (HPLC) analysis of the organic solvent metabolites showed that tetrols and B[a]P 9,10-diols were the major metabolites in all organs and only a small amount of the phenols were detected (Table 4). The results are expressed relative to B[a]P 7,8-diol that is considered the proximate carcinogenic form of B[a]P. The ultimate carcinogenic form is the B[a]P 7,8-dihydrodiol-9,10-epoxide that reacts with cellular DNA under the forma-

Table 1
Binding Levels of Benzo[a]pyrene to DNA in Cultured Human Tissues and Cells

	No. of modifications per 10^6 nucleotides		References
Human oral mucosa (cells)	1.4	(3)[a]	Autrup et al. (1985)
Human trachea (explants)	0.7	(4)	Autrup et al. (1980)
Human bronchus (explants)	1.0	(26)	Autrup and Harris (1983)
Human peripheral lung (explants)	2.4	(7)	Stoner et al. (1978)
Human pulmonary macrophages	2.0	(10)	Autrup et al. (1978)
Human esophagus (explants)	0.7	(11)	Autrup and Harris (1983)
Human bladder (explants)	6.4	(35)	Stoner et al. (1982)
(cells)	1.5	(3)	Autrup et al. (1981)
Nontarget organs			
Human liver (explants)	0.4	(6)	Autrup et al. (1984)
Human colon (explants)	0.3	(27)	Autrup and Harris (1983)

[a]Number of cases

Table 2
Interindividual Variation in B[a]P-DNA Binding in Cultured Human Tissues and Cells

	Fold variation	References
Human oral mucosa (cell)	2	Autrup et al. (1985)
Human trachea	6	Harris et al. (1984)
Human bronchus (explant)	75	Harris et al. (1984)
(cells)	2	Lechner et al. (1981)
Human peripheral lung	5	Stoner et al. (1978)
Human esophagus	99	Harris et al. (1984)
Human bladder (explant)	68	Harris et al. (1984)
(cells)	3	Autrup et al. (1981)

tion of a covalently formed adduct. HPLC analysis of the enzyme-digested DNA (Jeffrey et al. 1977) revealed that the major adduct was formed in the reaction between this metabolite and the exocyclic 2-amino group of guanine. This adduct was the major adduct in all human tissues investigated (Table 5); but minor adducts were also formed by the reaction with adenine and possibly cytosine. The binding of 7,12-dimethylbenz(a)anthracene to DNA (DMBA) in human bronchial explants was a DMBA dihydrodiol epoxide-deoxyguanosine adduct.

The metabolism of B[a]P is influenced by several exogenous factors including cigarette smoke constituents (Conney 1982). However, when we studied the metabolism of B[a]P in bronchial explant from nonsmokers and smokers, no significant difference in binding between the two groups was observed (Table 6).

DISCUSSION

The results suggest that human tissues exposed to tobacco-related carcinogens in vivo activate the PAH to their ultimate carcinogenic form. The binding level was

Table 3
Water Soluble B[a]P Metabolites of Total Metabolites

	(%) Total metabolites	References
Target organs		
Human trachea	28.4	Autrup et al. (1980)
Human bronchus	33.4	Autrup et al. (1980)
Human esophagus	24.9	Harris et al. (1979)
Human bladder (cell)	18.3	Autrup et al. (1981)
Nontarget organs		
Human liver	74.6	Autrup et al. (1984)
Human colon	50.0	Autrup (1979)

Table 4
Relative Distribution of B[a]P Metabolites Formed in Human Tissues and Cells (B[a]P 7,8-Diol = 1)

Human	Tetrols	9,10-diol	4,5-diol	Quinone	Phenol	References
Oral mucosa	5.5	1.4	0.4	0.1	0.4	H. Autrup et al., in prep.
Trachea	4.4	5.8	0.8	5.4	1.3	Autrup et al. (1983)
Bronchus (cells)	4.2	8.0	0.1	ND	0.5	Autrup et al. (1983)
(explants)	4.2	5.6	0.8	5.2	1.2	Autrup et al. (1983)
Peripheral lung	4.5	0.4	0.0	0.4	0.3	Autrup et al. (1983)
Esophagus	0.9	2.5	0.8	4.0	1.1	Harris et al. (1979)
Bladder cells	0.3	1.1	0.1	0.2	0.5	Autrup et al. (1981)
Nontarget organs						
Liver	ND					Autrup et al. (1984)
Colon	0.4	2.1	ND	ND	3.2	Autrup et al. (1982)

ND - not detectable

Table 5
Relative Distribution of B[a]P-DNA Adducts in Cultured Human Cells and Tissues

			Adducts (%)			
	Unknown I	Unknown II	BPDEI-Gua	BPDEII-Gua	BPDE-Ade	References
Bronchus (explants)	9	8	77	7	ND	Autrup and Harris (1983)
Esophagus (explants)	—	28	64	6	ND	Autrup and Harris (1983)
Oral mucosa (cells)	9	4	65	13	3	H. Autrup et al., in prep.
Liver (explants)	3	2	73	9	3	Autrup et al. (1984)

ND - not detectable

Table 6
Binding of B[a]P to Human Bronchial DNA (Effect of Smoking)

	pmoles B[a]P per 10 mg DNA	No. of cases
Whole group	41 +/- 50[a]	(34)
Never smoked	41 +/- 58	(14)
Smokers		
Years smoking		
< 20	57 +/- 81	(13)
20-49	32 +/- 40	(7)
> 50	—	
Number of cigarettes smoked		
< 20	31 +/- 36	(6)
20-29	61 +/- 10	(3)
> 30	41 +/- 51	(3)
Do not know	50 +/- 46	(3)

[a] mean +/- SEM

significantly higher in those organs with an increased risk of cancer, such as bronchus and oral mucosa, than in nontarget organs for B[a]P carcinogenesis. When the metabolism of different carcinogenic PAHs was investigated in human bronchial explants, the compound of the highest carcinogenic potency also exhibited the highest level of binding to DNA (Harris et al. 1974). A similar observation has been made in mouse skin in vivo in relation to skin tumor-initiating activity (Slaga et al. 1982). The binding level of B[a]P to human bronchial DNA corresponded to the level in hamster, a species highly susceptible to the carcinogenic action of B[a]P (Autrup et al. 1980). However, a wide interindividual variation, more than 75-fold, in the binding of B[a]P to DNA has been observed in human bronchus although the binding levels had a unimodal distribution without any subpopulation being present.

Culture of the tissues prior to incubation with carcinogens appears to be important for two reasons: (1) to minimize the effect of any exogenous exposure to inducers of mixed-function oxidases, e.g., cigarette smoking (Lodovici et al. 1983) and polychlorinated biphenyls (Wong et al. 1985); and (2) reversal of cellular ischemia and recovery of cytochrome P-450-associated enzyme activity (Autrup and Harris 1983). The ability of the target cells to activate PAH in cigarette smoke has also been demonstrated by induction of unscheduled DNA synthesis in bronchial (Doolittle et al. 1985) and oral mucosa cells (Ide et al. 1982) and by using human bronchial epithelial cells as the activating cells in a cell-mediated mutagenesis assay (Hsu et al. 1978). The cell-mediated mutagenesis approach may be useful in predicting the organ specificity of chemical carcinogens (Langenbach and Nesnow 1983).

When the metabolism of B[a]P was investigated in different segments of the human respiratory tract, the highest level of activity was found in the peripheral lung; and studies with isolated cells from the rabbit lung suggest that the Clara cells have the highest cytochrome P-450-related activities (Devereux et al. 1985). Pulmonary alveolar macrophages that may play an important role in tobacco-induced lung carcinogenesis also metabolized B[a]P extensively (Autrup et al. 1978). Cultured human tissues do also metabolize other classes of tobacco carcinogens, e.g., N-nitrosamines and aromatic amines (Autrup 1982), but the highest level of activation as measured by binding to DNA was observed with B[a]P.

CONCLUSION

Cultured human tissues from organs susceptible to tobacco-related carcinogens can metabolically convert these compounds into their ultimate carcinogenic and mutagenic forms. In the case of B[a]P, the binding to DNA appears to be higher than in organs not susceptible to tobacco carcinogens. The effect of several other factors that may increase the incidence of lung cancer in smokers can be investigated in in vitro systems using human tissues. Asbestos has been found to influence the uptake and metabolism of B[a]P in hamster tracheal cells (Eastman et al. 1983). It has been demonstrated that a noncarcinogenic component of cigarette smoke, e.g., benzo(e)pyrene, modified the tumor-inducing activity of B[a]P and altered the binding of B[a]P to DNA in hamster embryo cells (Smolarek and Baird 1984); and a tobacco smoke fraction has been found to inhibit B[a]P metabolism in isolated perfused lung (Bialer et al. 1984). Because of these conflicting observations, a careful study of the role of tobacco smoke condensate and its component in the metabolism of tobacco carcinogens in human target tissues is a high priority.

ACKNOWLEDGMENT

The author would like to thank his coworkers and collaborators, Drs. C.C. Harris, R.C. Grafstrom, A.M. Jeffrey, J.F. Lechner, G.D. Stoner, and B.F. Trump for valuable contributions to the various projects, as well as Dr. Leisgaard Christensen for valuable criticism of the manuscript. The Fibiger Institute is sponsored by a grant from the Danish Cancer Society.

REFERENCES

Autrup, H. 1979. Separation of water-soluble metabolites from cultured human colon. *Biochem. Pharmacol.* **28**: 1727.
———. 1982. Metabolism of chemical carcinogens by human tissues. *Drug Metab. Rev.* **13**: 603.

Autrup, H. and C.C. Harris. 1983. Metabolism of chemical carcinogens by human tissues and cells. In *Human carcinogenesis* (ed. C.C. Harris and H. Autrup), p. 169. Academic Press, New York.

Autrup, H., R. Grafström, and C.C. Harris. 1983. Metabolism of chemical carcinogens by tracheobronchial tissues. *Basic Life Sci.* **24**: 473.

Autrup, H., R.C. Grafström, B. Christensen, and J. Kieler. 1981. Metabolism of chemical carcinogens by cultured human and rat bladder epithelial cells. *Carcinogenesis* **2**: 763.

Autrup, H., R.C. Grafström, M. Brugh et al. 1982. Comparison of benzo(a)pyrene metabolism in bronchus, colon, esophagus and duodenum from the same individual. *Cancer Res.* **42**: 934.

Autrup, H., C.C. Harris, G. Stoner et al. 1978. Metabolism of ^{3}H-benzo(a)pyrene by cultured human bronchus and pulmonary alveolar macrophages. *Lab. Invest.* **38**: 217.

Autrup, H., C.C. Harris, S.-M. Wu et al. 1984. Activation of chemical carcinogens by cultured human fetal liver, esophagus and stomach. *Chem. Biol. Interact.* **50**: 15.

Autrup, H., T. Seremet, D. Arenholt et al. 1985. Metabolism of benzo(a)pyrene by cultured rat and human buccal mucosa cells. *Carcinogenesis* (in press).

Autrup, H., F.C. Wefald, A.M. Jeffrey et al. 1980. Metabolism of benzo(a)pyrene by cultured tracheobronchial tissues from mice, rats, hamsters, bovine and humans. *Int. J. Cancer* **25**: 293.

Bialer, M., S.D. Sloneker, and H.B. Kostenbauder. 1984. Isolation of a cigarette smoke fraction responsible for the inhibition of benzo(a)pyrene metabolism in the isolated perfused rabbit lung. *Chem. Biol. Interact.* **51**: 309.

Boyd, M.R., J.J. Grygiel, and R.F. Minchin. 1983. Metabolic activation as a basis for organ selective toxicity. *Clin. Exp. Pharmacol. Physiol.* **10**: 87.

Conney, A.H. 1982. Induction of microsomal enzymes by foreign chemicals and carcinogenesis by polycyclic aromatic hydrocarbons. *Cancer Res.* **42**: 4875.

Devereux, T.R., J.J. Diliberto, and J.R. Fouts. 1985. Cytochrome P-450 monooxygenase, epoxide hydrolase and flavin monooxygenase activities in Clara cells and alveolar type II cells isolated from rabbit. *Cell. Biol. Toxicol.* **1**: 57.

Doolittle, D.J., J.W. Furlong, and B.E. Butterworth. 1985. Assessment of chemically induced DNA repair in primary cultures of human bronchial epithelial cells. *Toxicol. Appl. Pharmacol.* **79**: 28.

Eastman, A., B.T. Mossman, and E. Bresnick. 1983. Influence of asbestos on the uptake of benzo(a)pyrene and DNA alkylation in hamster tracheal epithelial cells. *Cancer Res.* **43**: 1251.

Harris, C.C., H. Autrup, K. Vahakangas, and B.F. Trump. 1984. Interindividual variations in carcinogen activation and DNA repair. *Banbury report 16: Genetic variability in responses to chemical exposure* (ed. G.S. Omenn and H.V. Gelboin), p. 157. Cold Spring Harbor Laboratory, Cold Spring Harbor, New York.

Harris, C.C., B.F. Trump, R.G. Grafström, and H. Autrup. 1982. Differences in metabolism of chemical carcinogens in cultured human epithelial tissues. *J. Cell. Biochem.* **18**: 285.

Harris, C.C., H. Autrup, G.D. Stoner et al. 1979. Metabolism of benzo(a)pyrene, nitrosomethylamine and N-nitrosopyrrolidine and identification of the major carcinogen-DNA adducts formed in cultured human esophagus. *Cancer Res.* **39**: 4401.

Harris, C.C., V. Genta, A. Frank et al. 1974. Carcinogenic polynuclear hydrocarbons bind to macromolecules in cultured human bronchi. *Nature* **252**: 68.

Hecht, S.S., E. LaVoie, A. Amin et al. 1980. On the metabolic activation of the benzofluoranthenes. In *Polynuclear aromatic hydrocarbons: Chemistry and biological effects* (ed. A. Bjørseth and A.J. Dennis), p. 417. Battelle Press, Ohio.

Hodgson, R.M., K. Pal, P.L. Grover, and P. Sim. 1982. The metabolic activation of chrysene by hamster embryo cells. *Carcinogenesis* **3**: 1051.

Hoffmann, D., I. Schmeltz, S.S. Hecht, and E.L. Wynder. 1978. Tobacco carcinogenesis. In *Polycyclic hydrocarbons and cancer*, vol. I, p. 85. Academic Press, New York.

Hsu, I-C., G.D. Stoner, H. Autrup et al. 1978. Human bronchus-mediated mutagenesis of mammalian cells by carcinogen polynuclear aromatic hydrocarbons. *Proc. Natl. Acad. Sci. U.S.A.* **75**: 2003.

Ide, F., T. Ishikawa, M. Takagi et al. 1982. Unscheduled DNA synthesis in human oral mucosa treated with chemical carcinogens in short-term organ culture. *J. Natl. Cancer Inst.* **69**: 557.

Ittah, Y., D.R. Thakker, W. Levin et al. 1983. Metabolism of benzo(a)phenanthrene by rat liver microsomes and by a purified monooxygenase system reconstituted with different isozymes of cytochrome P-450. *Chem. Biol. Interact.* **45**: 15.

Jeffrey, A.M., I.B. Weinstein, K.W. Jennette et al. 1977. Structures of benzo(a)pyrene-nucleic acid adducts formed in human and bovine bronchial explants. *Nature* **269**: 348.

Kuroki, T., J. Hosomi, K. Munakata et al. 1982. Metabolism of benzo(a)pyrene in epidermal keratinocytes and dermal fibroblasts of humans and mice with reference to variation among species, individuals, and cell types. *Cancer Res.* **42**: 1859.

Langenbach, R. and S. Nesnow. 1983. Cell mediated mutagenesis, an in vitro approach to study organ specificity of chemical carcinogens. In *Safety evaluation and regulation of chemicals* (ed. F. Hamburger), p. 142. S. Karger, Basel, Switzerland.

LaVoie, E.J., S.S. Hecht, V. Bedenko, and D. Hoffmann. 1982. Identification of the mutagenic metabolites of fluoranthene, 2-methylfluoranthene, and 3-methylfluoranthene. *Carcinogenesis* **3**: 841.

Lechner, J.F., A. Haugen, H. Autrup et al. 1981. Clonal growth of epithelial cells from normal adult human bronchus. *Cancer Res.* **41**: 2294.

Lodovici, M., P. Dolara, G. Caderni et al. 1983. The effect of cigarette smoke on aryl hydrocarbon hydroxylase (AHH) activity of the human kidney. *Eur. J. Cancer Clin. Oncol.* **19**: 1565.

Mass, M.J., and D.G. Kaufman. 1983. A comparison between the activation of benzo(a)pyrene in organ cultures and microsomes from the tracheal epithelium of rats and hamsters. *Carcinogenesis* **4**: 297.

Melikian, A.A., E.J. LaVoie, S.S. Hecht, and D. Hoffmann. 1983. 5-methylchrysene metabolism in mouse epidermis *in vivo*, diolepoxide DNA adduct persistence, and diol epoxide reactivity with DNA. *Carcinogenesis* 4: 843.

Miller, E.C. 1978. Some current perspectives on chemical carcinogenesis in humans and experimental animals. *Cancer Res.* 38: 1479.

Nakayama, J., S.H. Yuspa, and M.C. Poirier. 1984. Benzo(a)pyrene DNA adduct formation and removal in mouse epidermis *in vivo* and *in vitro*: Relationship of DNA binding to initiation of skin carcinogenesis. *Cancer Res.* 44: 4087.

Perin-Roussel, O., S. Saquem, B. Ekert, and F. Zajdela. 1983. Binding to DNA of bay region and pseudo bay region diol epoxides of dibenzo(a,e)fluoranthene and comparison with adducts obtained with dibenzo(a,e)fluoranthene or its dihydrodiols in the presence of microsomes. *Carcinogenesis* 4: 27.

Slaga, T.J., S.M. Fischer, C.E. Weeks et al. 1982. Studies on the mechanisms involved in multistage carcinogenesis in mouse skin. *J. Cell. Biochem.* 18: 99.

Smolarek, T.A. and W.M. Baird. 1984. Benzo(a)pyrene induced alterations in the binding of benzo(a)pyrene to DNA in hamster embryo cell cultures. *Carcinogenesis* 5: 1065.

Stampfer, M.R., J.C. Bartholomew, H.S. Smith, and J.C. Bartley. 1981. Metabolism of benzo(a)pyrene by human mammary epithelial cells: Toxicity and DNA adduct formation. *Proc. Natl. Acad. Sci. U.S.A.* 78: 6251.

Stoner, G.D., F.B. Daniel, K.M. Schenck et al. 1982. Metabolism and DNA binding of benzo(a)pyrene in cultured human bladder and bronchus. *Carcinogenesis* 3: 195.

Stoner, G.D., C.C. Harris, H. Autrup, B.F. Trump, E.W. Kinesbury, and G. Myers. 1978. Explant culture of human peripheral lung. I. Metabolism of benzo(a)pyrene. *Lab. Invest.* 38: 685.

Theall, G., G. Hatch, I.B. Weinstein et al. 1982. Quantitative relationship between DNA adduct formation and biological effects. *Banbury report 13: Indicators of genotoxic exposure* (ed. B.A. Bridges, B.E. Butterworth, and I.B. Weinstein), p. 231. Cold Spring Harbor Laboratory, Cold Spring Harbor, New York.

van Bladeren, P.J., R.N. Armstrong, D.R. Thakker et al. 1982. Stereoselective formation of benz(a)anthracene (+) (55,6R) oxide and (+) (8R,9S)oxide by a highly purified and reconstituted system containing cytochrome P450c. *Biochem. Biophys. Res. Commun.* 106: 602.

Vigny, P., M. Spiro, R.M. Hodgson et al. 1982. Fluorescence spectral studies on the metabolic activation of chrysene by hamster embryo cells. *Carcinogenesis* 3: 1491.

Vyas, K.P., W. Levin, H. Yagi et al. 1982. Stereoselective metabolism of the (+) and (−) enantiomers of *trans* 1,2 dihydroxyl, 2 dihydrochrysene to bay region 1,2 diol 3,4 epoxide diastereomers by rat liver enzymes. *Mol. Pharmacol.* 22: 182.

Wong, T.K., R.B. Everson, and S.T. Hsu. 1985. Potent induction of human placental monooxygenase activity by previous dietary exposure to polychlorinated biphenyls and their thermal degradation products. *Lancet* i: 721.

COMMENTS

HOFFMANN: You find great variation in the binding of B[a]P in your explants. Do you have the case histories of the donors of these explants?

AUTRUP: Yes, we have case histories, and the binding data of B[a]P to bronchial DNA is being analyzed with respect to the case histories. We have obtained fetal liver from identical twins, and there were no differences in the binding of B[a]P to DNA in these two individuals. B[a]P-DNA adduct patterns were also completely identical.

HOFFMANN: In other words, do you think the recorded differences are primarily due to underlying genetic factors?

AUTRUP: Yes, it is genetic; and there's nothing methological in it. We have reported a coefficient of variation of 0.94. Furthermore, in the case of colonic tissues, we have happened to get a slice of colon from the same patient at a 2-month interval. When we did the metabolism studies there, we found no difference in the binding level.

CONNEY: Clearly, the environment is important—even with cultured cells which have an environment of culture medium. This system is a long way from living people. Doing assays with fresh tissues before culturing them could give results closer to what is observed in vivo.

AUTRUP: Yes, but for all the studies you will use the same cell environment, and we are using chemical defined media. There's no serum or anything that might influence the P-450 system. You can create different kinds of environments in the cell culture medium, and you can add an inducer as well.

HOFFMANN: In other words, treat the medium with serum from smokers and nonsmokers, is that what you feel? Do you see differences then?

AUTRUP: A few years ago there was a paper in *Biochemical Pharmacology* that reported the induction of the metabolism in animal cell culture by various batches of human serum and found that various batches of human serum induced the metabolism to a different extent. I haven't seen any paper in that area since then. We are able to induce the enzyme activity in our explant cultures when treated with traditional inducers, such as benz[a]-anthracene. We would like to extend these types of studies. Recently we studied the metabolism in human bladder cells. When you keep cells in culture for extended periods, they appeared to lose their metabolic activity and that is caused by deficiencies in the media composition. But when we supplement the media with components that are required for the synthesis of the P-450 enzyme, then we are able to increase the metabolic rate, even without induction. Then, on top of that, we can induce the P-450 more than in the nonsupplemented media.

HALEY: Are these cells subcultured?

AUTRUP: They are primary cultures.

TANNENBAUM: But you said that they are fibroblasts.

AUTRUP: They are both. You can get either fibroblastic or epithelial cultures.

TANNENBAUM: I thought you said that from many of those tissues you only got fibroblasts.

AUTRUP: No, no. We can get both.

TANNENBAUM: Isolated from one another.

AUTRUP: Oh, yes.

TANNENBAUM: But I think that you showed a clear example of the difficulties of going to less organized systems; and that if you looked at the tetrols, there was a gradient going from microsomes through cells to explants. One of the problems with all of the in vitro studies is just the limitation of the whole approach: One tends to have to work with higher substrate concentrations than one ever encounters under physiological conditions.

AUTRUP: Correct. If you look at the adduct pattern using the subcellular system, it is quite different from the one we see in the intact cell; it is much more complicated.

GRAFSTRÖM: Another reason for interindividual variation is that these experiments are not done at concentrations that saturate the involved enzymes. The concentrations are usually at 1.5 μM, which does not saturate the cytochrome P-450 system and indicates that some of the variation is dependent on the enzyme kinetics.

YOAKUM: Since you mentioned the activation of the *ras* genes, would you care to comment on the chemistry that led you to take a look at that?

AUTRUP: The *ras* gene activation at the 12 codon involves a $G \cdot C \rightarrow AT$ transversion.

Pathobiological Effects of Tobacco Smoke-related Aldehydes in Cultured Human Bronchial Epithelial Cells

ROLAND C. GRAFSTROM,* JAMES C. WILLEY,† KRISTINA SUNDQVIST,*
AND CURTIS C. HARRIS†
*Department of Toxicology
Karolinska Institute
S-10401 Stockholm
Sweden
†Laboratory of Human Carcinogenesis
National Cancer Institute
Bethesda, Maryland 20892

OVERVIEW

The causal relationship between smoking of tobacco products and the induction of bronchial carcinoma is well established. More than 6000 chemicals have been identified in tobacco smoke. These compounds represent different chemical classes, some of which may cause pathobiological effects associated with the multistep process of carcinogenesis. We have recently investigated the effects of the tobacco smoke-related aldehydes, e.g., formaldehyde, acetaldehyde, and acrolein, in epithelial cells and fibroblasts from human bronchus. These aldehydes each cause a different spectrum of biological effects in these normal human cells, including inhibition of proliferation, enhanced terminal squamous differentiation of the epithelial cells, DNA damage, mutation, and inhibition of DNA repair. We conclude that tobacco smoke-related aldehydes directly cause effects that relate to both the initiation and promotion stages of the carcinogenesis process. Furthermore, we speculate that aldehydes may function as cocarcinogens in tobacco smoke by inhibiting the repair of smoke-induced DNA damage.

INTRODUCTION

One approach to the extrapolation of experimental animal data to humans is the development of in vitro model systems using human tissues and cells. Remarkable progress has been made during the last few years in establishing conditions for culturing normal human epithelial tissues and cells. Isolated epithelial cells can now be transferred at clonal density for three or more times and grown for more than 30 cell generations in serum-free media (Lechner et al. 1986). Using this system, we are presently studying the pathobiological effects of many environmentally and endogenously occurring agents that may be cytotoxic or carcinogenic to the lung. Parameters measured relate to cell survival, changes of growth and differentiation, metabolism of chemical carcinogens, DNA damage and repair, and malignant transformation (Harris et al. 1985a,b).

Several reactive and volatile aldehydes are found in the gaseous phase of tobacco smoke and are interesting because of their potential carcinogenicity in the human respiratory tract. In particular, formaldehyde, acrolein, and acetaldehyde are present in amounts ranging from μg to mg per cigarette (Wynder and Hoffmann 1979). Such aldehydes are also metabolites of xenobiotics, e.g., N-nitrosodimethylamine, cyclophosphamide, and ethanol, and are formed endogenously as products of normal intermediary metabolism.

In this study we have investigated the effects of these aldehydes on different biological parameters including colony survival, clonal growth, morphology, crosslinked envelope formation, content of cellular thiols, DNA damage, mutations, and effects on O^6-methylguanine (O^6-mG) repair in cultured human bronchial cells. The potency of and mechanism by which these aldehydes cause different cyto- and genotoxic effects are compared and discussed.

RESULTS

The effects of acrolein, formaldehyde, and acetaldehyde on cell survival, cellular content of glutathione (GSH), and O^6-methylguanine-DNA methyltransferase (O^6-MT) activity in human bronchial fibroblasts are summarized in Table 1. The survival of fibroblasts was measured as the colony-forming efficiency (CFE) of cells cultured at clonal density. Clearly, acrolein was substantially more cytotoxic than formaldehyde, which in turn was markedly more toxic than acetaldehyde. The dose required to reduce CFE to 50% of control after a 1-hour exposure was about 2 μM for acrolein, 400 μM for formaldehyde, and 10 mM for acetaldehyde. However, mass cultures of quiescent fibroblasts maintained at confluency were less sensitive to aldehyde-induced cytotoxicity. When confluent cells were subcultured 48 hours after exposure to either formaldehyde or acrolein, approximately fivefold higher concentrations were required to inhibit CFE to an extent similar to that of exponentially growing cells (data not shown).

The cellular content of thiols, mainly GSH, protects the cell against cytotoxic effects by reacting with electrophilic compounds. As shown in Table 1, exposure of cells to acrolein markedly depleted the cellular GSH content. Formaldehyde or acetaldehyde only slightly decreased GSH. All three aldehydes affected survival and GSH content of cultured bronchial epithelial cells (data not shown) and fibroblasts similarly.

The repair of O^6-methylguanine (O^6-mG) is catalyzed by O^6-MT and involves the direct removal and transfer of the methyl group from guanine in DNA to a cysteine residue at the O^6-MT protein (Yarosh 1985). Because of the high reactivity of aldehydes towards thiols, we investigated their effects on O^6-MT. When cell extracts were isolated subsequent to the exposure of fibroblasts to either acrolein

Table 1
Effects of Tobacco Smoke-related Aldehydes on Colony-forming Efficiency, Glutathione Content, and O^6-methylguanine-DNA Methyltransferase Activity of Human Bronchial Fibroblasts[a]

Aldehyde (mM)	Colony-forming efficiency[b]	GSH content[c]	O^6-MT activity[d]
Acrolein			
0.001	92	NT	NT
0.003	45	91	NT
0.010	5	46	79
0.030	<1	11	60
0.100	<1	6	35
Formaldehyde			
0.1	76	97	89
0.3	58	82	84
1.0	8	71	NT
3.0	<1	71	NT
Acetaldehyde			
1.0	80	106	NT
3.0	75	99	NT
10.0	48	76	NT

[a] Cells were exposed to the various concentrations of the respective aldehyde for 1 hr in serum-free LHC medium.

[b] Mean CFE was assayed as described (Lechner et al. 1986), expressed as percent of control (220 colonies), and determined from colonies containing at least 12 cells after 7-day post-treatment culture of 500 fibroblasts per dish. The variation between data points obtained from duplicate dishes was less than 10%.

[c] Cells were assayed for their content of GSH as described by Cotgreave et al. (1986). The results are the mean of three independent determinations and expressed as percent of control. Untreated fibroblasts contained 52 ± 10 nmole GSH per 10^6 cells.

[d] Extracts were prepared subsequent to exposure of cells to the respective aldehyde, and O^6-methyltransferase activity assayed in vitro and expressed as percent of control as described (Krokan et al. 1985).

NT - not tested

or formaldehyde, the O^6-MT activity was markedly inhibited by acrolein and to a lesser degree with formaldehyde (Krokan et al. 1985) (Table 1). Neither of these aldehydes significantly affected the uracil-DNA glycosylase activity (date not shown).

Squamous differentiation of cultured epithelial cells is characterized by decreased clonal growth rate, formation of cross-linked envelopes, and flattening of cells, leading to an increased surface area (Willey et al. 1984a). As assayed by the clonal growth assay, the aldehydes were all growth-inhibitory in a dose-dependent fashion. Inhibition of the growth rate to approximately 50% was obtained at the concentration of 10 μM acrolein, 200 μM formaldehyde, or 30 mM acetaldehyde (Table 2). At these doses all aldehydes markedly increased the formation of cross-

Table 2
Effects of Tobacco Smoke-related Aldehydes on Growth and Differentiation of Human Bronchial Epithelial Cells

Aldehyde	Colony-forming efficiency[a] (mM)	Clonal growth rate[b] (mM)	Cell surface area[c] (μ^2)	Cross-linked envelope formation[d] (%)
Control	—	—	930 ± 270	2 ± 1
Acrolein	0.002	0.01	2550 ± 840	23 ± 3
Formaldehyde	0.40	0.20	983 ± 400	12 ± 2
Acetaldehyde	10.0	30.0	3200 ± 680	7 ± 2

[a]The concentration that produced a 50% reduction in colony survival after a 1-hr exposure of cells to the respective aldehyde in serum-free LHC-medium

[b]The concentration that produced a 50% reduction in clonal growth rate after 6-hr exposure. Assays were performed as described (Lechner et al. 1986).

[c]The median cell planar surface area was calculated from 250 randomly selected cells after exposure to the representive aldehydes for 6 hr. Assays were performed as described (Saladino et al. 1985).

[d]The mean cross-linked envelope frequency in the total cell population after exposure to the respective aldehyde for 6 hr at the concentration that inhibited the clonal growth to 50%. Assays were performed as described (Willey et al. 1984a).

linked envelopes, an event considered to occur late in terminal squamous differentiation. The median cell surface area was increased approximately threefold by exposure to acetaldehyde or acrolein, but insignificantly changed by formaldehyde.

Cigarette smoke in phosphate-buffered saline was recently shown to produce high levels of DNA single-strand breaks (SSB) in cultured human lung carcinoma cells (Nakayama et al. 1985). The ability of cigarette smoke condensate (CSC) and aldehydes to cause DNA damage in cultured human bronchial epithelial cells was measured by the sensitive alkaline elution technique (Table 3).

Table 3
DNA Single-strand Breaks and DNA Protein Cross-links Caused by Different Aldehydes or Cigarette Smoke Condensate in Human Bronchial Epithelial Cells

Agents	Dose	SSB/10^{10} daltons	DPC/10^{10} daltons
Formaldehyde	100 μM	1.4	10.8
Acrolein	100 μM	6.9	6.8
Acetaldehyde	1000 μM	<1.0	<2.0
CSC	100 μg/ml	2.1	<2.0

[a]Cells were exposed to the indicated aldehyde for 1 hr or CSC for 3 hr in serum-free LHC medium and subsequently assayed for DNA damage by the alkaline elution technique as described (Kohn et al. 1981; Grafstrom et al. 1984a).

Cigarette smoke condensate produced only low levels of SSB and no detectable DNA protein cross-links (DPC) at a concentration of 100 μg/ml, a highly cytotoxic dose to human bronchial epithelial cells (J.C. Willey et al., unpubl.). Exposure of cells to 100 μM of either acrolein or formaldehyde for 1 hour caused substantial DNA damage, whereas as much as 1 mM of acetaldehyde caused no detectable DNA damage. Formaldehyde caused substantially higher levels of DPC than SSB, whereas the level of both types of lesions was similar from exposure to acrolein. Nonsignificant levels of DNA-DNA cross-links were induced by these aldehydes at the tested concentrations.

Because formaldehyde easily reacts with cysteine in vitro, the potential effect of formaldehyde on O^6-mG repair was further investigated. Bronchial cells were exposed to N-methyl-N-nitrosourea (MNU), an agent known to cause the formation of O^6-mG in DNA (Fig. 1). Only about 20% of the initial MNU-induced levels of O^6-mG remain in DNA 5 hours following a 1-hour exposure of the cells to 200 μM MNU. However, when the MNU-treated cells were incubated in the presence of either 100 μM or 300 μM formaldehyde, a significantly slower rate of removal of O^6-mG was observed in three independent experiments (Grafstrom et al. 1985).

To further study the pathobiological consequences of formaldehyde exposure and inhibition of O^6-mG repair, we investigated the cytotoxic and mutagenic effects of formaldehyde and MNU separately and in combination (Table 4). The decrease in cell survival from the combination of formaldehyde and MNU was additive rather than synergistic when compared to the effects of each of these agents separately. Although the exposure times differed, formaldehyde was three times more mutagenic on a molar basis than MNU. However, addition of 50 μM or 75 μM formaldehyde to 200 μM MNU-treated cells resulted in a mutation frequency that was significantly greater than that found with either agent alone (Grafstrom et al. 1985).

DISCUSSION

Human bronchial epithelial cells or fibroblasts in serial culture provide useful in vitro model systems for studying the pathobiological effects of tobacco-smoke fractions and constituents. As a broad endpoint, cytotoxicity, in terms of reproductive sterilization, can be quantitated by measuring the colony-forming ability of cells passaged at low density. Exposure of cells to any of the three tobacco smoke-related aldehydes caused a different pattern of pathobiological response. Acrolein markedly reduced the cell survival at 3 μM, whereas, one or two orders of magnitude higher concentrations of either formaldehyde or acetaldehyde were required to significantly decrease the survival. As compared to the effective dose required to inhibit colony survival, threefold higher concentrations of acrolein were required to significantly decrease the clonal growth rate of a small number of surviving cells. In contrast, formaldehyde significantly decreased the clonal growth

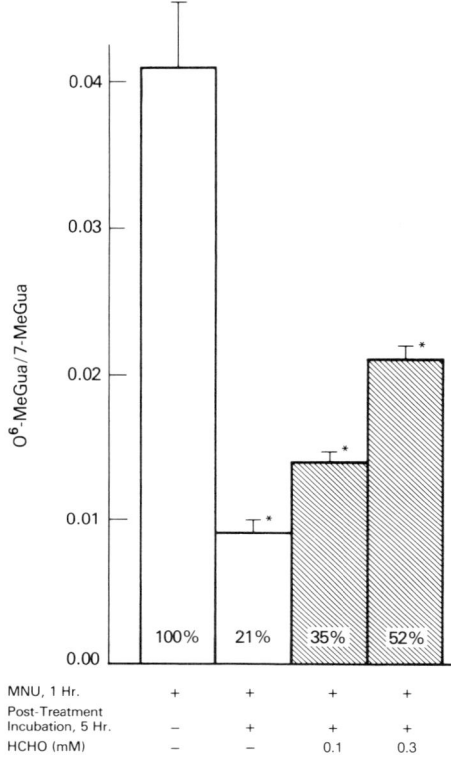

Figure 1
Effect of formaldehyde on the repair of O^6-mG in DNA of human fibroblasts exposed to MNU. Cells were initially exposed to 200 μM MNU. Values are ratios of O^6-mG to 7-methylguanine (7-mG) which can, over short periods of time, be used as a measure of O^6-mG repair. Experiments were performed as described in detail in Grafstrom et al. (1985).

rate at concentrations that only slightly affected colony survival. Acetaldehyde caused a response pattern of decreasing both colony survival and clonal growth rates only at very high concentrations, i.e., at least 10-30 mM.

Terminal squamous differentiation of epithelial cells is an important response from several aspects. Terminal differentiation is an active, synthetic process that is not triggered simply by inhibiting cell growth. Ultimately leading to cell death, differentiation causes a requirement for epithelial cell renewal in vivo. Another aspect of differentiation involves mechanisms of importance in multistep carcinogenesis. Resistance to inducers of terminal differentiation is regarded as one of

Table 4
Enhancement by Formaldehyde of the Mutagenicity of N-methyl-N-nitrosourea in Human Fibroblasts

Treatments		Colony forming efficiency (%)	6-Thioguanine-resistant colonies[b]	Mutation frequency (per 10^6 surviving cell)
MNU[a] (μM)	HCHO[a] (μM)			
0	0	100	0	< 2.2
0	50	82	1	1.7
0	75	40	0	< 1.8
200	0	78	3	5.4
200	50	37	24	41.9
200	75	16	28	84.6

[a] Exposure time to MNU (1 hr) and HCHO (5 hr)
[b] The expression time was 9 days. The mutation frequency was assayed as described (Grafstrom et al. 1985).
HCHO, formaldehyde

several potential clonal expansion advantages that could lead to selective survival and growth of carcinogen-initiated, preneoplastic or neoplastic cells (Yuspa and Morgan 1981; Harris et al. 1985a). Selective growth of these cells may be facilitated by induction of differentiation of the normal noninitiated cells. Because epidemiological and laboratory studies suggest that tobacco smoke has tumor-promoting activity in mouse skin carcinogenesis, (Wynder and Hoffmann 1979), it is interesting to note that the tobacco smoke-related aldehydes induced terminal differentiation as indicated by the formation of cross-linked envelopes. The concept of enhanced terminal differentiation of normal cells as a selection mechanism for preneoplastic cells is strongly supported by the fact that agents with tumor-promoting activity in the mouse skin carcinogenesis model, such as aplysiatoxin, 12-O-tetradecanoylphorbol-13-acetate (TPA), or teleocidin B, are the most potent inducers of terminal differentiation of normal human bronchial epithelial cells currently known (Willey et al. 1984a; Harris et al. 1985). Furthermore, lung carcinoma cell lines are relatively resistant to TPA-induced terminal differentiation (Willey et al. 1984b).

Conjugation with GSH constitutes a major cellular defense mechanism against toxic compounds as well as many electrophilic products of metabolic activation. To indicate the degree of chemical reactivity and the extent that tobacco smoke-related aldehydes pose a cellular challenge, the intracellular GSH content following exposure to aldehydes was investigated in bronchial cells. Exposure to acrolein markedly depleted cells of GSH in a dose-dependent manner, whereas exposure to formaldehyde or acetaldehyde only caused a minor decrease in the thiol content. The sulfhydryl group of GSH reacts with acrolein at the unsaturated β-carbon. Although formaldehyde dehydrogenase-catalyzed oxidation of formaldehyde to formate also requires reversible binding of GSH to the aldehyde group, formaldehyde is known to readily and irreversibly react with cysteine to give thiazolidinecarboxylic acid (Schauenstein et al. 1977). Thus, it should be noted that the reduced thiol components in the cell culture media could variably affect the biological effects exerted by reactive aldehydes.

Aldehydes are also generated from metabolism of N-nitrosamines, including those found in tobacco smoke. For example, N-nitrosodimethylamine is metabolically activated to yield alkyldiazonium ion and formaldehyde in equal amounts (Fig. 2). Whereas, the alkyldiazonium ion formed in this reaction is thought to be responsible for the carcinogenicity of N-nitrosamines, the possible effects of aldehydes has been largely neglected. In addition to directly damaging DNA (Table 3), formaldehyde inhibits repair of DNA damage caused by different chemical and physical carcinogens, including ionizing radiation, UV-radiation, benzo[a]pyrene diol epoxide (Grafstrom et al. 1983), or MNU (Fig. 1) (Grafstrom et al. 1985). The repair of O^6-mG and the resealing of ionizing radiation-induced SSB seem to be preferentially sensitive to formaldehyde.

A number of mechanisms may be involved in the inhibition of DNA repair by formaldehyde. The high reactivity of the chemical probably causes methyolation and cross-linking of chromatin or other proteins, including the enzymes critical to DNA repair processes. In cultured human bronchial epithelial cells or fibroblasts, there were 25-30,000 O^6-MT molecules per cell (Grafstrom et al. 1984b),

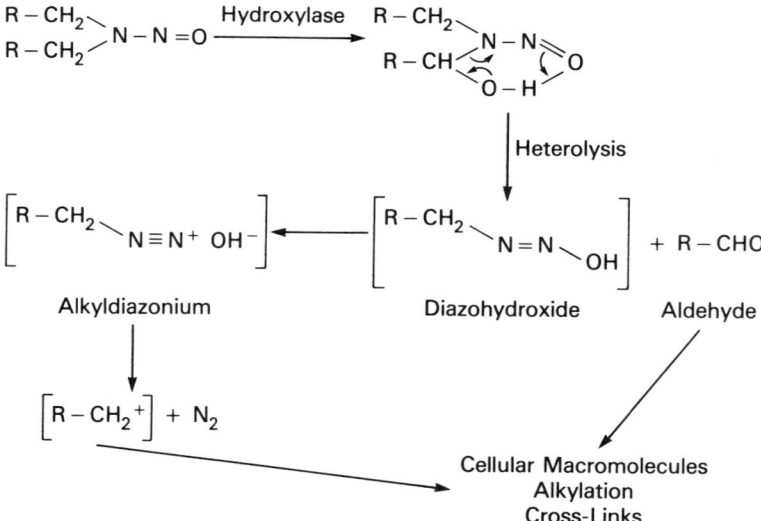

Figure 2
Metabolic activation of N-nitrosamines

which may have become partly inactivated by formaldehyde. Formaldehyde markedly inhibited the repair of O^6-mG in intact cells, whereas only a slight effect was observed on the O^6-MT activity in extracts of cells that had been previously exposed to formaldehyde. A stronger effect in intact cells may be explained by a loss of formaldehyde-induced, unstable, and reversible mono-adducts during preparation of the extracts for the in vitro assay for O^6-MT activity.

Independent of the mechanisms that may be involved, the effects of formaldehyde on DNA repair occur concomitant with potentiation of the mutagenicity of MNU in normal human fibroblasts (Grafstrom et al. 1985). Thus, the combination of MNU and formaldehyde had a higher mutagenic efficiency than did either agent alone. This result is to be expected if the persistence of the O^6-mG lesion had a more significant effect on induced mutation than it did on cell-killing. This is also further indirect evidence that O^6-mG is a promutagenic DNA lesion. In addition, MNU may inhibit the repair of promutagenic lesions caused by formaldehyde.

SUMMARY

Acrolein, acetaldehyde, or formaldehyde each cause a distinct pattern of pathobiological consequences in cultured human bronchial cells. Among these aldehydes the cytotoxicity differs by orders of magnitude; acrolein is more cytotoxic than formaldehyde, which in turn is more cytotoxic than acetaldehyde. Aldehydes cause terminal squamous differentiation of epithelial cells as indicated from the cessation of growth and increased formation of cross-linked envelopes. Of several genotoxic endpoints investigated, marked effects are induced in human cells by exposure to μM concentrations of either acrolein or formaldehyde. Induction of differentiation, DNA damage, mutation, and inhibition of DNA repair in human cells by formaldehyde seem particularly relevant because these effects occur at moderately low levels of cytotoxicity. We conclude that the aldehydes of the gaseous phase of tobacco smoke may contribute to the many pathological effects seen in the lungs of smokers. The synergistic mutation induction from the combined exposure to MNU and formaldehyde in human cells emphasize the need for further investigations of the interactive effects of the many genotoxic components of tobacco smoke. Finally, because aldehydes are also generated endogenously from metabolism of *N*-nitrosamines, more attention should be given to the potential influence of aldehydes in *N*-nitrosamine carcinogenesis.

ACKNOWLEDGMENT

We thank Drs. R.D. Curren, J. Harris, H.K. Krokan, A. Pegg, A.J. Saladino, and Li.L. Yang for valuable contributions to this work. R.C.G. and K.S. were supported in part by the Swedish Cancer Society, the Swedish Medical Research Council, the National Board of Laboratory Animals, the Swedish Work-Environment Health Fund, and the Swedish Tobacco Company.

REFERENCES

Cotgreave, I.C. and P. Moldeus. 1986. Methodologies for the application of monobromobimane to the simultaneous analysis of soluble and protein thiol components of biological systems. *J. Biochem. Biophys. Methods* (in press).

Grafstrom, R.C., A.J. Fornace, Jr., and C.C. Harris. 1984a. Repair of DNA damage caused by formaldehyde in human cells. *Cancer Res.* **44**: 4323.

Grafstrom, R.C., A.E. Pegg, B.F. Trump, and C.C. Harris. 1984b. O^6-alkylguanine-DNA alkyltransferase activity in normal human tissues and cells. *Cancer Res.* **44**: 2855.

Grafstrom, R.C., R.D. Curren, L.L. Yang, and C.C. Harris. 1985. Genotoxicity of formaldehyde in cultured human bronchial fibroblasts. *Science* **228**: 89.

Grafstrom, R.C., A.J. Fornace, Jr., H. Autrup, J.F. Lechner, and C.C. Harris. 1983. Formaldehyde damage to DNA and inhibition of DNA repair in human bronchial cells. *Science.* **220**: 216.

Harris, C.C., J.C. Willey, A.J. Saladino, and R.C. Grafstrom. 1985a. Effects of tumor promotors, aldehydes, peroxides and tobacco smoke condensate on growth and differentiation of cultured normal and transformed human bronchial cells. In *Cancer of the respiratory tract: Predisposing factors* (ed. M. Mass et al.), p. 159. Plenum Press, New York.

Harris, C.C., J.F., Lechner, G.H. Yoakum, P. Amstad, B.E. Korba, E. Gabrielson, R.C. Grafstrom, A. Shamsuddin, and B.F. Trump. 1985b. In vitro studies of human lung carcinogenesis. In *Carcinogenesis 9* (ed. J.C. Barrett and R. Tennet), p. 257. Raven Press, New York.

Kohn, K.W., L.C. Ewig, L.C. Ericson, and L.A. Zwelling. 1981. Measurement of strand breaks by alkaline elution. In *DNA repair, a laboratory manual of research procedures* (ed. E.C. Friedberg and P.C. Hanawalt), p. 379. Marcel Dekker, New York.

Krokan, H., R.C. Grafstrom, K. Sundqvist, H. Esterbauer, and C.C. Harris. 1985. Cytotoxicity, thiol depletion and inhibition of O^6-methylguanine-DNA methyltransferase by various aldehydes in cultured human bronchial fibroblasts. *Carcinogenesis.* **6**: 1755.

Lechner, J.F., G.D. Stoner, A. Haugen, J.C. Willey, B.F. Trump, and C.C. Harris. 1986. In vitro human bronchial epithelial model systems for carcinogenesis studies. In *In vitro models for cancer research* (ed. M. Webber et al.). CRC Press, New York. (In press).

Nakayama, T., M. Kaneko, M. Kodama, and C. Nagata. 1985. Cigarette smoke induces DNA single strand breaks in human cells. *Nature* **314**: 462.

Saladino, A.J., J.C. Willey, J.F. Lechner, R.C. Grafstrom, M. LaVeck, and C.C. Harris. 1985. Effects of formaldehyde, acetaldehyde, benzoyl peroxide and hydrogen peroxide on cultured normal human bronchial epithelial cells. *Cancer Res.* **45**: 2522.

Schauenstein, E., H. Esterbauer, and H. Zollner. 1977. *Aldehydes in biological systems*, Pion, London.

Willey, J.C., A.J. Saladino, J.F. Lechner, and C.C. Harris. 1984. Acute effects of 12-O-tetradecanoylphorbol-13-acetate, teleocidin, or 2,3,7,8-tetrachlorodibenzo-p-dioxin on cultured normal human bronchial epithelial cells. *Carcinogenesis.* **5**: 209.

Willey, J.C., C.E. Moser, Jr., J.F. Lechner, and C.C. Harris. 1984. Differential effects of 12-O-tetradecanoylphorbol-13-acetate on cultured normal and neoplastic human bronchial epithelial cells. *Cancer Res.* **44**: 5124.

Wynder, E.L. and D. Hoffmann. 1979. Tobacco and health. A social challenge. *N. Engl. J. Med.* **300**: 894.

Yarosh, D.B. 1985. The role of O^6-methylguanine-DNA methyltransferase in cell survival, mutagenesis and carcinogenesis. *Mutat. Res.* **145**: 1.

Yuspa, S.H. and D.L. Morgan. 1981. Mouse skin resistant to terminal differentiation associated with initiation of carcinogenesis. *Nature* **293**: 72.

COMMENTS

TANNENBAUM: It wasn't clear how you got into the 4-hydroxyalkenals, but there was a paper in *Science* very recently which has proposed these as the putative toxic metabolites, derived from the pyrolizidine alkaloids. I don't know if you saw that.

GRAFSTRÖM: No, I had not seen that. *Science* is delivered in Sweden more than one month later than it is in the United States. Our interest in these aldehydes arises from the fact that they are very similar to acrolein in their structure and because they are generated during lipid peroxidation, a process that may be important during tumor promotion. These lipid peroxidation aldehydes are formed as a consequence of the generation of active oxygen and lipid decomposition which has been proposed by Dr. Cerutti to be important in tumor promotion. The ability of these aldehydes to deplete thiols may further enhance lipid peroxidation and production of aldehydes.

PEGG: Roland [Grafström], are your cells growing, in culture, or are they stable?

GRAFSTRÖM: I am glad you asked that question because I would like to discuss it. In the clonal growth assay, about 5,000 cells are seeded on the dish, and the colony-forming efficiency and clonal growth rate of these cells is quantitated subsequent to exposure to your agent. In the alkaline elution assay or for measuring cellular thiols, between 100,000 cells to 200,000 cells are present on the dish. When you study these reactive aldehydes, the magnitude of the effects will depend on the number of cells that are present on your dish. In fact, I have calculated that the number of molecules of acrolein in 5 ml of medium is quite similar to the number of total thiol groups, in terms of molecules present in 100,000 cells. Accordingly, the magnitude of your result will be different if you have 50,000 instead of 100,000 cells per dish, or if you add 2 ml instead of 5 ml of acrolein solution to the dish. Therefore, it is difficult to directly correlate the viability in the clonal growth assay with other biological effects seen in mass cultures.

HECK: I guess what I'm not clear on is whether you are dealing with a dish that's full of cells, so that they can't divide further.

GRAFSTRÖM: For the clonal growth assay, or colony-forming efficiency assay, of course the cells divide because we are measuring their rate of division. The cells can also divide at the cell densities used for the alkaline elution and thiol assays. However, I think you are bringing up an important point. For example, marked cytotoxicity of acrolein is already seen at 2 μM in the clonal growth assay, whereas if confluent cells are initially exposed to acrolein, and then released from confluence 48 hours later, up to 30 μM acrolein will cause no significant cytotoxicity. Thus, both cell numbers and growth status of the cells will affect the quantitative but not the qualitative outcome of the experiment.

PEGG: I think the obvious point is that the rate of cell division is going to affect the susceptibility to these aldehydes, and your negative data with acetaldehyde may reflect the rate of cell division here.

GRAFSTRÖM: We are now studying the biological effects of higher concentrations of acetaldehyde, but it is still too early for us to present this work.

HECHT: I think I should mention that we became interested in crotonaldehyde because of our nitrosopyrrolidine work. We recently carried out a bioassay of crotonaldehyde given in drinking water and it did induce liver tumors in rats.

CONNEY: Has anyone studied the possible tumorigenic interaction between aldehydes and dimethylnitrosamine, which is a carcinogen that gives rise to an O^6-methylguanine adduct?

GRAFSTRÖM: Yes, I think acetaldehyde has been studied in combination with diethylnitrosamine.

TANNENBAUM: Is the reaction between glutathione and the aldehydes enzymatically modulated or is it simply a chemical reaction? Or is there a glutathione transferase enzyme involved in the reaction with the aldehydes?

GRAFSTRÖM: As Dr. Heck showed us earlier this morning, formaldehyde is metabolized in a three-step reaction sequence involving a reversible binding of formaldehyde to glutathione. In the cell there are several cytosolic or mitochondrial aldehyde dehydrogenases present that oxidize aldehydes to acids.

TANNENBAUM: So it is happening in the course of the metabolism of the aldehydes.

GRAFSTRÖM: Acrolein is conjugated directly to GSH and the mercapturate acid is excreted in urine. Formaldehyde binds reversibly to glutathione during its oxidation.

TANNENBAUM: Does that mean that in the reaction of acrolein with glutathione there is no enzymatic component?

GRAFSTRÖM: I don't know if glutathione transferases are involved but certainly they are not required.

TANNENBAUM: Does anybody know?

HECHT: Yes, aldehydes react very quickly with thiols.

GRAFSTRÖM: Formaldehyde is a normal cellular intermediate and participates in the tetrahydrofolate pathway for the synthesis of proteins and nucleic acids. Since it is a normal metabolite, the cells certainly have ways to detoxify formaldehyde. One can argue about the concentrations that can be reached in the cell; they are supposedly very low. During N-nitrosamine metabolism, the aldehydes are generated simultaneously with the carbonium ions. Since we get DNA adducts from the presumed carbonium ions, aldehydes may also escape detoxification.

HECK: The other thing is the problem of peroxides. I did not mention it and Roland [Grafström] hasn't alluded to it either, but aldehydes form peroxide very readily. It should be noted that this could be a complication in any in vitro study, not to mention an in vivo study. What we had to do to avoid this problem when we first discovered it was to purify the aldehyde by displacing it with nitrogen and rigorously avoid any air. Of course you can't do that when you're doing an in vivo study, but to the extent that you can, you avoid any contact of the aldehyde with air.

GRAFSTRÖM: As I showed you, our results with acetaldehyde were mostly negative. I agree that we should always consider a possible contamination with peroxides. It is a problem.

Factors Affecting O^6-Alkylguanine-DNA-alkyltransferase Activity

ANTHONY E. PEGG
Department of Physiology and Cancer Research Center
Pennsylvania State University College of Medicine
Hershey Medical Center
Hershey, Pennsylvania 17033

OVERVIEW

O^6-Alkylguanine is an important product of the reaction of alkylating agents with DNA, which may lead to mutations or to the potential initiation of tumors unless it is repaired before DNA replication. It is repaired by the action of a protein termed O^6-alkylguanine-DNA-alkyltransferase (AGT), which catalyzes the transfer of the alkyl group from the DNA to a cysteine residue in its amino acid sequence. This process restores the DNA structure in a single step, but the active site of the AGT is not regenerated. Therefore cells can only remove rapidly as many O^6-alkylguanine residues as there are molecules of the AGT. Additional damage saturates the repair system and provides an increased risk. This paper describes the cellular and species variations in AGT activity, the specificity of the AGT reaction, and factors influencing AGT activity. An ultrasensitive assay procedure for the AGT is also described.

INTRODUCTION

A number of compounds that represent potential human cancer hazards, including some which are present in tobacco products, are converted into alkylating agents (Pegg 1983; Bartsch and Montesano 1984; Hoffmann and Hecht 1985). At least 12 different products are formed when simple alkylating agents interact with DNA (Pegg 1977; Singer and Kusmierek 1982; Bartsch and Montesano 1984). The adducts formed by reaction at oxygen atoms may be of particular importance in the initiation of tumors and of mutations (Pegg 1984; Singer 1984). The rapid and efficient repair of such lesions may protect against mutagenesis and carcinogenesis.

Studies with *E. coli* have shown that a protein, which is highly inducible in response to damage caused by alkylating agents, is able to repair these lesions by a unique mechanism (Demple et al. 1982; Lindahl 1982; McCarthy et al. 1984; Margison et al. 1985; McCarthy and Lindahl 1985). This process involves the transfer of the alkyl group from these residues in DNA to a cysteine acceptor site on the protein. The protein (which is not strictly an enzyme since it acts only once because the cysteine is not regenerated from the alkylcysteine) is referred to as O^6-alkylguanine-DNA-alkyltransferase (AGT).

A protein which resembles the *E. coli* AGT in some but not all respects has been isolated from a variety of mammalian sources. Although it has not been purified to homogeneity, it appears that the mammalian protein also acts in this stoichiometric manner (Pegg 1983; Bartsch and Montesano 1984; Yarosh 1985). The substrate specificity, cellular and species variations in activity, and factors influencing the activity of this AGT protein are described in this paper.

RESULTS AND DISCUSSION

Cellular Distribution

There is a wide variation in the levels of AGT in different species and cell types. Human tissues and cells have much higher amounts than the equivalent rodent cells (Pegg 1983; Bartsch and Montesano 1984; Grafstrom et al. 1984; Myrnes et al. 1984a,b; Wiestler et al. 1984; Yarosh 1985). There are striking differences in the amounts of AGT activity found in extracts from different organs with liver having the highest activity and brain the least (Pegg 1983; Craddock and Henderson 1984; Grafstrom et al. 1984). The expression of AGT activity per unit of protein extracted gives only an approximate estimation of the activity per cell because mammalian cells differ substantially in size. Large cells with a high protein content are therefore underestimated in such comparisons and it is better to express the AGT activity on a per cell basis. However, comparisons of activity in separate organs which consist of mixtures of cell types may be somewhat misleading since the AGT content differs significantly from one cell type to another. For example, the high level of AGT in the rat liver is due to the fact that hepatocytes have high AGT content whereas the nonparenchymal cells in the liver have much lower amounts similar to cells in other organs (Swenberg et al. 1982). Similarly, the activity in Clara cells in the lung was much lower than that of alveolar type II cells or macrophages (Deilhaug et al. 1985).

The factors regulating mammalian AGT activity are not well understood. In rat hepatocytes the activity is increased by up to threefold in response to exposure to alkylating carcinogens and other hepatotoxins (Swenberg et al. 1982; Pegg 1983). There is also evidence that the rat liver AGT is under endocrine control and that it changes in response to partial hepatectomy and during development (Pegg 1983; Pegg and Wiest 1983). However, the AGT activity in livers of other rodents, including mice, gerbils, and hamsters, did not increase in response to partial hepatectomy or carcinogens (Bamborschke et al. 1983; Lindamood et al. 1983; Pegg 1983). There are directly conflicting results on the induction of AGT in cultured cells by exposure to alkylating agents (Waldstein et al. 1982; Pegg 1983; Foote and Mitra 1984; Laval and Laval 1984; Yarosh 1985). The substantial range in AGT activities between samples from different humans might be partially related to differences in the exposure to inducers, but individual genetic variations are likely to be primarily responsible for these differences.

There is general agreement that human cell lines differ greatly in AGT activity (Day et al. 1983; Scudiero et al. 1984; Yarosh 1985). A significant number of transformed lines show a lack or almost complete lack of AGT activity. These lines have been described as having a mer$^-$ or mex$^-$ phenotype. The biochemical basis underlying the absence of AGT activity responsible for this phenotype is unknown, but it confers a much greater sensitivity to mutagenesis and cell killing by alkylating agents (Day et al. 1983; Domoradzki et al. 1984; Yarosh 1985). Although most of the mer$^-$ cells so far described have been transformed (Day et al. 1983; Yarosh 1985), this is not an absolute requirement since at least two human fibroblast lines which are not transformed were also found to fit into this class (Domoradzki et al. 1984). Cells deficient in the AGT activity are also much more sensitive to killing by certain cancer-therapeutic bifunctional nitrosource derivatives such as 1-(2-chloroethyl)-1-nitroso-3-cyclohexylurea (CCNU) (Zlotogorski and Erickson 1984; Yarosh 1985). These compounds form a lethal cross link in the cellular DNA via a process which commences with an attack on the O^6 position of guanine. If the adduct at this position can be removed by the AGT before the chemical rearrangement which leads to the cross link occurs, the formation of this lesion is prevented.

Inhibitors of AGT Activity

The rat liver AGT does not require any cofactors for activity but is very unstable in the absence of thiol reducing agents such as dithiothreitol. It is readily inactivated by reaction with alkylating agents such as N-methyl-N-nitrosourea (MNU) (Pegg et al. 1983). This presumably results from the direct alkylation of the cysteine acceptor site and could contribute towards the saturation of repair after high doses of alkylating agents (Pegg 1983).

The AGT activity is strongly inhibited by certain metals. Complete loss of activity occurs in the presence of 100 μM Cd^{2+} or Cu^{2+} and Hg^{2+}; Zn^{2+} and Ag^{2+} were only slightly less effective (D. Scicchitano and A. Pegg, unpubl.). High levels of dithiothreitol protect the protein against inactivation by these metals.

When human cells in culture were exposed to 0.4 mM O^6-methylguanine (O^6-mG) or O^6-n-butylguanine, there was a substantial loss of the AGT activity, which declined by 75% or more within 4 hours (Dolan et al. 1985a; Karran and Williams 1985). This reduction appeared to be brought about by the free base's acting as a substrate (albeit a very weak one) for the AGT. Incubation of the AGT protein with 0.4 mM O^6-methyl[8-^{3}H]guanine for 2-3 hours results in the production of [8-^{3}H]guanine and the loss of the AGT activity (Dolan et al. 1985a).

The decrease in AGT activity brought about by exposure of cells to O^6-methylguanine is accompanied by an increased sensitivity of human fibroblasts to mutagenesis by N-methyl-N'-nitro-N-nitrosoguanidine (Domoradzki et al. 1985), an increased sensitivity to killing by CCNU of Hela cells (Dolan et al. 1985b) and human colon tumor cells (M. Dolan and A. Pegg, unpubl.), but not Raji cells (Karran and Williams 1985). The reason that Raji cells showed this anomalous behavior is not clear, but it may relate to the rate of synthesis of the AGT in these cells. It was reported that the AGT activity was fully restored within 4 hours of removal of the O^6-mG (Karran and Williams 1985) whereas full restoration in Hela cells took at least 36 hours (Dolan et al. 1985a). If these results reflect the relative rate of synthesis of the new AGT protein, it is possible that the AGT is produced de novo in Raji cells sufficiently rapidly to remove the lesions at the O^6-position of guanine before a lethal cross link is formed. It should be noted that the AGT protein is inactivated by reaction with the free base O^6-mG with an affinity and a rate many thousands of times slower than the reaction with O^6-alkylguanine in DNA. Therefore, the newly formed AGT will preferentially react with lesions in the DNA if these are present, even if the free base is still there.

Further experiments using the exposure of cells to O^6-alkylguanine to reduce AGT activity are clearly needed to investigate its importance in protecting against the toxic effects of alkylating agents, including carcinogenesis, mutagenesis, and cell killing. If such studies confirm the role of the AGT in reducing the toxicity of the therapeutic nitrosourea derivatives towards mer$^+$ human tumor cells (Scudiero et al. 1984; Zlotogorski and Erickson 1984), it is conceivable that the combined treatment with O^6-alkylguanines and these drugs might bring about an increased benefit.

It is possible that the factors such as metals which are described above could act as cocarcinogens by reducing the capacity of the cell to repair critical alkylation damage. Similarly, factors preventing or retarding the resynthesis of the AGT after its exhaustion by alkylating agents could increase the probability of the initiation of a tumor. The model system in which the AGT is depleted experimentally by the use of O^6-alkylguanines could be used to investigate this possibility.

Specificity of the AGT Reaction

The mammalian AGT differs significantly from the *E. coli* AGT in a number of important respects. Both proteins will remove larger adducts than methyl groups from the O^6 position of guanine, but the bacterial protein does so at a very much slower rate (e.g., ethyl and n-propyl groups are removed at least 100 times more slowly than methyl). The rat or human AGT removes ethyl or n-propyl groups at a rate only 3-4 times more slowly than methyl. The rate of removal decreases with the size of the adduct and branched chain adducts are removed much more slowly than the linear alkyl groups. The relative rates of repair of alkyl groups are in the order methyl > ethyl, n-propyl > n-butyl ≫ iso-propyl, iso-butyl, 2-hydroxyethyl (Pegg et al. 1984; Morimoto et al. 1985).

A second major difference between the *E. coli* and the mammalian AGTs is that the latter do not remove methyl groups from the O^4 position of thymine (Dolan et al. 1984; Dolan and Pegg 1985; Yarosh et al. 1985) or from methylphosphate triesters (Pegg et al. 1983; Yarosh et al. 1985). Therefore, in tissues which have a significant AGT activity, the rapid repair of O^6-alkylguanine, while O^4-alkylthymine is diminishing at a slower rate, may lead to a significant buildup of the relatively minor thymine adduct; and this could be important in the initiation of tumors (Singer 1984; Swenberg et al. 1984; Richardson et al. 1985).

The rate of repair of O^6-alkylguanine is much greater when it is contained within a double-stranded DNA; but single-stranded DNA (Pegg et al. 1983) and short oligodeoxynucleotides that contain O^6-mG are also substrates. The dodecamers that were synthesized by Gaffney et al. (1984), which are double-stranded and contain two O^6-alkylguanine residues (one in each strand), are very good substrates and are repaired completely within 1-2 minutes (D. Scicchitano and A. Pegg, unpubl.). The tetranucleotide, 5'-dTpm^{6}GpCpA-3' (Green et al. 1984), which is single-stranded, is also repaired but much more slowly, needing 1.5 hours for a complete reaction (D. Scicchitano and A. Pegg, unpubl.).

These oligonucleotides can be used for the assay of alkyltransferase activity. The methylated form can readily be separated from the demethylated form of these substrates either by HPLC or by precipitation of the methylated oligonucleotide with antibodies specific for O^6-mG. Since it is a simple procedure to label these oligonucleotides at very high specific activity with ^{32}P by reaction with [^{32}P-γ]ATP and polynucleotide kinase, these results form the basis of a very convenient and sensitive assay for the alkyltransferase activity (D. Scicchitano et al., unpubl.). This assay should be sensitive enough to use on very small samples such as biopsy material and on small samples of purified cell types obtained from some complex tissues.

SUMMARY

The amount of AGT present varies greatly according to the species and cell type with hepatocytes having the greatest activity and cells in the nervous system having the least. Human cells have considerably higher activity than their rodent equivalents. Some cultured human cell lines have little or no activity and are very sensitive to the toxic effect of alkylating agents. AGT is inactivated by certain metals such as Cd^{2+}, by direct alkylation, or by reaction with O^6-mG. Exposure to this free base can be used to deplete AGT activity and provide an experimental model to examine the importance of the AGT activity. The mammalian AGT is specific for adducts at the O^6-position of guanine and does not remove alkyl groups from the O^4 position of thymine or from alkylphosphate triesters in DNA. In these important respects it differs from the *E. coli* AGT. Larger alkyl groups are also removed from the O^6-position of guanine by the mammalian AGT although the rate of reaction decreases with increasing size of the adduct. Short oligodeoxynucleotides containing O^6-mG are substrates for the AGT. These can be labeled with ^{32}P and used for a rapid, extremely sensitive and convenient assay for the activity.

ACKNOWLEDGMENTS

Research on this topic in the author's laboratory was supported by grant CA-18137 from the National Cancer Institute.

REFERENCES

Bamborschke, S., P.J. O'Connor, G.P. Margison, P. Kleihues, and G.B. Maru. 1983. DNA methylation by dimethylnitrosamine in the Mongolian gerbil. *Cancer Res.* 43: 1306.
Bartsch, H. and R. Montesano. 1984. Relevance of nitrosamines to human cancer. *Carcinogenesis* 5: 1381.
Craddock, V.M. and A.R. Henderson. 1984. Repair and replication of DNA in rat and mouse tissues in relation to cancer induction by N-nitroso-N-alkylureas. *Chem.-Biol. Interact.* 52: 223.
Day, R.S., D.A. Scudiero, M.R. Mattern, and D.B. Yarosh. 1983. Repair of O^6-methylguanine by normal and transformed human cells. *Proc. Am. Asson. Cancer Res.* 29: 335.
Deilhaug, T., B. Myrnes, T. Aune, H. Krokan, and A. Haugen. 1985. Differential capacities for DNA repair in Clara cells, alveolar type II cells and macrophages of rabbit lung. *Carcinogenesis* 6: 661.
Demple, B., M. Jacobsson, P. Olsson, P. Robins, and T. Lindahl. 1982. Repair of alkylated DNA in E. coli: Physical properties of O^6-methylguanine-DNA-methyltransferase. *J. Biol. Chem.* 257: 13776.
Dolan, M.E. and A.E. Pegg. 1985. Extent of formation of O^4-methylthymine in calf thymus DNA methylated by N-methyl-N-nitrosourea and lack of repair of this product by rat liver O^6-alkylguanine-DNA-alkyltransferase. *Carcinogenesis* 6: 1611.
Dolan, M.E., K. Morimoto, and A.E. Pegg. 1985a. Reduction of O^6-alkylguanine-DNA-alkyltransferase activity in HeLa cells treated with O^6-alkylguanines. *Cancer Res.* 45: 6413.
Dolan, M.E., C.D. Corsico, and A.E. Pegg. 1985b. Exposure of Hela cells to O^6-alkylguanine increases the sensitivity to the cytotoxic effects of alkylating agents. *Biochem. Biophys. Res. Commun.* 132: 178.
Dolan, M.E., D. Scicchitano, B. Singer, and A.E. Pegg. 1984. Comparison of repair of methylated pyrimidines in poly(dT) by extracts from rat liver and *Escherichia coli. Biochem. Biophys. Res. Commun.* 123: 324.
Domoradzki, J., A.E. Pegg, M.E. Dolan, V.M. Maher, and J.J. McCormick. 1984. Correlation between O^6-methylguanine-DNA-methyltransferase activity and resistance of human cells to the cytotoxic and mutagenic effect of N-methyl-N'-nitro-N-nitrosoguanidine. *Carcinogenesis* 5: 1641.
———. 1985. Depletion of O^6-methylguanine-DNA-methyltransferase in human

fibroblasts increases the mutagenic response to N-methyl-N'-nitro-N-nitrosoguanidine. *Carcinogenesis* **6**: 1823.

Foote, R.S. and S. Mitra. 1984. Lack of induction of O^6-methylguanine-DNA methyltransferase in mammalian cells treated with N-methyl-N'-nitro-N-nitrosoguanidine. *Carcinogenesis* **5**: 277.

Gaffney, B.L., L.A. Marky, and R.A. Jones. 1984. Synthesis and characterization of a set of four dodecadeoxyribonucleoside undecaphosphates containing O^6-methylguanine opposite adenine, cytosine, guanine and thymine. *Biochemistry* **23**: 5686.

Grafstrom, R.C., A.E. Pegg, B.F. Trump, and C.C. Harris. 1984. O^6-Alkylguanine-DNA-alkyltransferase activity in normal human tissues and cells. *Cancer Res.* **44**: 2855.

Green, C.L., E.L. Loechler, K.W. Fowler, and J.M. Essigmann. 1984. Construction and characterization of extrachromosomal probes for mutagenesis by carcinogens. *Proc. Natl. Acad. Sci. U.S.A.* **81**: 13.

Hoffmann, D. and S.S. Hecht. 1985. Nicotine-derived N-nitrosamines and tobacco-related cancer: Current status and future directions. *Cancer Res.* **45**: 935.

Karran, P. and S.A. Williams. 1985. The cytotoxic and mutagenic effects of alkylating agents on human lymphoid cells are caused by different DNA lesions. *Carcinogenesis* **6**: 789.

Laval, F. and J. Laval. 1984. Adaptive response in mammalian cells: Cross reactivity of different pretreatments on cytotoxicity as contrasted to mutagenicity. *Proc. Natl. Acad. Sci. U.S.A.* **81**: 1062.

Lindahl, T. 1982. DNA repair enzymes. *Annu. Rev. Biochem.* **51**: 61.

Lindamood, C., M.A. Bedell, K.C. Billings, M.-C. Dyroff, and J.A. Swenberg. 1983. O^6-alkylguanine alkyl acceptor protein activity in hepatocytes of C3H and C57BZ mice during dimethylnitrosamine exposure. *Chem.-Biol. Interact.* **45**: 381.

Margison, G.P., D.P. Cooper, and J. Brennand. 1985. Cloning of the *E. coli* O^6-methylguanine and methylphosphotriester methyltransferase gene using a functional DNA repair assay. *Nucl. Acid Res.* **13**: 1939.

McCarthy, T. and T. Lindahl. 1985. Methyl phosphotriesters in alkylated DNA are repaired by the Ada regulatory protein of *E. coli. Nucl. Acid Res.* **13**: 2683.

McCarthy, T.V., P. Karran, and T. Lindahl. 1984. Inducible repair of O-alkylated pyrimidines in *Escherichia coli. Eur. Mol. Biol. Organ. J.* **3**: 545.

Morimoto, K., M.E. Dolan, D. Scicchitano, and A.E. Pegg. 1985. Repair of O^6-propylguanine and O^6-butylguanine in DNA by O^6-alkylguanine-DNA-alkyltransferases from rat liver and *E. coli. Carcinogenesis* **6**: 1027.

Myrnes, B., K. Norstrand, K.-E. Giercksky, C. Sjunneskog, and H. Krokan. 1984a. A simplified assay for O^6-methylguanine-DNA methyltransferase and its application to human neoplastic and non-neoplastic tissues. *Carcinogenesis* **5**: 1061.

Myrnes, B., G. Eggset, G. Volden, and H. Krokan. 1984b. Enzymatic repair of premutagenic DNA lesions in human epidermis. *Mutat. Res.* **131**: 183.

Pegg, A.E. 1977. Formation and metabolism of alkylated nucleosides: Possible role in carcinogenesis by nitroso compounds and alkylating agents. *Adv. Cancer Res.* **25**: 195.

———. 1983. Alkylation and subsequent repair of DNA after exposure to dimethylnitrosamine and related carcinogens. *Rev. Biochem. Toxicol.* **5**: 83.

———. 1984. Methylation of the O^6-position of guanine in DNA is the most likely initiating event in carcinogenesis by methylating agents. *Cancer Invest.* **2**: 223.

Pegg, A.E. and L. Wiest. 1983. Regulation of O^6-methylguanine-DNA methyltransferase levels in rat liver and kidney. *Cancer Res.* **43**: 972.

Pegg, A.E., D. Scicchitano, and M.E. Dolan. 1984. Comparison of rates of repair of O^6-alkylguanines in DNA by rat liver and bacterial O^6-alkylguanine-DNA-alkyltransferase. *Cancer Res.* **44**: 3806.

Pegg, A.E., L. Wiest, R.S. Foote, S. Mitra, and W. Perry. 1983. Purification and properties of O^6-methylguanine-DNA transmethylase from rat liver. *J. Biol. Chem.* **258**: 2327.

Richardson, F.C., M.C. Dyroff, J.A. Boucheron, and J.A. Swenberg. 1985. Differential repair following exposure to methylating and ethylating hepatocarcinogens. *Carcinogenesis* **6**: 625.

Scudiero, D.A., S.A. Meyer, B.E. Clatterbuck, M.R. Mattern, C.H. Ziolkowski, and R.S. Day. 1984. Sensitivity of human cell strains having different abilities to repair O^6-methylguanine in DNA to inactivation by alkylating agents including chloroethylnitrosoureas. *Cancer Res.* **44**: 2467.

Singer, B. 1984. Alkylation of the O^6 of guanine is only one of many chemical events that may initiate carcinogenesis. *Cancer Invest.* **2**: 233.

Singer, B. and J.T. Kusmierek. 1982. Chemical mutagenesis. *Annu. Rev. Biochem.* **52**: 655.

Swenberg, J.A., M.A. Bedell, K.C. Billings, D.R. Umbenhauer, and A.E. Pegg. 1982. Cell specific differences in O^6-alkylguanine DNA repair activity during continuous carcinogen exposure. *Proc. Natl. Acad. Sci. U.S.A.* **79**: 5449.

Swenberg, J.A., M.C. Dyroff, M.A. Bedell, J.A. Popp, N. Huh, U. Klrstein, and M.F. Rajewsky. 1984. O^4-ethyldeoxythymidine, but not O^6-ethyldeoxyguanosine, accumulates in hepatocyte DNA of rats exposed continuously to diethylnitrosamine. *Proc. Natl. Acad. Sci. U.S.A.* **81**: 1692.

Waldstein, E.A., E.-H. Cao, and R.B. Setlow. 1982. Adaptive resynthesis of the O^6-methylguanine acceptor protein can explain the differences between mammalian cells proficient and deficient in methyl excision repair. *Proc. Natl. Acad. Sci. U.S.A.* **79**: 5117.

Wiestler, O., P. Kleihues, and A.E. Pegg. 1984. O^6-alkylguanine-DNA alkyltransferase activity in human brain and brain tumors. *Carcinogenesis* **4**: 199.

Yarosh, D.B. 1985. The role of O^6-methylguanine-DNA methyltransferase in cell survival, mutagenesis and carcinogenesis. *Mutat. Res.* **145**: 1.

Zlotogorski, C. and L.C. Erickson. 1984. Pretreatment of human colon tumor cells with DNA methylating agents inhibit their ability to repair chloroethylmonoadducts. *Carcinogenesis* **5**: 83.

COMMENTS

RANDERATH: What is the current idea about why cells have this enzyme in the first place?

PEGG: That's a very good question and any answer I give you is speculation, but I'd be happy to speculate about it. One possibility is that it has been shown by a number of people that S-adenosylmethionine acts as a chemical methylating agent. So over the lifetime of any cell, you would expect to get a few molecules of methylated bases produced by a chemical reaction with S-adenosylmethionine. It's the price you pay for having this nucleoside in the cell to act as a methyl donor for enzymatic reactions. The chemical methylation reaction goes predominantly via an SN2 reaction and the O^6 adduct is a very minor component of that. So probably you'd only get one or two molecules of O^6-methylguanine per cell and just having a few molecules of this protein around would enable you to take care of that. In some ways, I like that explanation because it helps to explain why there's such a big difference in the relative rates with longer aklyl groups between the *E. coli* and the mammalian protein. If it's really designed to deal with methyl groups, there wouldn't be any selective pressure to have it be good or bad on ethyl or longer groups and this might vary considerably from one species to another. However, this doesn't explain—at least I don't think it explains—why there is so much more of it in liver, particularly of hepatocytes than there is in other cells. That seems to point more toward some function related to repair of DNA damage caused by exogenous agents since this damage may be greatest in liver. Finally, it's also not inconceivable (and you may have data on this) that there are other alkylated bases formed in DNA in very small amounts, which play some role in differentiations.

RANDERATH: On our ^{32}P-fingerprints, we have some indication of tissue-specific "background" patterns. This could be an artifact of some sort or could indicate some real differences intrinsic to the DNAs. We are investigating this.

PEGG: There are many possibilities. The other possibility, which has been raised by a number of people, is that this protein really does something else and it's just purely by chance that it happens to repair DNA since it's not really an enzyme. They suggest that it is really designed to carry out some other reaction and have told me to find out what it really does. We've looked at a number of things and have not been very successful at them. One thing I would point out is that this protein has a very high affinity for double-stranded DNA. It's very convenient to purify it like that, suggesting that it has some function that is related to DNA.

HARRIS: If you alter the levels of O^6-methyltransferase in mammalian cells by the procedure that you just suggested is the spontaneous mutation frequency altered at all? Is there any correlation between the spontaneous mutation frequency and the level of O^6-methyltransferase activity in mammalian cells?

PEGG: I don't know the answer. Within the only mutation study we've done, where we altered it, there was no significant increase in the basal mutation frequency, only in the cells treated with MNNG. However, the basal rate is so low that we didn't really have enough cells to measure the rate accurately.

TANNENBAUM: I was going to ask a similar question. What would happen if you fed O^6-methylguanine? Would it be taken up by the liver?

PEGG: Yes. It is.

TANNENBAUM: So then over a long period of time, it would cause the accumulation of lesions, and it could be a carcinogen.

PEGG: Why would it cause the accumulation of lesions? It would reduce the level of the alkyltransferase protein, but there would have to be some other endogenous process which was putting the lesions into DNA.

TANNENBAUM: But you just told us that there are probably several endogenous processes which lead to alkylation of O^6-methylguanine in DNA in the liver.

PEGG: I think that's true, but I don't know whether these would be enough to see an effect in carcinogenesis. One can certainly do the experiment by reducing the alkyltransferase in this way and then treating deliberately with some alkylating agent and see what happens. I'm doing that now.

MAGEE: You said that you are in the process of doing carcinogenesis tests in which the enzymes have been "knocked out"?

PEGG: Yes.

MAGEE: How are you knocking that enzyme out?

PEGG: In the way I just described—by injecting O^6-methylguanine. Let me make it clear to everybody who's interested in this what is actually going on here. It is very important that you understand the way in which this works. The free base is a very weak substrate for the protein. So you can eliminate the activity as I suggested by treating with O^6-methylguanine. However, if you then administer an alkylating agent, which alkylates DNA in the cell, the newly synthesized alkyltransferase, which is being made all the time, will repair the DNA. The newly synthesized alkyltransferase would much rather react with damaged DNA than it would with a free base. So for that reason, as demonstrated earlier, there was a much greater effect on killing by CCNU than there was on killing by MNNG. The reason is that it takes quite a long time for the lethal mutations caused by MNNG to actually become apparent in these experiments. During that time, the protein which has been resynthesized can repair some of the lesions. With CCNU, the initial attack is on the O^6 position, and then you get a rearrangement which forms a lethal cross link. After about 1 or 2 hours, the lethal cross link has been formed. Whether the alkyltransferase can come back or not makes no difference. Thus, in order to design the carcinogenicity test which I just described, you have to use something where you get tumors with a single shot.

CONNEY: What are the factors that increase or decrease the level of the alkyltransferase DNA repair enzyme? Why does it go up more extensively in *E. coli* than in mammalian cells? Are there safe ways that this enzyme could be increased 100-fold in mammalian cells?

PEGG: Obviously the strategy is to use the same strategy that was used in *E. coli*; but this protein is not nearly as inducible in response to alkylation damage as it is in *E. coli*. Now some people have argued with me when I said that, and said, "How do you know that the mammalian cells that you're looking at are not already 80% or 90% induced because of some endogenous production of alkylated lesions?" It is possible that that is correct.

CONNEY: Is anyone studying the genes that regulate the synthesis of the alkyltransferase in *E. coli*?

PEGG: Yes. We are trying. It is quite difficult because there isn't all that much of this protein, even in the mammalian cells that have the highest activity; but there are a number of different strategies which various groups are trying. The most promising one is to take cells which do not have the alkyltransferase and transfect them with DNA, and then use CCNU or some other killing agent as a selective pressure to find ones which are expressing the gene. That seems to be working, but that's all I can say.

E. RANDERATH: Have you ever observed a C^5-de-methylase in addition to your dealkylase?

PEGG: Yes. It depends on your interests and what you think is more important, but I have not looked specifically for that. However, this protein does not remove methyl groups from O^4-methylthymine or 3-methylthymine. Some of those experiments were done by a person in my laboratory who was working with a very crude preparation, and there wasn't anything else in this crude preparation that removed methyl groups from methylated pyrimidines either.

In Vitro Carcinogenesis Studies of Human Bronchial Epithelial Cells

TOHRU MASUI,* GEORGE H. YOAKUM,* JOHN F. LECHNER,* JAMES C. WILLEY,* PAUL AMSTAD,* BENJAMIN F. TRUMP,† AND CURTIS C. HARRIS*
*Laboratory of Human Carcinogenesis
Division of Cancer Etiology
National Cancer Institute
Bethesda, Maryland 20892
†Department of Pathology
University of Maryland School of Medicine
Baltimore, Maryland 21201

OVERVIEW

An in vitro model using normal human bronchial epithelial cells allows investigators to bridge the gap between epidemiological studies and animal model system studies. Chemical and physical carcinogens (i.e., cigarette smoke condensate and its subfractions, nickel ion, and asbestos) cause phenotypic changes in bronchial epithelial cells in vitro, including aberrations in pathways controlling their growth and differentiation. The *ras, myc,* and *raf* families of oncogenes are associated with lung cancer. Transfection of v-Ha-*ras* into normal human bronchial epithelial cells initiates the multistep process of malignant transformation.

INTRODUCTION

Tobacco smoke has been clearly identified as the major cause of human lung cancer. It is also an example of a complex mixture of chemical and physical agents in which more than 40 are known carcinogens (Table 1). The tumorigenicity of tobacco smoke can be enhanced by cocarcinogenic agents, including radon daughters (Lundin et al. 1971) and asbestos (Selikoff et al. 1968). Lung carcinogenesis is considered to occur in multiple steps, i.e., tumor initiation, promotion, conversion, and progression (Fig. 1), all of which could be influenced by the various components of tobacco smoke (Harris 1983).

Understanding the processes that control the growth and differentiation of normal human epithelial cells and elucidating how those controlling mechanisms differ in carcinoma cells is an important part of understanding carcinogenesis. The majority of human cancers are derived from epithelial cells which terminally differentiate (Green 1977), and diminished response to differentiation inducers is a common phenotypic marker of malignant cells (Rheinwald and Beckett 1980; Yuspa and Morgan 1981; Wille et al. 1982; Lechner et al. 1983; Kawamura et al. 1985;

Table 1
Examples of Identified Carcinogens and Cocarcinogens in Tobacco Smoke

Gas phase
  N-nitrosodimethylamine, N-nitrosodiethylamine, N-nitrosomethylethylamine, N-nitrosopyrrolidine, N-nitrosopiperidine, N-dibutylnitrosamine, formaldehyde, acetaldehyde
Particulate phase
  Carcinogens
    Benzo[a]pyrene, dibenz[a,h]acridine, dibenz[a,c]anthracene, dibenz[a,j]acridine, dibenzo[c,g]carbazone, β-naphthylamine, benzo[a]fluoranthene, aminostilbene, dibenzo[a,e]fluoranthene, benzo[j]fluoranthene, methylfluoranthene, benz[a]anthracene, chrysene, idento[1,2,3-cd]pyrene, 5-methylchrysene, 2-,3-dimethylchrysene, N-nitrosoanabasine, benzo[c]phenanthrene, N-nitrosonornicotine, polonium 210, arsenic, cadmium, nickel compounds
  Cocarcinogens
    Pyrene, fluoranthene, benzo[g,h,i]perylene, benzo[e]pyrene, naphthalenes, 1-methylindoles, 9-methylcarbazoles, 4,4'-dichlorostilbene, catechol

Compounds, such as N-nitrosamines, may be found in both the gas and particulate phases.

Scott and Maercklein 1985; Willey et al. 1985a; Masui et al. 1986). Aberrations in differentiation-inducing pathways (as have been repeatedly noted in carcinomas) could affect the balance between proliferation and terminal differentiation, resulting in a permanent tilt towards multiplication. In this paper, therefore, we will briefly review our studies concerning the effects of tobacco smoke components mainly on growth and differentiation controls of human bronchial epithelium in vitro. Since carcinogens found in tobacco smoke may activate certain oncogenes and such oncogenes have been isolated from human lung cancers (Perucho et al. 1981; Yuasa et al. 1983; Nakano et al. 1984), we will also discuss the effects of transfected oncognes on the growth, differentiation, and neoplastic potential of normal human bronchial epithelial (NHBE) cells in vitro. For the most part, we used an in vitro culture system for the NHBE cells described previously (Lechner et al. 1982, 1983, 1985; Lechner and LaVeck 1985). Other methods employed will be discussed in Results and Discussion.

RESULTS AND DISCUSSION

The Biochemical and Morphological Effects of Cigarette Smoke Condensate and Its Fractions on NHBE Cells In Vitro

Epidemiologic studies have established that cigarette smoking markedly increases the risk of developing bronchial carcinoma (U.S. Department of Health, Education

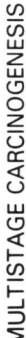

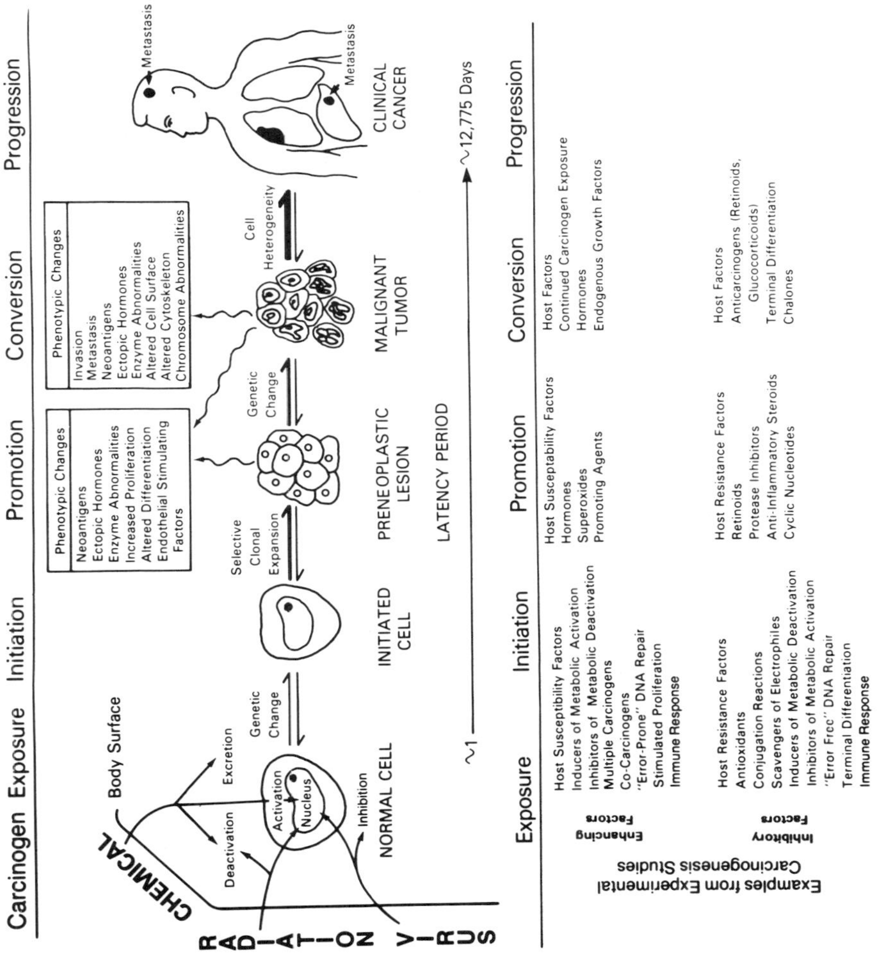

Figure 1
Schematic representation of multistage carcinogenesis in the human lung. Examples of factors that may either enhance or inhibit carcinogenesis are taken from studies of experimental carcinogenesis.

and Welfare 1979) and that this increased risk is at least in part due to tumor promotion (Armitage and Doll 1961). By using the mouse skin two-stage carcinogenesis model, as well as inhalation studies in a variety of animals, it has been determined that much of the tumor initiators is in the basic fraction of cigarette smoke condensate (CSC) (Fig. 2) and includes several 4- and 5-ring aromatic hydrocarbons (Wynder and Hoffmann 1967). CSC-derived tumor promoters for mouse skin reside primarily in the strongly polar neutral subfraction (N_{Meoh}) (Bock et al. 1970), the weakly acidic fraction (WA_e), and the phenolic fraction (Hoffmann et al. 1983).

Since it is not known what compounds may serve as tumor promoters for NHBE or what their effects might be, we initially investigated the effects of representative compounds from three different chemical classes of tumor promoters that had been identified in the mouse skin carcinogenesis model (Willey et al. 1984b, 1984c). Teleocidin B, 12-O-tetradecanoyl phorbol-13-acetate (TPA), aplysiatoxin, and debromoaplysiatoxin induce terminal squamous differentiation in NHBE cells in culture. In order to determine if compounds in CSC would have similar effects on NHBE cells, we studied the effects of CSC, N_{Meoh}, WA_e, BI_a, and BI_b on the differentiation markers (i.e., a decrease in clonal growth rate,

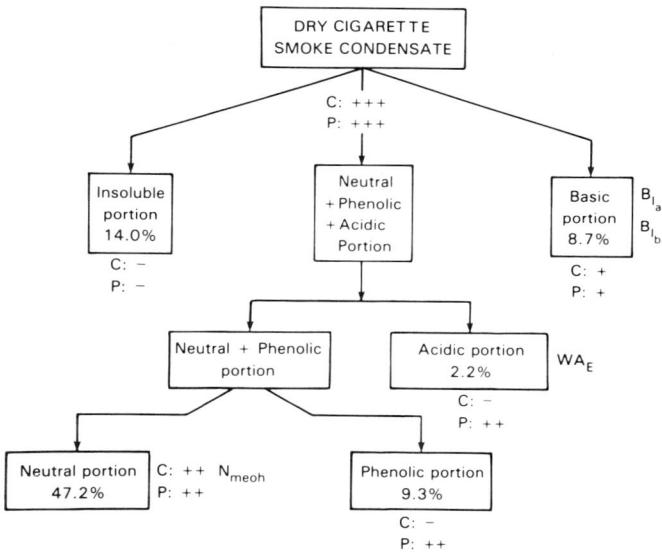

Figure 2
Fractionation scheme of CSC and relative carcinogenic and promoter activities of major fractions on mouse skin (Wynder and Hoffmann 1967). (C) Relative carcinogenic activity; (P) relative tumor-promoting activity.

an increase in plasminogen activator (PA), an increase in cross-linked envelope (CLE) formation, and an increase in cell surface area) (Willey et al. 1984c) and ornithine decarboxylase (ODC) activity (Yuspa et al. 1976). One of the early effects of TPA and other tumor promoters in many epithelial cell culture systems, including NHBE cells, is inhibition of epidermal growth factor (EGF) binding (Brown et al. 1979; Shoyab et al. 1979; Horowitz et al. 1983). Therefore, we observed the effect of CSC and CSC fractions on EGF binding in NHBE cells. Measurement of intracellular thiol levels provides a sensitive indication of the effects of electrophiles, such as reactive aldehydes and peroxides, on cells. From previous investigations it is known that CSC decreases thiol levels in isolated suspensions of rat liver or lung cells (Moldeus et al. 1985). In addition, the inhibitory effects of CSC on clonal growth of cultured human bronchial fibroblasts were partially prevented when the cells were coincubated with N-acetylcysteine, a compound with nucleophile properties similar to glutathione. Therefore, we measured the effects of CSC and CSC fractions on thiol levels in NHBE cells. Finally, since CSC has been reported to be mutagenic (DeMarini 1983) and clastogenic (Leuchtenberger et al. 1973) and cigarette smoke caused DNA single-strand breaks (SSB) (Nakayama et al. 1985) in other systems, we measured CSC effects on DNA SSB formation.

Neither CSC nor any of the fractions was mitogenic over the range 0.01–100 μg/ml. All were growth inhibitory at higher concentrations. The 50% growth inhibitory concentrations (IC_{50}) for CSC, BI_a, BI_b, WA_e, and N_{Meoh} were 10, 10, 10, 3 and 1 μg/ml, respectively. Effects on differentiation markers, ODC activities, EGF binding, and thiol levels were evaluated using IC_{50} concentrations. We found that CSC and all fractions tested caused an increased formation of CLEs from a baseline of 0.5% in the untreated cells to an increase of 20% induced by N_{Meoh}, a squamous morphological change was observed within 1 hour after exposure to N_{Meoh}, WA_e, and CSC. The BI_a and BI_b fractions had little effect on morphology. Only N_{Meoh} increased PA significantly, i.e., twofold. CSC, WA_e, and N_{Meoh} ($N_{Meoh} > WA_e > $ CSC) fractions caused a decrease in EGF binding, in each case reaching a maximum effect after a 10- to 12-hour incubation. At the IC_{50} neither CSC nor any of the fractions significantly affected intracellular thiol levels. CSC caused significant DNA SSB only at a concentration of 100 μg/ml levels. CSC and any of the fractions were not effective on ODC activity. Due to the effects of the N_{Meoh} fraction on differentiation markers and EGF binding, we consider it to be the likeliest portion of CSC to contain compounds with actions similar to those of the phorbol ester, indole alkaloid, and polyacetate tumor promoters.

Effects of Nickel Sulfate on Growth and Differentiation of NHBE Cells

In addition to chemical carcinogens, tobacco smoke contains several physical carcinogens including metals such as nickel (Table 1). To determine the effects of nickel ion, cultured NHBE cells were continuously exposed to a dose (5-20 ug/ml) of Ni_2SO_4 that reduced their colony-forming efficiency 30-80%. After 40 days of incubation, the cultures consisted of large, squamous cells, and mitotic cells were not observed. The cells were then maintained in medium without Ni_2SO_4. After 40-75 total days of incubation, colonies of mitotic cells appeared at a rate of one colony per 100,000 cells originally at risk. On the other hand, no colonies appeared in control cultures or in cultures exposed to < 5 µg Ni_2SO_4/ml for 90 days. Twelve Ni_2SO_4-altered cell cultures isolated from five experiments have been expanded into mass cultures. Most of the cell populations recovered have an increased population-doubling potential. Some exhibit aberrations in the terminal squamous differentiation process whereas others have lost the requirement for EGF for clonal growth. Aneuploidy and marker chromosomes have also been noted. However, none of these Ni_2SO_4-altered cell cultures was anchorage-independent nor produced tumors upon injection into athymic nude mice (Lechner et al. 1984a).

Therefore, in contrast to these reported results with rodent cells (DiPaolo and Casto 1979), we found that the long-term exposure of NHBE cells to Ni_2SO_4 did not result in malignantly transformed cells. Instead, we have found that the cells, after prolonged exposure to Ni_2SO_4-altered cultures, have reduced growth factor requirements and an extended culture population-doubling potential, reduced responsiveness to differentiation inducers, i.e., blood-derived serum (BDS) and TPA, and chromosomal abnormalities. Although these properties are found in carcinoma cells, the altered cells have also retained normal cell characteristics, i.e., they do not recognize BDS factors as mitogens, are anchorage-dependent, and are not tumorigenic.

Cellular Ingestion, Toxic Effects, and Lesions Observed in Human Bronchial Epithelial Tissue and Cells Cultured with Asbestos and Glass Fibers

Although exposure to asbestos has been shown to synergistically increase the risk of bronchogenic carcinoma for cigarette smokers in epidemiological studies (Selikoff et al. 1968), the pathobiological mechanisms responsible for the cocarcinogenic action of asbestos are not known. Therefore, the effects of asbestos fibers on normal human tracheobronchial epithelium were studied (Haugen et al. 1982). Asbestos fibers, i.e., amosite, crocidolite, and chrysotile (UICC samples) and glass fibers were initially assayed for their cytotoxicity. NHBE cells exposed to either asbestos or glass fibers displayed inhibition of cell growth as a function of fiber concentration. When compared to glass fibers, asbestos fibers caused a statistically significant ($P < 0.05$) decrease in clonal growth rate. Chrysotile was approximately ten times more cytotoxic than either amosite or crocidolite and more than 100 times more cytotoxic than the glass fibers. NHBE cells were 10-15 times more sensitive to the cytotoxic effects of asbestos fibers than bronchial fibroblasts from the same donor. By using electron microscopy, asbestos fibers were seen to be ingested by epithelial cells. After exposure for 2 hours, short fibers ($< 12\ \mu m$) were found both in the cytoplasm and within phagosomes. High-voltage electron microscopy, combined with stereo microscopy, revealed asbestos fibers in the cytoplasmic matrix. A single exposure to amosite asbestos (100-1000 $\mu g/ml$) was found to induce focal hyperplasia and epidermoid metaplasia with cellular atypia in human tracheobronchial explants. Surface fine-structure observations revealed asbestos fibers protruding from these lesions. Intracytoplasmic and intranuclear fibers of amosite were identified in these focal lesions using x-ray microanalysis in combination with transmission electron microscopy. With increasing time, fibers were also seen deposited within the submucosa of the explants. The preferential cytotoxicity of asbestos for epithelial cells and the metaplastic response of bronchial epithelium may be important in the cocarcinogenic action of asbestos.

Malignant Transformation of Human Bronchial Epithelial Cells by Transfected Harvey ras Oncogene

Three families of oncogenes, *ras*, *myc* and *raf*, have so far been associated with human lung cancer. Approximately 10% of the carcinoma cell lines have yielded *ras*-mutated proto-oncogene sequences when their DNA has been transfected into mouse NIH-3T3 cells (Land et al. 1983). The *myc* family of proto-oncogenes has been found to be activated by amplification in many cell lines established from small-cell carcinoma of the lung (Nau et al. 1985, 1986). The third family, *raf*, is also found to be overexpressed in small-cell carcinomas (G. Mark et al., unpubl.).

Since these proto-oncogenes may play an intrinsic role in human lung carcinogenesis and/or the maintenance of the malignant phenotype, the above mentioned associations are particularly interesting. Initially, we considered it important to determine the phenotypic alterations caused by these oncogenes following their transfection into NHBE cells in vitro. Our strategy for these investigations is outlined in Table 2. NHBE cells were chosen for these studies because they are the progenitor cells of bronchogenic carcinoma.

We chose the *ras* family of oncogenes to initiate our investigations (Yoakum et al. 1985) for three reasons: (1) their frequent association with human carcinomas, including those of the lung (Perucho et al. 1981; Yuasa et al. 1983; Nakano et al.

Table 2
Strategy for Studying Neoplastic Transformation of NHBE Cells by Transfected Oncogenes

A. Select oncogenes associated with lung cancer.
B. Use progenitor epithelial cells of bronchogenic carcinoma.
C. Develop and use high frequency gene transfection method.
D. Develop and use conditions to select preneoplastic and neoplastic cells.
E. Establish criteria to identify preneoplastic and neoplastic cells.

1984), (2) their genetic dominance in the transformation of murine cells (Spandidos and Wilkie 1984), and (3) the well-defined point mutations in the structural gene. The native form of v-Ha-*ras* was selected because of its small size, its strong Moloney long-terminal repeat (LTR) transcriptional promoter, and its readily identifiable phosphorylated protein, p21 (Shih et al. 1980; Furth et al. 1982). We consider the introduction of v-Ha-*ras* to be a direct genetic test of the transforming potential of Ha-*ras* p21 in NHBE cells.

Since high concentrations of calcium ions in the calcium-phosphate method of Graham and van der Eb (1973) are cytotoxic to human epithelial cells and a moderate concentration (i.e., 500 μM) enhances pathways of terminal squamous differentiation (Lechner et al. 1984b), we developed an alternative method (Yoakum et al. 1983; Yoakum 1984). A plasmid was constructed to contain the oncogene(s) and a positive selectable marker gene (e.g., *gpt* or *neo*). Protoplasts then formed, sedimented onto the surface of the epithelial cells by centrifugation and in the presence of purified polyethylene glycol. The membranes of the protoplasts and epithelial cells fused, permitting access of the plasmids into NHBE cells. The frequency of stable integration of genes transfected in human epithelial cells by this method is as high as that achieved by the calcium-phosphate method in rodent fibroblasts (i.e., approximately $1-5 \times 10^{-3}$).

Selection pressures to isolate presumptive neoplastic cells were based on the hypothesis that premalignant or malignant cells have a defect in their differentiation pathways. Whereas the normal cells are responsive to these inducers of differentiation, human carcinoma cell lines are relatively resistant and continue to grow in the presence of TPA, an exogenous inducer, or BDS, which contains type β transforming growth factor (TGF-β), an endogenous inducer of terminal squamous differentiation (Lechner et al. 1983; Willey et al. 1984a,c; Masui et al. 1986). In addition, maintenance of the NHBE cells either at confluence or in suspension causes terminal differentiation. These observations are consistent with the hypothesis and formed the foundation for our experimental design.

Selection of differentiation-resistant transfected NHBE cells was initiated in the presence of 2% BDS. Then the cells were maintained at confluence as a second selective pressure, and after 2 months, four multilayered cellular foci (TBE-1, -2, -3, and -4) appeared. These four foci were subcultured as individual cultures and have continued to grow indefinitely (i.e., > 120 cell generations). One of these cell lines (TBE-1) has been extensively studied (Yoakum et al. 1985).

The phenotypic properties of the NHBE cells, TBE-1 cells, TBE-1SA (anchorage-independent TBE-1 cells), and TBE-1SAT (cells isolated from tumors formed by TBE-1SA cells injected into irradiated athymic nude mice), are listed in Table 3. The v-Ha-*ras*-transfected cells are not induced to terminally differentiate by either 2% BDS or 100 nM TPA. TBE-1 cells rarely grow in semisolid medium and make progressing tumors after 9-12 months in athymic nude mice (see Table 3). In contrast, cells isolated from colonies of TBE-1 cells growing in agar (TBE-1SA) have a

Table 3
Summary of the Phenotypic Properties of NHBE Cells and v-H-a-ras-Transfected HBE Cells (TBE-1, TBE-1SA, and TBE1-SAT Cells)

Cell name	Differentiation response[a]		Anchorage independence	Tumorigenicity in athymic nude mice (subcutaneous)		Type IV collagenase activity
	BDS	TPA		Frequency	Metastasis	
NHBE	+	+	−		−	+
TBE-1	−	−	+[b]	+[r] (2/16)	+	++
TBE-1SA	−	−	+	+ (13/14)	++	+++
TBE-1SAT	−	−	+	+ (9/10)	++	nd

[a]Column indicates the differentiation response of NHBE grown in serum-free medium supplemented with 2% BDS or 100 nM TPA.
[b]The ability to form colonies during growth in soft agar was used to isolate TBE-1 derivatives capable of anchorage-independent growth (TBE-1SA). Early passage TBE-1 cells did not form colonies during growth in soft agar when seeded at 10^6 cells/60 mm dish.
+[r] indicates that after 14 days the nodules regressed when 10^6 or 2×10^7 TBE-1 cells were injected subcutaneously in irradiated athymic nude mice. Tumors reappeared in a few animals at 7-9 months.
(+) positive; (−) negative; nd, test not done

higher activity of type IV collagenase and produce progressively growing tumors with a latency period of approximately 2 months. These tumor cells (TBE-1SAT) have been shown to be of human origin on the basis of their isoenzyme patterns and the chromosomal analysis of the cultured cells. When TBE-1SAT cells are injected into athymic nude mice, they again display their tumorigenic properties. When analyzed by immunoperoxidase staining, these anaplastic tumors contain small amounts of keratin marker of epithelial cells (the presence of which has been confirmed by immunoprecipitation using antiserum to total keratin purified from human stratum corneum).

The transfected v-Ha-*ras* oncogene apparently caused NHBE cells to become immortal and malignant as judged by their continued growth, aneuploidy, and tumorigenicity in athymic nude mice. The mechanism by which the v-Ha-*ras* p21 initiates this multistage process is unknown. The possibility was tested that a secondary alteration causing increased expression of a non-*ras* oncogene might have occurred. Total cell RNA was extracted from TBE-1, TBE-1SA, and TBE-1SAT cells. This RNA was screened by "dot-blot" hybridization with probes specific for H-*ras*, N-*myc*, c-*myc*, and *raf*. In no case was increased expression observed relative to a NHBE cell control.

It is interesting that although TPA was not used as a selective pressure in their isolation, the transformed cells nonetheless acquired a resistance to induction of differentiation by TPA. This observation implies a more generalized defect in the differentiation program of these transformed cells. We noted that Cholera toxin and epinephrine which activate the GTP binding protein system (Gilman 1984) antagonized differentiation-inducing stimuli, i.e., BDS and TGF-β (Lechner et al. 1984b; Masui et al. 1986). Therefore, aberration in GTP binding protein systems that might be caused by v-Ha-*ras* p21 may be responsible for the insensitivity of v-Ha-*ras*-transfected NHBE cells to differentiation-inducing reagents.

The data noted above are consistant with the hypothesis that preneoplastic and neoplastic human bronchial epithelial cells have an imbalance in their growth and differentiation programs. Such an imbalance would provide these cells with a selective growth expansion advantage over the normal epithelial cells. In vitro carcinogenesis studies using cells from experimental animals have also provided data supporting this hypothesis. Defects in control of cellular differentiation have been associated with the initiation phase of carcinogenesis in mouse epidermal cells (Yuspa and Morgan 1981; Kawamura et al. 1985) and 3T3 T proadipocytes (Scott and Maercklein 1985).

CONCLUSION

An in vitro model system has been used to explore the pathophysiological responses of human bronchial epithelium to tobacco smoke and cocarcinogens, i.e., asbestos and nickel. These studies demonstrate the promoter-like activity in tobacco smoke, preferential epithelial cytotoxicity of asbestos, and the altered growth factor requirement of NHBE cells caused by nickel ion. The protoplast fusion method for transfecting oncogenes into human cells allows the examination of possible linkages between oncogenes and human cancer. Three multigene families of oncogenes, *myc*, *raf*, and *ras*, have been associated with human lung cancer. Transfected *ras* oncogene initiated the neoplastic transformation of NHBE cells. These results suggest that oncogenes may play an important role in human lung carcinogenesis.

REFERENCES

Armitage, P. and R. Doll. 1961. Stochastic models for carcinogenesis. In *Proceedings of the fourth Berkeley symposium on mathematical statistics and probability* (ed. J. Neyman), vol. 4, p. 19. University of California Press, Berkeley, California.

Bock, F.G., A.P. Swain, and R.L. Stedman. 1970. Composition studies on tobacco. XLI. Carcinogenesis assay of subfractions of the neutral fraction of cigarette smoke condensate. *J. Natl. Cancer Inst.* **44**: 1305.

Brown, K.D., P. Dicker, and E. Rozengurt. 1979. Inhibition of epidermal growth factor binding to surface receptors by tumor promoters. *Biochem. Biophys. Res. Commun.* **86**: 1037.

DeMarini, D.M. 1983. Genotoxicity of tobacco smoke and tobacco smoke condensate. *Mutat. Res.* **114**: 59.

DiPaolo, J.A. and B.C. Casto. 1979. Quantitative studies of *in vitro* morphological transformation of Syrian hamster cells by inorganic metal salts. *Cancer Res.* **39**: 1008.

Furth, M.E., L.J. Davis, B. Fleurdelys, and E.M. Scolnick. 1982. Monoclonal antibodies to the p21 products of the transforming gene of Harvey murine sarcoma virus and of the cellular *ras* gene family. *J. Virol.* **43**: 294.

Gilman, A.G. 1984. G proteins and dual control of adenylate cyclase. *Cell* **36**: 577.

Graham, F.L. and A.J. van der Eb. 1973. A new technique for the assay of infectivity of human adenovirus 5 DNA. *Virology* **52**: 456.

Green, H. 1977. Terminal differentiation of cultured human epidermal cells. *Cell* **11**: 405.

Harris, C.C. 1983. Concluding remarks: Role of carcinogens, cocarcinogens, and host factors in cancer risk. In *Human carcinogenesis* (ed. C.C. Harris and H. Autrup), p. 941. Academic Press, New York.

Haugen, A., P.W. Schafer, J.F. Lechner, G.D. Stoner, B.F. Trump, and C.C. Harris. 1982. Cellular ingestion, toxic effects, and lesions observed in human bronchial epithelial tissue and cells cultured with asbestos and glass fibers. *Int. J. Cancer* **30**: 265.

Hoffmann, D., S.S. Hecht, and E.L. Wynder. 1983. Tumor promoters and cocarcinogens in tobacco carcinogenesis. *Environ. Health Perspect.* **50**: 247.

Horowitz, A.D., H. Fujiki, I.B. Weinstein, A. Jeffrey, E. Okin, R.E. Moore, and T. Sugimura. 1983. Comparative effects of aplysiatoxin, debromoaplysiatoxin, and teleocidin on receptor binding and phospholipid metabolism. *Cancer Res.* **43**: 1529.

Kawamura, H., J.E. Strickland, and S.H. Yuspa. 1985. Association of resistance to terminal differentiation with initiation of carcinogenesis in adult mouse epidermal cells. *Cancer Res.* **45**: 2748.

Land, H., L.F. Parada, and R.A. Weinberg. 1983. Cellular oncogenes and multistep carcinogenesis. *Science* **222**: 771.

Lechner, J.F. and M.A. LaVeck. 1985. A serum-free method for culturing normal human bronchial epithelial cells at clonal density. *J. Tissue Culture Methods.* **9**: 43.

Lechner, J.F., A. Haugen, I.A. McClendon, and E.W. Pettis. 1982. Clonal growth of normal adult human bronchial epithelial cells in a serum-free medium. *In Vitro* **18**: 633.

Lechner, J.F., T. Tokiwa, I.A. McClendon, and A. Haugen. 1984a. Effects of nickel sulfate on growth and differentiation of normal human bronchial epithelial cells. *Carcinogenesis* **5**: 1697.

Lechner, J.F., A. Haugen, I.A. McClendon, and A.M. Shamsuddin. 1984b. Induction of squamous differentiation of normal human bronchial epithelial cells by small amounts of serum. *Differentiation* **25**: 229.

Lechner, J.F., I.A. McClendon, M.A. LaVeck, A.M. Shamsuddin, and C.C. Harris. 1983. Differential control by platelet factors of squamous differentiation in normal and malignant human bronchial epithelial cells. *Cancer Res.* **43**: 5915.

Lechner, J.F., G.D. Stoner, A. Haugen, H. Autrup, J.C. Willey, B.E. Trump, and C.C. Harris. 1986. *In vitro* human bronchial epithelial model systems for carcinogenesis studies. In *In vitro models for cancer research* (ed. M. Webber and L. Sekely). CRC Press, Boca Raton, Florida. (In press).

Leuchtenberger, C., R. Leuchtenberger, and A. Schneider. 1973. Effects of marijuana and tobacco smoke on human lung physiology. *Nature* **241**: 137.

Lundin, F.E., J.K. Wagoner, and G. Archer. 1971. *Radon daughter exposure and respiratory cancer: Quantitative and temporal aspects.* U.S. Technical Information Service, U.S. Department of Commerce, Springfield, Virginia.

Masui, T., L.M. Wakefield, J.F. Lechner, M.A. LaVeck, M.B. Sporn, and C.C. Harris, 1986. Type β transforming growth factor is the primary differentiation-inducing serum factor for normal human bronchial epithelial cells. *Proc. Natl. Acad. Sci. U.S.A.* **83**: 2438.

Moldeus, P., M. Berggren, and R. Grafstrom. 1985. N-acetylcystein protection against the toxicity of cigarette smoke and cigarette smoke condensates in various tissues and cells *in vitro*. *Eur. J. of Respir. Dis.* **66** (Suppl.) **139**: 123.

Nakano, H., F. Yamamoto, C. Neville, D. Evans, T. Mizuno, and M. Perucho. 1984. Isolation of transforming sequences of two human lung carcinomas: Structural and functional analysis of the activated c-K-*ras* oncogenes. *Proc. Natl. Acad. Sci. U.S.A.* **81**: 71.

Nakayama, T., M. Kaneko, M. Kodama, and C. Nagata. 1985. Cigarette smoke induces DNA single-strand breaks in human cells. *Nature* **314**: 462.

Nau, M.M., B.J. Brooks, J. Battey, E. Sausville, A.F. Gazdar, I.R. Kirsch, O.W. McBride, V. Bertness, G.F. Hollis, and J.D. Minna. 1985. L-*myc*, a new *myc*-related gene amplified and expressed in human small cell lung cancer. *Nature* **318**: 69.

Nau, M.M., B.J. Brooks, Jr., D.N. Carney, A.F. Gazdar, J.F. Battey, E.A. Sausville, and J.D. Minna. 1986. Human small-cell lung cancers show amplification and expression of the N-*myc* gene. *Proc. Natl. Acad. Sci. U.S.A.* **83**: 1092.

Perucho, M., M. Goldfarb, K. Shimizu, C. Lama, J. Fogh, and M. Wigler. 1981. Human-tumor-derived cell lines contain common and different transforming genes. *Cell* **27**: 467.

Rheinwald, J.G. and M.A. Beckett. 1980. Defective terminal differentiation in culture as a consistent and selectable character of malignant human keratinocytes. *Cell* **22**: 629.

Scott, R.E. and P.B. Maercklein. 1985. An initiator of carcinogenesis selectively and stably inhibits stem cell differentiation: A concept that initiation of carcinogenesis involves multiple phases. *Proc. Natl. Acad. Sci. U.S.A.* **82**: 2995.

Selikoff, I.J., E.C. Hammond, and J. Churg. 1968. Asbestos exposure, smoking, and neoplasia. *J. Am. Med. Assoc.* **204**: 104.

Shih, T.Y., A.G. Papageorge, P.E. Stokes, M.O. Weeks, and E.M. Scolnick. 1980. Guanine nucleotide-binding and autophosphorylating activities associated with the p21^{src} protein of Harvey murine sarcoma virus. *Nature* **287**: 686.

Shoyab, M., J.E. DeLarco, and G.J. Todaro. 1979. Biologically active phorbol esters specifically alter affinity of epidermal growth factor membrane receptors. *Nature* **279**: 387.

Spandidos, D.A. and N.M. Wilkie. 1984. Malignant transformation of early passage rodent cells by a single mutated human oncogene. *Nature* **310**: 470.

U.S. Department of Health, Education and Welfare. 1979. *Smoking and Health, a report of the Surgeon General*, chp. 5 and 14, Publ. (PHS) 79-50066. U.S. Government Printing Office, Washington, D.C.

Wille, J.J., Jr., P.B. Maercklein, and R.E. Scott. 1982. Neoplastic transformation and defective control of cell proliferation and differentiation. *Cancer Res.* **42**: 5139.

Willey, J.C., C.E. Moser, Jr., J.F. Lechner, and C.C. Harris. 1984a. Differential effects of 12-*O*-tetradecanoylphorbol-13-acetate on cultured normal and neoplastic human bronchial epithelial cells. *Cancer Res.* **44**: 5124.

Willey, J.C., C.E. Moser, Jr., and C.C. Harris. 1984b. Effects of aplysiatoxin and debromoaplysiatoxin on growth and differentiation of normal human bronchial epithelial cells. *Cell Biol. Toxicol.* **1**: 145.

Willey, J.C., A.J. Saladino, C. Ozanne, J.F. Lechner, and C.C. Harris. 1984c. Acute effects of 12-*O*-tetradecanoylphorbol-13-acetate, teleocidin B, or 2,3,7,8-tetrachlorodibenzo-*p*-dioxin on cultured normal human bronchial epithelial cells. *Carcinogenesis* **5**: 209.

Wynder, E.L. and D. Hoffmann. 1967. *Tobacco and tobacco smoke. Studies in experimental carcinogenesis*. Academic Press, New York.

Yoakum, G.H. 1984. Protoplast fusion: A method to transfect human cells for gene isolation, oncogene testing and construction of specialized cell lines. *Biotechniques* **2**: 24.

Yoakum, G.H., B.E. Korba, J.F. Lechner, T. Tokiwa, A.F. Gazdar, T. Seeley, M. Siegel, L. Leeman, H. Autrup, and C.C. Harris. 1983. High-frequency transfection and cytopathology of the hepatitis B virus core antigen gene in human cells. *Science* **222**: 385.

Yoakum, G.H., J.F. Lechner, E.W. Gabrielson, B.E. Korba, L. Malan-Shibley, J.C. Willey, M.G. Valerio, A.M. Shamsuddin, B.F. Trump, and C.C. Harris. 1985. Transformation of human bronchial epithelial cells transfected by Harvey *ras* oncogene. *Science* **227**: 1174.

Yuasa, Y., S.K. Srivastava, C.Y. Dunn, J.S. Rhim, E.P. Reddy, and S.A. Aaronson. 1983. Acquisition of transforming properties by alternative point mutations within c-*bas/has* human proto-oncogene. *Nature* **303**: 775.

Yuspa, S.H. and D.L. Morgan. 1981. Mouse skin cells resistant to terminal differentiation associated with initiation of carcinogenesis. *Nature* **293**: 72.

Yuspa, S.H., U. Lichti, T. Ben, E. Patterson, H. Hennings, T.J. Slaga, N. Cclburn, and W. Kelsey. 1976. Phorbol esters stimulate DNA synthesis and ornithine decarboxylase activity in mouse epidermal cell cultures. *Nature* **262**: 402.

COMMENTS

PEGG: Out of the hundreds of human lung cancers, how many of them were surveyed for these oncogenes?

HARRIS: I suppose that if you look at the world's literature, there are less than 20 cases in which *ras* oncogenes have been identified in human carcinomas. However, only a small number of tumors have been tested.

POIRIER: Do you envision a role of chemical carcinogens acting in combination with oncogenes? Have you thought about trying a combination of oncogenes and chemical carcinogens?

HARRIS: I mentioned the studies to date in the literature in which chemical and physical carcinogens have been shown in a variety of systems to cause activation of oncogenes. In none of these reported studies have lung tumors been investigated. I think there is a real opportunity to ask the question: Is there activation of oncogenes in any of these tobacco-related carcinogenesis experiments?

YOAKUM: Specifically to that point, Alan Balbain and Mario Barbacid's system for looking at chemical activation of the Harvey *ras* oncogene turned up at least one very good chemical model in which about 85% of the end-product carcinomas were carrying a specific mutation in the Harvey *ras* gene. I'm sure he probably screened through a couple of chemical models to find one that behaved that way; however, I think that if you went the other way and took a chemical model and then screened through a series of oncogenes, you might find a relevant oncogene the same way he did. In response to your question about people expressing percents, some oncogene alterations have been interpreted to account for about 20% of non-small cell lung carcinomas—

that's based on restriction polymorphism data as well as transfection experiments. However, others may not be willing to make claims from these observations. Still, it's not a trivial percentage, and one cannot expect it to account for everything.

PEGG: Aren't you saying that you think that 20% is a reasonable number?

YOAKUM: I think they have data to support their claims. I don't know what's reasonable yet. I don't think enough is known.

HARRIS: I agree with that.

GRAFSTRÖM: At what stage do you see if p21 is produced in these transfected cells?

HARRIS: p21 production and aneuploidy occur very early, within the second passage of the transfected cells. We're doing experiments to determine how rapidly aneuploidy occurs in the cells, that is within two- or three-cell division.

YOAKUM: I think that in the transduction experiment, the p21 expression is immediate. The selection permits many cross-feeding effects; so you're carrying along many normal cells and you don't see very high levels of phosphorolated p21 product in your first passage of cells. But then those experiments were not run with a plasmid that carries, or neomycin, or a guanine phosphoribosyltransferase marker; so the normal cells were not eliminated. By the time you get to passage two, as Curt [Harris] says, there is a measurable level of phosphorylated p21 produced from the transfected Harvey *ras* oncogene.

HARRIS: Yes, because the normal cells have terminally differentiated by that time.

MAGEE: Do you think that the protoplast fusion method would work better than the standard transfection method?

HARRIS: To use the protoplast fusion method, you have to construct plasmids that contain genes you want to test. So it will not work very efficiently in terms of taking tumor DNA and trying to put it into cells. There are other methods—other than calcium phosphate—that one can think of. I suspect that one of the reasons that the results with NIH3T3 cells are frequently negative when you transfect DNA is that it's related to the recipient cell. These cells are exquisitely sensitive to the *ras* family of oncogenes. In fact that's how they were initially selected for testing as recipient cells.

STELLMAN: I feel somewhat overwhelmed sitting back here, as an epidemiologist and chemist. Listening to details of the role of nitrosamines, polycyclic hydrocarbons, aldehydes, and oncogenes, I wonder if someone could help us out a little by synthesizing a bigger picture of the collective role of all of these various factors in tobacco-induced human cancer.

HARRIS: I'll make a few brief comments. A number of various chemical carcinogens, including some of those which would produce lesions similar to those produced by tobacco-smoke compounds, have led to the activation of the *ras* family of oncogenes. Presumably through damaging DNA, predominantly guanines has led to miscoding, and this has led to the activation of oncogenes. Another possibility is that these agents damage DNA and cause chromosomal breaks and chromosomal rearrangements; the micronuclei tests that were previously discussed are examples of this.

YOAKUM: There are some specific cases where I think that is an arguable case; for instance if you were to look at retinoblastoma or at Wilm's tumors, there are now definite findings. Those cancers can be attributed to the loss of definable genes. In addition, there are claims that people can diagnose these cancers prenatally by restriction fragment length polymorphism. I think this will shortly be published and applied by Cavence et al., so I think the answer that you're giving here is yes and no. In some limited cases, where enough genetic information about specific types of cancers has been accrued, specific diagnostic inferences can be made from the structure of the DNA rearrangements that are found in identified genetic alleles, and the diagnostic indication will be right 99% of the time.

HARRIS: I think George [Yoakum] makes a good point in that if you are confused now, you are going to be more confused very soon because there is another class of genes which control the expression of oncogenes; and these genes, which suppress malignancy, are, in my opinion, much more interesting than the oncogenes we have heard about so far. Wilm's tumor and retinoblastoma are the two cases in which I think these genes will be first isolated.

Factors Involved in the Induction of Urinary Bladder Cancer by Aromatic Amines

FREDERICK A. BELAND AND FRED F. KADLUBAR
National Center for Toxicological Research
Jefferson, Arkansas 72079

OVERVIEW

Aromatic amines, which are components of cigarette smoke, are known to induce urinary bladder cancer in man. This paper considers the role of specific metabolic and pharmacodynamic factors in determining an individual's susceptibility to bladder tumor induction by aromatic amines. These factors include hepatic N-oxidation, urinary pH, urothelial prostaglandin H synthase, and acetylation pharmacogenetics.

INTRODUCTION

Cigarette smoking has long been associated with the induction of bladder cancer in man with an estimated 40-85% of all cases being attributed to tobacco exposure (Wynder et al. 1963; Hoover and Cole 1971; Wynder and Goldsmith 1977; Wigle et al. 1980; Moolgavkar and Stevens 1981; Mommsen and Aagaard 1983). The increased risk of bladder cancer in smokers is calculated to be two- to tenfold, and is correlated with both average daily cigarette consumption and cumulative cigarette usage. Although a wide variety of carcinogens have been detected in tobacco smoke (Hoffmann et al. 1982), it is the aromatic amines that are generally associated with bladder tumor induction in man. These compounds, which were originally discovered to be bladder carcinogens as a result of industrial exposure (Case et al. 1954), are found in nanogram quantities in mainstream smoke and even higher concentrations in sidestream smoke (Masuda and Hoffmann 1969; Patrianakos and Hoffmann 1979). In this paper, we consider the metabolic activation of tobacco-related aromatic amines. In particular, we emphasize which factors may potentially increase or decrease an individual's susceptibility to the induction of bladder cancer by aromatic amines as a result of exposure to tobacco products.

HEPATIC OXIDATION AND GLUCURONIDATION

As with most xenobiotics, the liver is the primary site for the metabolism of aromatic amines. With regard to bladder cancer, three hepatic biotransformations are particularly important: N-oxidation, C-oxidation, and N-glucuronidation.

Hepatic N-oxidation of primary arylamines is catalyzed by the cytochrome P-450 monooxygenases and in some cases by the flavin-containing monooxygenase (Fig. 1) (Hammons et al. 1985). The resultant N-hydroxy arylamines, which are mutagenic and carcinogenic per se (Kadlubar et al. 1977; Dooley et al. 1984), are converted into stable N-hydroxy arylamine N-glucuronides by hepatic glucuronyl transferases and are then transported via the circulation to the kidney where they are filtered into the urinary bladder lumen. Although these conjugates are stable at neutral pH, they can be hydrolyzed to release N-hydroxy arylamines under the slightly acidic conditions that are found in the urine of certain species susceptible to bladder tumors (Young and Kadlubar 1982). An alternative pathway is hepatic N-glucuronidation of the parent arylamines (Fig. 1) (Lilienblum and Bock 1984; Wang et al. 1985) followed by transport of the arylamine N-glucuronides to the bladder. Under acidic conditions these conjugates are hydrolyzed to yield free arylamines which can undergo subsequent peroxidative activation in the bladder epithelium (Yamazoe et al. 1985).

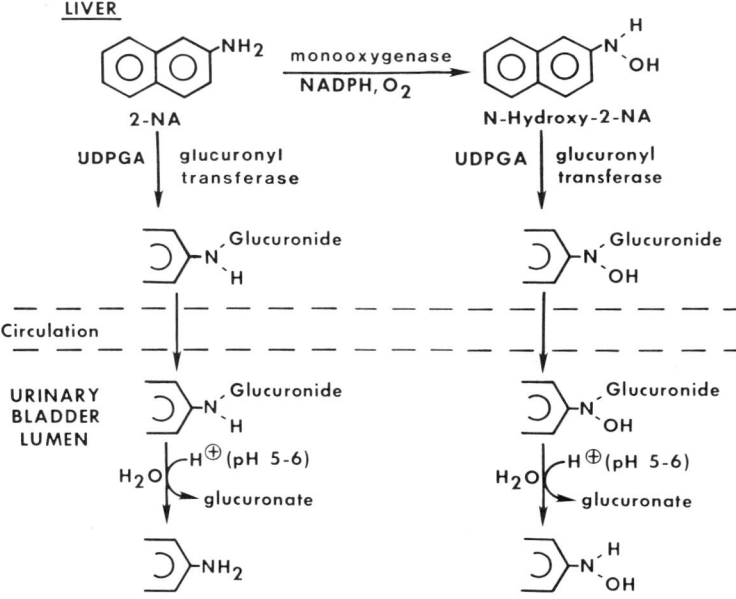

Figure 1
Hepatic N-oxidation and/or N-glucuronidation of aromatic amines. Primary aromatic amines (e.g., 2-naphthylamine [2-NA]) are N-oxidized in the liver by monooxygenases. The resultant N-hydroxy arylamines are N-glucuronidated and transported to the bladder where under slightly acidic conditions the conjugates are hydrolyzed to release free N-hydroxy arylamines. Alternatively, the arylamines can be directly N-glucuronidated to conjugates which are also acid-labile. (*UDPGA*) Uridine-5′ diphosphoglucuronic acid.

Since hepatic N-oxidation is catalyzed by cytochrome P-450, the specificity of particular cytochrome P-450 isozymes for the N-oxidation of individual aromatic amines may be a critical factor in determining the carcinogenic potential of these compounds. This specificity was investigated by examining the N- and C-oxidation of representative aromatic amines by purified cytochrome P-450 isozymes (Hammons et al. 1985). Nearly all of the isozymes could catalyze the oxidation of 1-naphthylamine. This proceeded entirely through hydroxylation of the carbon atom *ortho* to the amine function and no N-oxidation was detected (Fig. 2A). The same metabolic profile was observed when using hepatic microsomes from rats, dogs, and humans. It is this failure to N-oxidize 1-naphthylamine that probably accounts for the lack of carcinogenicity of 1-naphthylamine in any bioassay conducted to date (Radomski et al. 1980; Purchase et al. 1981).

In contrast to what was found with 1-naphthylamine, N-oxidized metabolites were the major products detected in in vitro incubations with the carcinogen, 2-aminofluorene. As shown in Figure 2B, a number of isozymes catalyzed the N-oxidation of 2-aminofluorene with the greatest rates being observed with the β-naphthoflavone-inducible P-450, BNF-B, and the isosafrole-inducible P-450, ISF-G. N-Oxidized metabolites were also the major products detected from incubations conducted with microsomes from rat, dog, and human liver.

The carcinogenic arylamine, 2-naphthylamine, differed from 2-aminofluorene in that it was N-oxidized by only a single isozyme, ISF-G (Fig. 2C). Whether or not a similar isozyme exists in human liver is presently not known. However, human liver microsomes were able to catalyze the N-oxidation of 2-naphthylamine, and interestingly, although the cytochrome P-450 content of these preparations varied less than threefold, the rate of 2-naphthylamine N-oxidation per nmole cytochrome P-450 varied more than thirtyfold (Hammons et al. 1985). Furthermore, there was no direct relationship between cytochrome P-450 levels and the rate of N-oxidation. These observations suggest that there may be specific inducers for isozymes which N-oxidize 2-naphthylamine and/or genetic heterogeneity for N-oxidation capacity in human populations. Both of these factors could be an important determinant of cancer risk from aromatic amine exposure.

URINARY pH

Humans, as well as dogs, have urinary pH values that are slightly acidic, with the average values being 5.9 and 6.3, respectively (Young and Kadlubar 1982). By comparison, the urinary pH of monkeys and rats is approximately one pH unit higher. This difference in pH appears to be an important factor in arylamine-induced bladder carcinogenesis since humans and dogs are much more susceptible to bladder tumor induction as a result of arylamine exposure than monkeys and rats (Young and Kadlubar 1982). The increased susceptibility of humans and dogs may be due to the chemical lability of the N-glucuronide conjugates because, as

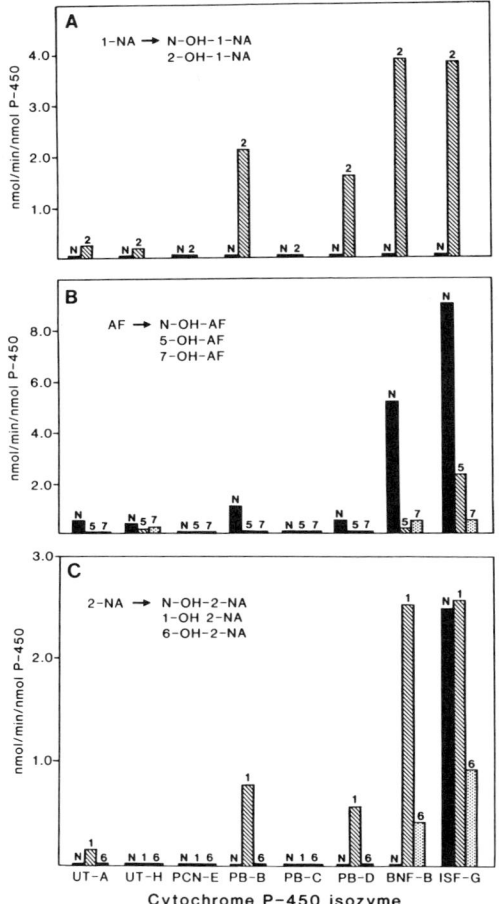

Figure 2
Oxidation of aromatic amines by purified rat liver cytochrome P-450 isozymes. The nomenclature for the individual isozymes is given in Guengerich et al. (1982). The number or letter above the histogram bars refers to the site of hydroxylation. (*NA*) Naphthylamine; (*AF*) 2-aminofluorene; (*OH*) hydroxy; (*UT*) untreated; (*PCN*) pregnenolone-16α-carbonitrile; (*PB*) phenobarbital; (*BNF*) β-naphthoflavone; (*ISF*) isosafrole.

previously shown in Figure 1, these undergo acid-catalyzed hydrolysis. In an experiment where the urinary pH of rats was decreased from pH 7.7 to pH 5.7, the total concentration of free and conjugated *N*-oxidized metabolites of 2-naphthylamine remained constant (Kadlubar et al. 1981a). However, the ratio of free to conjugated *N*-hydroxy-2-naphthylamine increased sixfold as the pH became more acidic. Thus, the exposure to reactive *N*-hydroxy arylamines was increased as the urinary pH decreased. This relationship was combined with other factors, such as voiding interval, urine volume, and resorption of arylamine metabolites, to develop a pharmacokinetic model that e imated the relative risk of exposure of the bladder epithelium to N-hydroxy-2-naṛ ıthylamine (Young and Kadlubar 1982). The model correctly predicted the relative usceptibility of various species to 2-naphthylamine-induced bladder tumors and ⌣uggested that factors which alter urinary pH in humans may significantly influence the relative risk for bladder cancer induction.

UROTHELIAL PROSTAGLANDIN H SYNTHASE

Although the primary site for aromatic amine oxidation appears to be the liver, it is also possible that a certain amount of N-oxidation of urinary arylamines could occur in the bladder epithelium itself. Cytochrome P-450 and the associated enzymatic N-oxidation of 4-aminobiphenyl were detected in bovine bladder (Poupko et al. 1983); however, similar monooxygenase activity for the N-oxidation of several arylamines was not found in dog epithelial preparations (Poupko et al. 1983; Wise et al. 1984). Although the dog bladder seems to be devoid of monooxygenase activity, it does contain high levels of prostaglandin H synthase (PHS) (Wise et al. 1984), which could catalyze the arachidonic acid-dependent peroxidation of aromatic amines. In in vitro studies, 2-naphthylamine was found to undergo PHS-catalyzed peroxidation, and analysis of the metabolites indicated that two reactive metabolites were formed: N-hydroxy-2-naphthylamine and 2-imino-1-naphthoquinone, the latter arising from further oxidation of the primary metabolite, 2-amino-1-naphthol (Fig. 3) (Kadlubar et al. 1982). In additional experiments, 2-naphthylamine was administered to dogs and the DNA adducts formed in bladder epithelium were examined (Kadlubar et al. 1981b; Yamazoe et al. 1985). Adducts indicative of both N-hydroxy-2-naphthylamine (80%) and 2-imino-1-naphthoquinone (20%) as reactive intermediates were detected. This suggested that a portion of the bladder epithelial DNA adducts could arise from PHS-mediated peroxidation in addition to those obtained from hepatic N-oxidation and N-glucuronidation of 2-naphthylamine (Fig. 3).

The contribution of urothelial PHS to the activation of aromatic amines in humans is presently not known. However, in preliminary in vitro experiments, human bladder microsomes did catalyze the arachidonic acid-dependent binding of aromatic amines to DNA. The relative order of this presumed PHS-mediated DNA binding was benzidine > 4-aminobiphenyl ~2-naphthylamine >Glu-P-1~ IQ~Trp-P-2 (F. Kadlubar, unpubl.).

ACETYLATION

The hepatic N-acetylation of aromatic amines is catalyzed by acetyl coenzyme A (AcCoA)-dependent N-acetyltransferases. In humans, as well as certain other

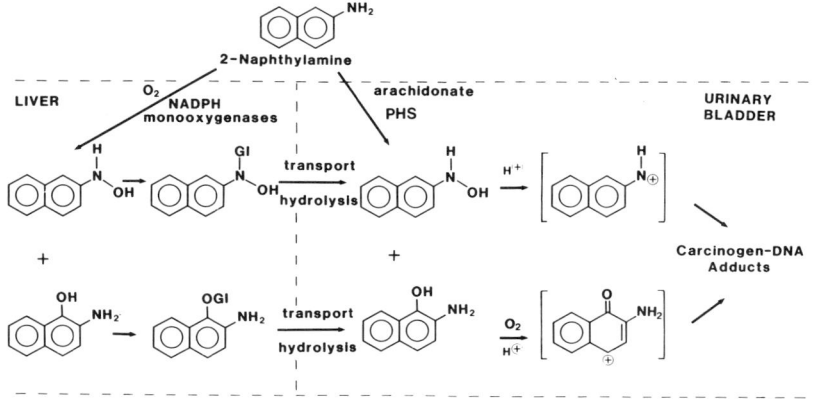

Figure 3
Prostaglandin H synthase (PHS)-mediated peroxidation of aromatic amines. Arylamines, such as 2-naphthylamine, are peroxidized by PHS to yield N-hydroxy and ortho-hydroxy derivatives. These metabolites can also be formed by hepatic oxidation and conjugation, transport to the bladder, and subsequent hydrolysis of the conjugate. N-hydroxy arylamines undergo acid-catalyzed reactions with DNA. Ortho aminophenols spontaneously oxidize to iminoquinones which also react with DNA.

species, the capability for N-acetylation is polymorphic with both rapid and slow phenotypes being observed (Weber and Hein 1985). The slow phenotype appears to be a homozygous autosomal recessive trait whereas rapid acetylators are either homozygous- or heterozygous-dominant. Within populations of European origin, there is nearly an equal distribution of fast and slow acetylators, and interestingly, among bladder cancer patients from low-risk groups, there is a slight excess of the slow-acetylator phenotype (Mommsen et al. 1985). The increased susceptibility of slow acetylators to bladder cancer has been attributed to the exposure of these individuals to a greater concentration of reactive N-hydroxy arylamines as compared to the rapid acetylator phenotype (Wolf et al. 1980). With fast acetylators, arylamine N-acetylation presumably precedes N-oxidation which would decrease the concentration of arylamine and N-hydroxy arylamine available for N-glucuronidation and eventual transport to the bladder.

In recent studies, we have been examining the ability of cytosolic acetylases to catalyze an AcCoA-dependent binding of N-hydroxy arylamines to DNA (Flammang et al. 1985a; Flammang and Kadlubar 1985; Djuric' et al. 1985; Djuric' et al. 1986; Flammang and Kadlubar 1986). This activity was found in a number of rat tissues, including the liver, intestine, mammary gland, and kidney (Flammang and Kadlubar 1985; Flammang and Kadlubar 1986). Although the mechanism of this activation requires further investigation, the data suggest that certain N-hydroxy arylamines are directly O-acetylated. The resultant N-acetoxy arylamines are highly reactive species which, at neutral pH, bind to DNA to a far greater extent than their parent N-hydroxy derivatives (Fig. 4). This AcCoA-dependent activation of N-hydroxy arylamines has also been detected in cytosolic preparations from a variety of species, including mouse, rat, rabbit, hamster, guinea pig, and human (Flammang and Kadlubar 1985; Flammang and Kadlubar 1986). However, it is notably absent in the liver and bladder cytsols of dogs, a species lacking N-acetyltransferase activity. These observations suggest that N-acetylation of aromatic amines and O-acetylation of N-hydroxy arylamines may be catalyzed by the same cytosolic AcCoA-dependent acetyltransferase. This conclusion is supported by recent experiments which demonstrated a correlation between arylamine N-acetylation and N-hydroxy arylamine O-acetylation with human liver cytosol (Flammang et al. 1985b).

These results indicate that acetylation may be viewed as a two-edged sword. If N-acetylation precedes N-oxidation, then detoxification may occur, whereas if the arylamine is initially N-hydroxylated, further activation may occur through O-acetylation. A number of factors will influence which metabolic pathway predominates, including the particular arylamine, the specific P-450 isozymes that are present, and the acetylator phenotype of the individual. The interplay of these factors may explain why only a slight excess of bladder cancers are observed in slow acetylator phenotypes from low-risk groups (Mommsen et al. 1985), whereas in populations exposed to specific types of aromatic amines, there appears to be a highly significant correlation between slow acetylator phenotype and bladder tumor induction (Cartwright et al. 1982).

ACKNOWLEDGMENT

We thank Cindy Hartwick for her help in preparing this manuscript.

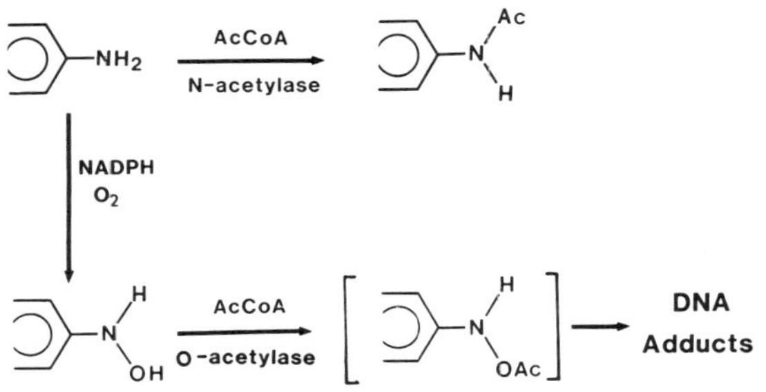

Figure 4
Acetylation of aromatic amines. Primary arylamines can be directly N-acetylated. Alternatively, the aromatic amine can be N-oxidized and the resultant N-hydroxy arylamine O-acetylated to yield a reactive N-acetoxy arylamine.

REFERENCES

Cartwright, R.A., R.W. Glashan, H.J. Rogers, R.A. Ahmad, D. Barham-Hall, E. Higgins, and M.A. Kahn. 1982. Role of N-acetyltransferase phenotypes in bladder carcinogenesis: A pharmacogenetic epidemiological approach to bladder cancer. *Lancet* ii: 842.

Case, R.A.M., M.E. Hosker, D.B. McDonald, and J.T. Pearson. 1954. Tumours of the urinary bladder in workmen engaged in the manufacture and use of certain dyestuff intermediates in the British chemical industry. I. The role of aniline, benzidine, alpha-naphthylamine and beta-naphthylamine. *Br. J. Ind. Med.* 11: 75.

Djuric, Z., E.K. Fifer, and F.A. Beland. 1985. Acetyl coenzyme A-dependent vinding of carcinogenic and mutagenic dinitropyrenes to DNA. *Carcinogenesis* 6: 941.

Djuric, Z., E.K. Fifer, P.C. Howard, and F.A. Beland. 1986. Oxidative microsomal metabolism of 1-nitropyrene and DNA-binding of oxidized metabolites following nitroreduction. *Carcinogenesis* (in press).

Dooley, K.L., F.A. Beland, T.J. Bucci, and F.F. Kadlubar. 1984. Local carcinogenicity, rates of absorption, extent and persistence of macromolecular binding, and acute histopathological effects of N-hydroxy-1-naphthylamine and N-hydroxy-2-naphthylamine. *Cancer Res.* 44: 1172.

Flammang, T.J. and F.F. Kadlubar. 1986. Acetyl coenzyme A-dependent metabolic activation of N-hydroxy-3, 2'-dimethyl-4-aminobiphenyl and several carcinogenic N-hydroxy arylamines in relation to tissue and species differences, other acyl donors, and arylhydroxamic acid-dependent acyltransferases. *Carcinogenesis* 7: 919.

———. 1985. Acetyl CoA-dependent, cytosol-catalyzed binding of carcinogenic N-hydroxy-arylamines to DNA. In *Microsomes and drug oxidations* (ed. A.R. Boobis, J. Caldwell, F. DeMatteis, and C.R. Elcombe), p. 190. Taylor and Francis, London.

Flammang, T.J., J.G. Westra, F.F. Kadlubar, and F.A. Beland. 1985a. DNA adducts formed from the probable proximate carcinogen, N-hydroxy-3,2'-dimethyl-4-aminobiphenyl, by acid catalysis or S-acetyl coenzyme A-dependent enzymatic esterification. *Carcinogenesis* 6: 251.

Flammang, T.J., Y. Yamazoe, F.P. Guengerich, and F.F. Kadlubar. 1985b. Relation between slow/fast acetylator phenotype and metabolic activation of aromatic amines. *Proc. Am. Assoc. Cancer Res.* 26: 108.

Guengerich, F.P., G.A. Dannan, S.T. Wright, M.V. Martin, and L.S. Kaminsky. 1982. Purification and characterization of liver microsomal cytochromes P-450: Electrophoretic, spectral, catalytic, and immunochemical properties and inducibility of eight isozymes isolated from rats treated with phenobarbital or β-naphthoflavone. *Biochemistry* 21: 6019.

Hammons, G.J., F.P. Guengerich, C.C. Weis, F.A. Beland, and F.F. Kadlubar. 1985. Metabolic oxidation of carcinogenic arylamines by rat, dog, and human hepatic microsomes and by purified flavin-containing and cytochrome P-450 monooxygenases. *Cancer Res.* 45: 3578.

Hoffmann, D., I. Hoffmann, S.E. Shackney, and E.K. Weisburger. 1982. Mechanisms of carcinogenesis. In *The health consequences of smoking. Cancer: A report of the Surgeon General* (ed. J. Luoto), p. 192. U.S. Department of Health and Human Services, Rockville, Maryland.

Hoover, R. and P. Cole. 1971. Population trends in cigarette smoking and bladder cancer. *Am. J. Epidemiol.* **94**: 409.

Kadlubar, F.F., J.A. Miller, and E.C. Miller. 1977. Hepatic microsomal N-glucuronidation and nucleic acid binding of N-hydroxy arylamines in relation to urinary bladder carcinogenesis. *Cancer Res.* **37**: 805.

Kadlubar, F.F., C.B. Frederick, C.C. Weis, and T.V. Zenser. 1982. Prostaglandin endoperoxide synthetase-mediated metabolism of carcinogenic aromatic amines and their binding to DNA and protein. *Biochem. Biophys. Res. Commun.* **108**: 253.

Kadlubar, F.F., L.E. Unruh, T.J. Flammang, D. Sparks, R.K. Mitchum, and G.J. Mulder. 1981a. Alteration of urinary levels of the carcinogen, N-hydroxy-2-naphthylamine, and its N-glucuronide in the rat by control of urinary pH, inhibition of metabolic sulfation, and changes in biliary excretion. *Chem. Biol. Interact.* **33**: 129.

Kadlubar, F.F., J.F. Anson, K.L. Dooley, and F.A. Beland. 1981b. Formation of urothelial and hepatic DNA adducts from the carcinogen 2-naphthylamine. *Carcinogenesis* **2**: 467.

Lilienblum, W. and K.W. Bock. 1984. N-Glucuronide formation of carcinogenic aromatic amines in rat and human liver microsomes. *Biochem. Pharmacol.* **33**: 2041.

Masuda, Y. and D. Hoffmann. 1969. Quantitative determination of 1-naphthylamine and 2-naphthylamine in cigarette smoke. *Anal. Chem.* **41**: 650.

Mommsen, S. and J. Aagaard. 1983. Tobacco as a risk factor in bladder cancer. *Carcinogenesis* **4**: 335.

Mommsen, S., N.M. Barfod, and J. Aagaard. 1985. N-Acetyltransferase phenotypes in the urinary bladder carcinogenesis of a low-risk population. *Carcinogenesis* **6**: 199.

Moolgavkar, S.H. and R.G. Stevens. 1981. Smoking and cancers of bladder and pancreas: Risks and temporal trends. *J. Natl. Cancer Inst.* **67**: 15.

Patrianakos, C. and D. Hoffmann. 1979. Chemical studies on tobacco smoke. LXIV. On the analysis of aromatic amines in cigarette smoke. *J. Anal. Toxicol.* **3**: 150.

Poupko, J.M., T. Radomski, R.M. Santella, and J.L. Radomski. 1983. Organ, species, and compound specificity in the metabolic activation of primary aromatic amines. *J. Natl. Cancer Inst.* **70**: 1077.

Purchase, I.F.H., A.E. Kalinowski, J. Ishmael, J. Wilson, C.W. Gore, and I.S. Chart. 1981. Lifetime carcinogenicity study of 1- and 2-naphthylamine in dogs. *Br. J. Cancer* **44**: 892.

Radomski, J.L., W.B. Deichmann, N.H. Altman, and T. Radomski. 1980. Failure of pure 1-naphthylamine to induce bladder tumors in dogs. *Cancer Res.* **40**: 3537.

Wang, C.Y., K. Zukowski, and M.-S. Lee. 1985. Glucuronidation of carcinogenic arylamine metabolites by rat liver microsomes. *Biochem. Pharmacol.* **34**: 837.

Weber, W.W. and D.W. Hein. 1985. N-Acetylation pharmacogenetics. *Pharmacol. Rev.* **37**: 25.

Wigle, D.T., Y. Mao, and M. Grace. 1980. Relative importance of smoking as a risk factor for selected cancers. *Can. J. Public Health* **71**: 269.

Wise, R.W., T.V. Zenser, F.F. Kadlubar, and B.B. Davis. 1984. Metabolic activation of carcinogenic aromatic amines by dog bladder and kidney prostaglandin H synthase. *Cancer Res.* **44**: 1893.

Wolf, H., G.M. Lower, Jr., and G.T. Bryan. 1980. Role of N-acetyltransferase phenotype in human susceptibility to bladder carcinogenic arylamines. *Scand. J. Urol. Nephrol.* **14**: 161.

Wynder, E.L. and R. Goldsmith. 1977. The epidemiology of bladder cancer: A second look. *Cancer* **40**: 1246.

Wynder, E.L., J. Onderdonk, and N. Mantel. 1963. An epidemiological investigation of cancer of the bladder. *Cancer* **16**: 1388.

Yamazoe, Y., D.W. Miller, C.C. Weis, K.L. Dooley, T.V. Zenser, F.A. Beland, and F.F. Kadlubar. 1985. DNA adducts formed by *ring*-oxidation of the carcinogen 2-naphthylamine with prostaglandin H synthase *in vitro* and in the dog urothelium *in vivo*. *Carcinogenesis* **6**: 1379.

Young, J.F. and F.F. Kadlubar. 1982. A pharmacokinetic model to predict exposure of the bladder epithelium to urinary N-hydroxyarylamine carcinogens as a function of urine pH, voiding interval, and resorption. *Drug Metab. Dispos.* **10**: 641.

COMMENTS

HECHT: How can you distinguish between the acetylation of the hydroxylamine and N, O-acyltransferase?

BELAND: The way we originally discovered O-acetylation was to examine the DNA binding of the hydroxamic acid of 3,2'dimethyl-4-aminobiphenyl (DMABP) in an N,O-acyltransferase assay. We did not detect DNA binding, which agrees with the observation of Charles King that arylhydroxamic acids with *ortho* or *peri* substituents are poor substrates for N,O-acyltransferase. In contrast, when incubations were conducted with the hydroxylamine of DMABP and acetyl coenzyme A, the binding to DNA was quite extensive.

HARRIS: How important do you think the peroxidase pathway is?

BELAND: At present, I am not sure how important PHS activation in bladder epithelium is. What I neglected to mention in my presentation is that *ortho* hydroxylation can also occur in the liver. These metabolites can be conjugated, transported to the bladder, and hydrolyzed to yield free *ortho*-aminophenols. We do not know the relative contribution of each pathway.

PHS activation may be quite important with benzidine because it is an excellent substrate for this enzyme and extensive DNA-binding results.

BARTSCH: How, by chance, did you find that this CoA-S-acetyl-dependent acetylation works so efficiently in vitro? In our early experiments, published in 1972, the acetyl transfer from CoA-S-acetyl to N-hydroxy-2-aminofluorene by rat liver cytosol was taking place, but at a slow rate.

BELAND: This was an oversight on my part; I did not mean to imply that we discovered O-acetylation but rather that it seemed to be the only pathway consistent with the adducts we found.

BARTSCH: Did you change the assay condition to see this CoA-S-acetyl-dependent acetylation?

BELAND: No, we didn't. When we conducted a standard N,O-acyltransferase assay with the hydroxamic acid of DMABP, we did not get any DNA binding. We knew that all of the adducts obtained in vivo were nonacetylated and we wondered how they could be formed. We considered N,O-acyltransferase to be the most plausible pathway, but, as I mentioned, it did not work. We also tried sulfotransferase activation with the hydroxylamine of DMABP, but again this did not work. This led to our experiments with acetyl coenzyme A.

CORREA: These 1700 cases that you referred to reflect the heterogeneity of human tumors. At one point there was a distinction between bladder cancer produced or associated with cigarette smoking, another group probably associated with industrial pollution, and then another one associated with infections. Dr. Harris' presentation may be telling us that the grouping of human tumors is just beginning to be sorted out or to get more confused. Because, for instance, with lung cancer, the so-called Krayberg's type I grouped small-cell and squamous cell carcinomas were produced by cigarettes. Adenocarcinoma was not really associated with cigarettes. Now with the oncogenes we have a different grouping with the small-cell and adenocarcinoma in one group. So I think that pooling all these studies together may not be a very good idea. You should separate people living in an area highly exposed to industrial pollution from smokers.

BELAND: That is what Cartwright did. He found a unique population which presumably had been exposed to one class of chemicals. This allowed him to obtain a very good relationship between slow acetylator phenotype and bladder cancer induction.

STELLMAN: I know of a case-control study on bladder cancer by Mommsen in rural Denmark; the one you showed has about ten times as many cases in it.

BELAND: Mommsen did not have a statistical difference between the groups he examined. However, when he combined his data with that of seven previous studies, he found a statistical difference between bladder tumor incidence and acetylator phenotype. This included Lower and Bryan's study of Danish populations.

STELLMAN: Are these all Danish?

BELAND: No, they are not all Danish. That is a combination of all those studies.

STELLMAN: He knows, at least for the Danish component, who is a smoker and who isn't. In fact, he knows about 20 variables, including artificial sweeteners, for which he found an effect in women. So one could easily produce a statistical means to separate out smoking.

TANNENBAUM: He did that in the Danish population. You're talking about two different things. You are talking about acetylator phenotype and you are talking about cigarette smokers versus nonsmokers.

STELLMAN: Right.

TANNENBAUM: Mommsen just published a paper for the Danish population in which he has measured the risk to cigarette smoking and he shows it does respond to relationship for cigarette smoking, up to an excess risk of about sevenfold in the group that smokes the most cigarettes.

STELLMAN: Right, he forgot the little Danish cheroots. My question is, does he do them all simultaneously in the same analysis?

BELAND: No, not in that paper. There has never been a single study in which a significant difference has been found between acetylator phenotype and bladder tumor incidence. Only when all eight studies were combined was a statistical difference observed.

TANNENBAUM: In smokers?

CORREA: That's very misleading because the difference between 59% and 65%, even if it is statistically significant, may not have much biologic value.

BELAND: I agree.

Session 4: New Associations of Tobacco Use and Cancer Risk

Cigarette Smoking and Cancer of the Uterine Cervix

WARREN WINKELSTEIN, JR.
Department of Biomedical and Environmental Health Sciences
School of Public Health
University of California
Berkeley, California 94720

OVERVIEW

An association between cigarette smoking and cancer of the uterine cervix was first noted in 1966 (Naguib et al. 1966). In 1977, a specific hypothesis regarding cervical cancer and smoking was advanced (Winkelstein 1977). To date, 15 of 18 published studies have demonstrated such an association. Both cohort and case-control studies have been implemented and many have shown a dose-response relationship as well as controlling for confounding variables.

INTRODUCTION

The hypothesis that cigarette smoking was causally associated with cancer of the uterus was first presented 8 years ago (Winkelstein 1977). In an editorial published in the July 22-29, 1983 issue of the *Journal of the American Medical Association*, the following statement appeared: "although the biochemical mechanism whereby cigarette smoking causes cervical dysplasia and neoplasia may not yet be identified, a pragmatist must conclude that the causal role is sufficiently clear to permit preventive measures to reduce the risk of the disease" (Austin 1983). Indeed, although a biochemical mechanism has been proposed, the evidence is no better than for other site-specific cancers presumed to be etiologically associated with chemical carcinogens (Winkelstein et al. 1984).

The hypothesis that cigarette smoking was causally associated with cervical cancer was based on the observation that cancer of the lung in men and of the uterine cervix in women had similar geographic distributions in the Third National Cancer Survey and on the knowledge that most, if not all, smoking-related site-specific cancers were predominantly of squamous cell histology (Kreyberg 1962; Winkelstein et al. 1977).

Prior to the publication of the hypothesis, four case-control and two cohort studies had reported data relevant to the relationship of cervical cancer and smoking (Naguib et al. 1966; Tokuhata 1967; Thomas 1973; Cederlof et al. 1975; Hirayama 1975; Williams and Horm 1977). All but one showed significantly elevated relative risks for smoking (Tokuhata 1967). In that study a number of smoking-related diseases were included among the controls, thereby biasing the results. Two of the studies controlled for confounding (Thomas 1973; Williams and Horm 1977). One investigator (Naguib et al. 1966) commented that the association might possibly be causal and another (Williams and Horm 1977) indicated that the finding was "suggestive." The studies are briefly summarized in Table 1.

Between publication of the hypothesis and the editorial (Austin 1983) recognizing that causal nature of the association between cigarette smoking and cervical cancer, eight publications reported relevant investigations (Wright et al. 1978; Harris et al. 1980; Stellman et al. 1980; Wigle et al. 1980; Buckley et al. 1981; Clarke et al. 1982; Lyon et al. 1983; Trevathan et al. 1983). All but one reported elevated relative risks for cigarette smoking (Stellman et al. 1980). The appropriateness of the controls in this study, as well as the statistical treatment of the data, have been questioned (Winkelstein and Levin 1981). Of the remaining seven studies, six provided information regarding a dose-response relationship and five of these demonstrated this phenomenon (Wright et al. 1978; Wigle et al. 1980; Buckley et al. 1981; Clarke et al. 1982; Trevathan et al. 1983).

One study from this group is particularly interesting (Buckley et al. 1981). Buckley and his colleagues at Oxford set out to study the risk of cervical epithelial abnormalities related to the sexual practices of husbands. To do this they identified a group of married women with such abnormalities who reported only one sexual partner, their husbands, and matched these women to women without cervical disease, who had also reported their husbands as their only sexual partner. They then ascertained characteristics of husbands and found a distinct excess of sexual partners among the husbands of patients as compared to those of controls. At the same time they obtained information regarding smoking practices of the cases and controls. The study design eliminated confounding by multiple sexual partners of cases and controls although it required adjustment for the number of sexual partners of the husbands. A strong dose-response was revealed for smoking among cases. The data are summarized in Table 2.

Despite the demonstration of elevated relative risks and a dose-response relationship for cigarette smoking and cervical cancer in the previous cohort and case-control studies reported by the Oxford Group (Wright et al. 1978; Harris et al. 1980), these investigators raised the possibility that the association was due to unknown confounders and questioned the biological plausibility of the association. Because of the eminence of these investigators and the pertinence of the issues which they raised, my colleagues and I reexamined these questions and reported our conclusions at the 1982 meeting of the International Epidemiological Association in Edinburgh. The substance of our remarks were subsequently published (Winkelstein et al. 1984).

With respect to biological plausibility, we first reexamined the assertion that the cancers which are most strongly associated with cigarette smoking are predominantly squamous cell in type. To do this, we selected for study the five most common site-specific cancers of women plus bladder cancer, an established cigarette-related

Table 1
Relative Risks for Smoking and Cervical Cancer Revealed by Various Investigations

References	Study type	RR	Confounders controlled	Conclusions of investigators
Before hypothesis				
Naguib et al. (1966)	Screening	2.6	No	Possibly causal
Tokuhata (1967)	Case-control	1.1	No	None
Thomas (1973)	Case-control	1.5	13 variables	None
Hirayama (1975)	Cohort	1.8–3.5	No	None
Cederlof et al. (1975)	Cohort	7.2	No	None
Williams and Horm (1977)	Case-control	1.2–1.8	7 variables	Suggestive
After hypothesis (1977) until Austin (1983)				
Wright et al. (1978)	Cohort	1.4–2.9	5 variables	Confounded
Wigle et al. (1980)	Case-control	1.2–2.7	No	Supportive
Stellman et al. (1980)	Case-control	1.2–1.3	2 variables	$P = 0.06$
Harris et al. (1980)	Case-control	2.2–2.1	3 variables	Implausible
Buckley et al. (1981)	Case-control	3.7–7.9	1 variable	Lending weight
Clarke et al. (1982)	Case-control	2.2	3 variables	Supportive
Lyon et al. (1983)	Cohort	3.5	2 variables	Further study
Trevathan et al. (1983)	Case-control	2.3–12.7	5 variables	Strong dose-response
Since Austin (1983)				
Berggren and Sjostedt (1983)	Case-control	3.0	No	A risk factor
Marshall et al. (1983)	Case-control	1.6	No	No dose-response
Martin and Hill (1984)	Case-control	1.3	2 variables	$P > 0.05$
Greenberg et al. (1985)	Cohort[a]	1.6–2.1	5 variables	$P < 0.001$

[a] Update of Wright et al. (1978)

Table 2
Matched Relative Risks for Smoking and Cervical Cancer among Cases and Controls with Lifetime History of One Sexual Partner (Adjusted for Number of Sexual Partners of Husbands)

Smoking status	Cases (n = 57) (RR)
Nonsmokers	1.00
Exsmokers	3.70
Current smokers	7.85
Trend chi-square	< 0.001

Adapted from Buckley et al. (1981)

neoplasm (Williams and Horm 1977). We then determined the percent of these site-specific cancers, which were designated as having squamous cell histology in the Third National Cancer Survey and arranged them in order from a high of 82% for cervical cancer to a low of 0.03% for uterine cancer. Next, we obtained relative risks for smokers of greater than 15 cigarettes per day compared to those who never smoked, from the Swedish prospective study of 28,000 women, and found a good correspondence. The data are shown in Table 3.

We also documented the fact that carcinogenic and mutagenic chemicals can be absorbed through the lungs of humans and experimental animals and transported to distant organs (Kotin et al. 1959; Yamasaki and Ames 1977; Petrakis et al. 1980). Recently, Sasson and colleagues at the American Health Foundation and Falu Hospital in Sweden, showed that nicotine and cotinine could be detected in the cervical fluids of smokers, providing additional evidence on this point (Sasson et al. 1985). Finally, we cited the analogy of multiple causation for lung cancer as consistent with multiple causation for cervical cancer, i.e., viral and chemical.

With respect to the question of an unknown confounder, a statistical model was developed to demonstrate the required relative prevalence and relative risk required

Table 3
Squamous Cell Type (%) and Relative Risk of Selected Cancers for Smokers

Cancer site (ICD No.)	Squamous cell (%)	RR
Cervix (180)	81.6	7.2
Lung (162)	21.1	4.8
Bladder (188–9)	3.2	1.7
Breast (174)	0.1	1.6
Colon (152–3)	0.05	0.9
Uterus (182)	0.03	0.7

Adapted from Winkelstein et al. (1984)

by an unknown confounder to account for the observed relative risk for smoking and cervical cancer observed in the Oxford studies. In those studies, the smoking prevalence was 32% and the relative risk was approximately two, after adjustment for age, number of sexual partners, history of pregnancy outside marriage, and years of oral contraceptive use. The parameters which describe the possible unknown relationships that are consistent with the observed relationships are prevalence of the high-risk level of the unknown explanatory factor, the relative prevalence of the high-risk level of the unknown explanatory factor with respect to cigarette smoking, and the relative risk of cervical cancer in those with the high-risk level of the unknown factor compared with those with its low-risk level. The combinations of values which show the smallest common values sufficient to explain the observed relative risks in the Oxford studies are shown in Table 4. The smallest possible common value is 3.4, realized when the prevalence of the high-risk level of the unknown factor is 50%, a level which would have been unlikely to go unnoticed by so many competent investigators. Note that when a small proportion of the population is at the high-risk prevalence level of the unknown factor, very large relative prevalence and relative risk values are needed to explain an observed smoking cervical cancer association with an adjusted relative risk of two. For example, if the prevalence of the high-risk level of the unknown factor is 0.1 (10%), then the smallest common explanatory value for relative prevalence and relative risk is seven.

After the publication of the editorial (Austin 1983) indicating the probable causal nature of the cervical cancer smoking association, four additional publications reported relevant data. Of these, three indicated elevated relative risks (Berggren and Sjostedt 1983; Marshall et al. 1983; Greenberg et al. 1985). The negative results were reported from a study in a black population in Southern Africa (Martin and Hill 1984). These studies are also summarized in Table 1.

Table 4
Combination of Least Common Values of Unknown Factor Sufficient to Explain an Observed Relative Risk of Two for Smoking and Cervical Cancer

Prevalence of high risk level of unknown factor	Lowest common relative prevalence and relative risk of unknown factor[a]
0.1 (10%)	6.9
0.2 (20%)	4.9
0.4 (40%)	3.8
0.5 (50%)	3.4

Adapted from Winkelstein et al. (1984)
[a]Compared to smoking and cervical cancer

In Table 5, the data from the latest publication are summarized (Greenberg et al. 1985). These come from an update of the cohort study of cervical cancer and contraceptive practices by the Oxford group (Wright et al. 1978). A dose-response relationship is shown for invasive and in situ cancer as well as for dysplasia. The relationships are strong and consistent and the investigators concluded that they are probably causal. However, they noted that the "adjusted estimates of risk with smoking were lower than the unadjusted estimates." Apparently they felt that this observation might weaken the causal interpretation of the associations.

If, however, both cigarette smoking and multiple sexual partners are independently associated with cervical cancer, then it is to be expected that adjustment for each factor would reduce the crude relative risk. This phenomenon is clearly demonstrated by unpublished data from Prague (V. Vonka, pers. comm.). The results are shown in Table 6. A relative risk of one is assigned to persons who never smoked and gave a lifetime history of ten or fewer sexual partners. For

Table 5
Relative Risks for Smoking and Cervical Neoplasia and Dyplasia in Women Grouped by Cigarette Smoking History at Study Entry

Diagnostic and smoking group	No. of cases	Incidence rate	RR[a]	Chi-square trend	P value
Invasive					
Never smoked	6	5.7	1.0		
Former	1	4.5	0.8	4.7	<0.05
1-14 cig/day	2	5.9	1.0		
>14 cig/day	8	31.7	5.6		
In situ					
Never smoked	32	30.4	1.0		
Former	9	40.3	1.3	7.3	<0.01
1-14 cig/day	24	71.1	2.3		
>14 cig/day	19	75.6	2.5		
Dyplasia					
Never smoked	37	35.2	1.0		
Former	17	76.4	2.2	6.6	<0.01
1-14 cig/day	16	47.4	1.4		
>14 cig/day	24	95.6	2.7		
All diagnoses					
Never smoked	75	71.5	1.0		
Former	27	121.4	1.7	18.0	<0.001
1-14 cig/day	42	124.7	1.8		
>14 cig/day	51	203.8	2.9		

Reprinted, with permission from Greenberg et al. (1985)
[a] Adjusted for age, social class, age at first marriage, contraceptive method, and duration of pill use

Table 6
Risk of Developing In Situ or Invasive Cervical Cancer According to Lifetime Number of Sexual Partners and Cigarette Smoking Status on Entry

Smoking status	Sexual partners	
	10 or less	> 10
−	1.0	2.5
+	3.5	6.6

V. Vonka, pers. comm.
Cohort > 46,000 person-years observation

nonsmokers with greater than ten sexual partners, the relative risk is 2.5, and for persons giving a history of ten or fewer sexual partners who are current smokers, the relative risk is 3.5. For smokers with greater than ten lifetime sexual partners, and who were current smokers, the relative risk is 6.6. Clearly, controlling for number of sexual partners or for smoking substantially reduces the crude relative risk. Interestingly, this is the only analysis which attempts to show the joint effects of both smoking and elevated number of sexual partners. This interaction was not directly examined in any of the 18 publications listed in Table 1.

There are several reasons why it is important to address the interaction of cigarette smoking and number of sexual partners directly. First, as long ago as 1938, Rous and Kidd showed that the simultaneous administration of a chemical carcinogen at one site potentiated the production of skin cancers by papilloma viruses applied at a distant site in rabbits (Rous and Kidd 1938). The possibility of an analogous chemical virus interaction in humans has not, as yet, been studied epidemiologically. Cervical cancer would appear to be an ideal model for such an investigation. The data provided by Vonka (V. Vonka, pers. comm.) suggestive as they are, are insufficient to answer this question. Second, failure to provide the complete data for both smoking and number of sexual partners makes it impossible to calculate the attributable risk for each factor independently. In other words, without the availability of joint distributions of prevalence, it is impossible to adjust for each factor in calculating the attributable risk proportion. Clearly, estimating the attributable risks without the joint distribution will overestimate this parameter.

Recently, Zunzunegui in the epidemiology program at the School of Public Health, University of California, Berkeley, completed a case-control study of male influences on cervical cancer risk (Zunzunegui 1986). The cases were selected from a high incidence group whose traditions and culture mediated against multiple sexual partners and cigarette smoking. Of the 39 cases only two gave a history of more than three lifetime sexual partners and only seven had ever smoked. However, as indicated in Table 7, more than twice as many husbands of cases than controls gave a history of 20 or more sexual partners and the adjusted odds ratio for

Table 7
Numbers of Lifetime Sexual Partners and Current or Past Cigarette Smoking Histories of Husbands of Cervical Cancer Cases and Controls

	Cases' husbands	Controls' husbands
No. of partners		
20+	24	10
< 20	15	29
	OR = 4.6 (P = < 0.01)	
Smoking		
+	31	24
−	8	15
	OR = 2.4	

Adapted from Zunzunegui (1985)
OR, adjusted for no. of partners = 3.4 (P= 0.10)

smoking among husbands of cases was 3.4. Although this odds ratio was not statistically significant, because of the small size of the sample, the results strongly suggest an association between cervical cancer risk and husbands' smoking habits. Presumably, the semen or prostatic fluid of the smoking husbands was carrying a carcinogenic agent or a factor which might promote the carcinogenicity of an infectious agent, or the wives were being affected by passive smoking.

DISCUSSION

It is now apparent that cancer of the uterine cervix is causally associated with an infectious agent and a chemical carcinogen contained in cigarette smoke. The evidence for the independent effects of these agents is plentiful. The most likely candidates for the infectious agents are herpes virus type II and human papilloma virus (zur Hausen 1982). As indicated earlier in this volume, it is not possible to designate a single chemical carcinogen in tobacco smoke as the responsible agent for neoplastic transformation of cells at various organ sites. Nevertheless, the ability to measure proxy indicators by chemical and biological methods has become very sophisticated. Thus, further epidemiological studies of cervical cancer should include appropriate laboratory involvement.

Perhaps the most effective approach to further elucidation of the etiological mechanism of viral and chemical carcinogenesis for cervical cancer is to undertake prospective studies in cohorts of high-risk women. The characteristics of such populations would be young age and low socioeconomic status. As soon as reliable in vitro systems are available for isolation of human papilloma viruses and for testing serologically for infection, such prospective studies should be established.

SUMMARY

The evidence for a causal association between cigarette smoking and cancer of the uterine cervix has been reviewed. Since 1966, 18 published studies have provided relevant data. In 15 of these studies, the association has been demonstrated; five of the 15 are cohort studies. Several studies have indicated that the association is stronger in young women. The demonstration of a causal association between a chemical carcinogen transmitted in cigarette smoke and cervical cancer is not inconsistent with a causal association between viral infection and cervical cancer. There is a need for further research to elucidate the possible interaction between viral and chemical carcinogens in cervical cancer.

REFERENCES

Austin, D.F. 1983. Smoking and cervical cancer (editorial). *J. Am. Med. Assoc.* 250: 516.

Berggren, G. and S. Sjostedt. 1983. Pre-invasive carcinoma of the cervix uteri and smoking. *Acta Obstet. Gynecol. Scand.* 62: 653.

Buckley, J.D., R.W.C. Harris, R. Doll, M.P. Vessey, and P.T. Williams. 1981. Case-control study of the husbands of the women with dysplasia or carcinoma of the cervix uteri. *Lancet* ii: 1010.

Cederlof, R., I. Friberg, Z. Hrubec, and U. Lorich. 1975. The relationship of smoking and some social covariables to mortality and cancer morbidity: A ten year follow-up of 55,000 Swedish subjects age 18–59. Department of Environmental Hygiene, Karolinska Institute, Stockholm, Sweden.

Clarke, E.A., R.W. Morgan, and A.M. Newman. 1982. Smoking as a risk factor in cancer of the cervix: Additional evidence from a case-control study. *Am. J. Epidemiol.* 115: 59.

Greenberg, E.R., M.P. Vessey, K. McPherson, and D. Yeats. 1985. Cigarette smoking and cancer of the uterine cervix. *Br. J. Cancer* 51: 139.

Harris, R.W.C., L.A. Brinton, R.H. Cowell, D.C.G. Skegg, D.G. Smith, M.P. Vessey, and R. Doll. 1980. Characteristics of women with dysplasia or carcinoma in situ of the cervix uteri. *Br. J. Cancer.* 42: 359.

Hirayama, T. 1975. Prospective studies on cancer epidemiology based on census population in Japan. *Excerpta Med.* 3: 26.

Kotin, E., H.L. Falk, and R. Busser. 1959. Distribution, retention, and elimination of C^{14}-3,4-benzypyrene after administration to mice and rats. *J. Natl. Cancer Inst.* 23: 541.

Kreyberg, L. 1962. Histological lung cancer types: A morphological and biological correlation. *Acta Pathol. Microbiol. Scand. Suppl.* 152: 1.

Lyon, J.L., J.W. Gardner, D.W. West, W.M. Stanish, and R.M. Herbertson. 1983. Smoking and carcinoma in situ of the uterine cervix. *Am. J. Public Health* 73: 558.

Marshall, J.R., S. Graham, S.T. Byers, M. Swanson, and J. Brasure. 1983. Diet and smoking in the epidemiology of cancer of the cervix. *J. Natl. Cancer Inst.* 70: 847.

Martin, P.M.D. and G.B. Hill. 1984. Cervical cancer in relation to tobacco and alcohol consumption in Lesotho, Southern Africa. *Cancer Detect. Prev.* **7**: 109.

Naguib, S.M., F.E. Lundin, Jr., and H.J. Davis. 1966. Relation of various epidemiologic factors to cervical cancer as determined by a screening program. *Obstet. Gynecol.* **28**: 451.

Petrakis, M.L., C.A. Maach, and R.E. Lee. 1980. Mutagenic activity in nipple aspirates of human breast fluid. *Cancer Res.* **40**: 188.

Rous, P. and J.G. Kidd. 1938. The carcinogenic effect of a papilloma virus on the tarred skin of rabbits. *J. Exp. Med.* **67**: 399.

Sasson, I.M., N.J. Haley, N.D. Hoffman, E.L. Wynder, D. Hellberg, and S. Nilsson. 1985. Cigarette smoking and neoplasia of the uterine cervix: Smoke constituents in cervical mucous (letter). *N. Eng. J. Med.* **312**: 315.

Stellman, S.D., H. Austin, and E.L. Wynder. 1980. Cervix cancer and cigarette smoking: A case-control study. *Am. J. Epidemiol.* **111**: 383.

Thomas, D.B. 1973. An epidemiologic study of carcinoma in situ and squamous dysplasia of the uterine cervix. *Am. J. Epidemiol.* **98**: 10.

Tokuhata, G.K. 1967. IV. Tobacco and cancer of the genitalia among married women. *Am. J. Public Health* **57**: 830.

Trevathan, E., P. Layde, L.A. Webster, J.B. Adams, B.E. Benigno, and H. Ory. 1983. Cigarette smoking and dysplasia and carcinoma in situ of the uterine cervix. *J. Am. Med. Assoc.* **250**: 499.

Wigle, D.T., Y. Mao, and M. Grace. 1980. Smoking and cancer of the uterine cervix: Hypothesis (letter). *Am. J. Epidemiol.* **111**: 125.

Williams, R.R. and J.W. Horm. 1977. Association of cancer sites with tobacco and alcohol consumption and socio-economic status of patients: Interview study from the Third National Cancer Survey. *J. Natl. Cancer Inst.* **58**: 525.

Winkelstein, W., Jr. 1977. Smoking and cancer of the uterine cervix: Hypotheses. *Am. J. Epidemiol.* **106**: 257.

Winkelstein, W., Jr. and L.I. Levin. 1981. Confounded confounding (letter). *Am. J. Epidemiol.* **113**: 99.

Winkelstein, W., Jr., S.T. Sacks, V.L. Ernster, and S. Selvin. 1977. Correlations of incidence rates for selected cancers in the nine areas of the Third National Cancer Survey. *Am. J. Epidemiol.* **105**: 407.

Winkelstein, W., Jr., E.J. Shillitoe, R. Brand, and K.K. Johnson. 1984. Further comments on cancer of the uterine cervix, smoking, and herpesvirus infection. *Am. J. Epidemiol.* **119**: 1.

Wright, N.H., M.P. Vessey, B. Kenward, K. McPherson, and R. Doll. 1978. Neoplasia and dysplasia of the cervix uteri and contraception: A possible protective effect of the diaphragm. *Br. J. Cancer.* **38**: 273.

Yamasaki, E. and B.N. Ames. 1977. Concentration of mutagens from urine by adsorption with the non-polar resin XAD-2: Cigarette smokers have mutagenic urine. *Proc. Natl. Acad. Sci. U.S.A.* **74**: 3555.

Zunzunegui, M.V., M.-C. King, C.F. Coria, and J. Charlet. 1986. Male influences on cervical cancer risk. *Am. J. Epidemiol.* **123**: 302.

zur Hausen, H. 1982. Human genital cancer: Synergism between two virus infections or synergism between a virus infection and initiating events? *The Lancet* ii: 1370.

COMMENTS

WINKELSTEIN: One of the most interesting observations regarding the smoking-cervical cancer association was made by three of the investigators, Cederlof, Lyon, and Berggren. All of these investigators found that the association was strongest in young women and essentially disappeared in the elderly. This observation cannot be explained by early diagnosis. It seems to me that the most parsimonious explanation for the association is that women who smoke absorb chemical carcinogens, which transported through the bloodstream differentially, affect the cervical epithelium.

STELLMAN: I don't want to argue about the data. The presentation is very nice. It displays a very plausible picture. There is one important piece that's missing from this picture. I have been struggling with it for a long time, and I still don't know what the answer is. It has to do with the trend over time in the incidence and mortality rates for invasive cervical cancer, which are declining in the United States, but at the same time the prevalence of cigarette smoking in women has been increasing. I just wonder if you have any information on this at all.

WINKELSTEIN: Evaluation of the time trend of cervical cancer incidence in the United States is complicated by regional and local differences in screening. The consensus, I believe, is that early diagnosis results in prevention of the progression of in situ lesions to invasive lesions so that where screening has been extensive, invasive cervical cancer rates have declined. However, in such places, in situ rates have increased. I would draw your attention to the data from the New York State Cancer Registry which clearly shows this trend. Whether or not the overall incidence is rising or declining is difficult to assess. Furthermore, a declining time trend of cervical cancer is no less consistent with a viral etiology than it is with a chemical etiology.

GRAFSTRÖM: Could the difference in incidence now or before be explained on the basis of the latency period?

STELLMAN: The incidence and mortality have been declining for four decades.

CORREA: It means that probably the main factor is not smoking, so that the other more potent factors may be responsible for the decline. In that case you will not see an effect on the death rates, but you will see one on the case-control study.

WINKELSTEIN: But there are others who disagree. There are those who argue strongly that the smear screening has not had the effect that we think it has. I agree.

CONNEY: Could cigarette smoking influence secondary factors such as hormone metabolism? Recent reports indicate lower plasma levels of testosterone in smokers than in nonsmokers. In addition, smokers have a lower urinary excretion of estrogens during the luteal phase of the menstrual cycle than do nonsmokers. An interesting report appeared last week indicating that cigarette smokers have a lower risk of endometrial cancer than nonsmokers. Would someone care to comment on these observations?

STELLMAN: Shapiro had a relevant paper this week in the *New England Journal of Medicine*. I was frustrated in my attempt to evaluate that paper, because there wasn't enough information in it to satisfy my curiosity about what was really going on. They found that the relative risk of endometrial cancer in women who smoke is approximately 70% of the risk in women who don't smoke.

WINKELSTEIN: That is the same as observed by Cederlof some years ago.

STELLMAN: And this is taking a number of other factors into account, including age, obesity (which is a major risk factor for endometrial cancer), and a variety of other things.

CORREA: Did it take the contraceptive into account?

STELLMAN: Yes, both use of oral contraceptives and of exogenous estrogens.

TANNENBAUM: One of the things I wish people would do is to put confidence intervals around things, I mean 0.7 plus or minus what?

WINKELSTEIN: The 0.7 is very stable because it is based on 23,000 persons observed over 10 years. Thus, the confidence interval will be very small. I don't usually consider relative risks increased until they are at least two. I also like to see a graded response when I am assessing the etiological role of a risk factor. Furthermore, the observation must have biological plausibility if it is to be accorded any validity. In my view, the question of statistical significance is relatively minor. It can only be useful when other study criteria have been satisfied.

TANNENBAUM: Okay, but how do you feel about a relative risk that's less than one? That's my question.

WINKELSTEIN: When relative risks are less than one, one must consider the restriction in scale. When the relative risk is over one, this is not a problem.

HOFFMANN: Nancy [Haley], you did the cervical fluid analysis.

HALEY: We have investigated nicotine and cotinine content of cervical aspirates and compared them to levels found in the urine and serum of these same women. The study groups contained both smokers and nonsmokers. These samples were collected by Dan Helberg in Sweden and analyzed in our laboratories. What we found was that relative to the levels found in serum, nicotine was concentrated in the cervical aspirates. The amounts of cotinine found were fairly consistent across the body fluids analyzed, but nicotine was much higher in the cervical mucus of smokers. This high content of nicotine could provide a necessary component for in vivo nitrosation and give rise to the formulation of nitrosamines at this anatomical site. This might provide biological evidence for the epidemiological observations on cigarette smoking and cervical cancer.

The Passive Smoking-Cancer Controversy

PELAYO CORREA
Department of Pathology
Louisiana State University Medical Center
New Orleans, Louisiana 70112

INTRODUCTION

It is important for our society to determine if involuntary exposure to tobacco smoke (passive smoking) causes cancer. If it does, the problem may be of large magnitude because tobacco smoke is probably the most ubiquitous indoor pollutant in the world.

To properly evaluate the present controversy, a brief critical review of the available evidence and a discussion of the outstanding issues are indicated.

REVIEW

Epidemiology

Some of the available results are summarized in Table 1. Although some reports raised the issue several years ago (Neutel and Buck 1971; Miller 1978), two relatively recent studies published almost simultaneously have brought it strikingly to the attention of health professionals. Trichopoulos and coworkers (1981) conducted a case-control study of cancer (excluding adenocarcinoma) of the lung in women from Athens, Greece. The original report was based on results for 51 cases and 163 controls, expanded later to 77 cases and 225 controls (1983). An estimated relative risk of 2.4 was reported for nonsmoking women whose husbands smoked less than one pack of cigarettes per day and 3.4 for those who smoked more than one pack per day. The limitations of this study, discussed by the investigators and other correspondents (Heller 1983), are several: (1) The number of cases is small; (2) 35% of the cases lacked histologic confirmation; (3) the controls were obtained from a different hospital than the cases. The authors presented their work not as a definitive answer to the question, but as a finding in need of corroboration and further research. They also noted that "the smoking habits of a woman's husband may be an index of a broader exposure to cigarette smoke than that which emanates from the husband himself."

Hirayama (1981) reported on a cohort study involving 91,540 Japanese nonsmoking women followed for 14 years. The risk of lung cancer for women whose husbands smoked more than 20 cigarettes per day was approximately double that of those whose husbands were nonsmokers. A smaller increase in the relative risk

Table 1
Summary of Epidemiologic Studies of Passive Smoking

Author	Results	Comments
Case-series		
Miller (1978) Pennsylvania	OR = 1.94; all cancers, deceased nonemployed wives' smoking husbands	Interview of next of kin
Knoth et al. (1983) W. Germany	61% of women with lung cancer lived with a smoker (X 3 expected)	66% Squamous
Case-control studies		
Trichopoulos et al. (1981) Greece	OR = 2.9 lung cancer	Positive linear trend. Excluded adenocarcinomas, orthopedic hospital controls.
Correa et al. (1983) Louisiana	OR = 2.0 lung cancer	Hospital controls. All histologic types.
Koo et al. (1983, 1985) Hong Kong	OR = 1.2 lung cancer	Mostly adenocarcinomas. Controls matched by residential district.
Kabat and Wynder (1984) Five states	OR = 1.0 lung cancer	Subset of on-going study. Hospital controls. All histologic types.
Sandler et al. (1985) North Carolina	OR = 1.5 all sites	Age: 15–59 years; controls: friends or telephone sample.
Wu et al. (1985) Los Angeles	OR = 1.2 lung cancer	Adenocarcinoma neighborhood controls

Table 1 (Continued)

Author	Results	Comments
Dalager et al., in prep., New Jersey, Texas and Louisiana	OR = 1.5 lung cancer	Population-based. All histologic types.
Garfinkel (1985) New Jersey and Ohio	OR = 1.3 lung cancer	Control: colon cancer. All histologic types.
Cohort studies		
Neutel and Buck (1971) Canada	OR = 1.3 all childhood cancers	Newborn 7–10 years follow-up
Hirayama (1981; 1984) Japan	OR = 2.0 lung cancer	No histology. 14-year follow-up.
Garfinkel (1981) United States	OR = 1.1 lung cancer	No histology. 12–15-year follow-up.
Vandenbroucke (1984) Holland	All causes of death. No effect.	No breakdown by cause of death
Gillis et al. (1984) West Scotland	OR = 3.2 lung cancer	No histology. 6–10-year follow-up.

OR = odds ratio

(1.49) was found for emphysema, but no increase in risk was detected for cervical or gastric cancer. The husband's alcohol usage did not influence the risk of these diseases in their wives. This report has been extensively criticized and defended in the medical literature. Points of criticism include the fact that the histological types of the tumors were not studied; the lack of consideration of other possible sources of indoor pollution such as heating and cooking equipment; the lack of consideration of the socioeconomic status; as well as other minor objections. Hirayama's responses to the criticism (1983), his additional data (1984), and the reanalysis by international experts (Hammond and Selikoff 1981) leave little doubt that passive smoking increases the risk of lung cancer and cancer of the paranasal sinuses in Japanese women. The question then becomes whether the Japanese experience can be extrapolated to the United States, given the marked differences in culture and housing patterns. These doubts were amplified by Garfinkel's report on the analysis of the American Cancer Society cohort (1981). In this study, 176,739 nonsmoking women were followed for 12 years and a relative risk of 1.37 was observed for women whose husbands smoked less than 20 cigarettes per day and of 1.04 for those whose husbands smoked more than 20 cigarettes per day, neither figure being statistically significant. Reanalysis of Garfinkel's data, correcting for the confounding effect of passive smoking at the workplace, produced results which are consistent with those of the Japanese cohorts (Repace 1984). The most serious criticism of Garfinkel's data, however, has been that data on smoking were not available for 73% of the husbands of the nonsmoking women (Weiss et al. 1983).

A study of 1338 subjects with lung cancer and 1393 cancer-free subjects (controls) has been reported in Louisiana (Correa et al. 1983). This population included eight men and 22 women who were nonusers of tobacco. The estimated relative risk of lung cancer was 1.48 for those whose spouse smoked 1-40 pack-years and 3.1 for those whose spouse smoked more than 40 pack-years. The latter relative risk was statistically significant at the 5% level. The most serious drawback of this study is the small number of cases.

Chinese women in several countries have a high risk to lung cancer and several epidemiologic studies on them are available (McLennan et al. 1977; Ho et al. 1982; Koo et al. 1983). These studies have contributed to our understanding of the role of nutrition and other factors, but have been inconclusive concerning involuntary exposure to cigarette smoke. A study of women in Hong Kong was published by Koo and her coworkers (1983). It reports on interviews with 120 female lung cancer patients and an equal number of controls matched by age, socioeconomic status, and residential district. To calculate the risk of passive smoking, a summation of total hours and years of exposure at home and work was estimated. The patients who were nonsmokers had an average excess exposure to passive smoking of 3156 hours or 3.8 years when compared with controls. This difference was not statistically significant. The study had 56 patients who were nonsmokers, 34 of whom were exposed to passive smoke at home, two at work, and four at home and at work. The method of analysis utilized in this study was based on the assumption that all hours of involuntary exposure to tobacco smoke can be accurately quantified and have equal weight as a carcinogenic influence. It disregarded the intimacy of the contact, the ventilation characteristics of the environment, and the age at exposure. A more orthodox analysis of the published data (Table IX in Koo et al. 1983) yielded an estimated relative risk of 1.9 associated with smoking by the husband and 2.5 with smoking by the parents. This table, however, appears to include smoking and nonsmoking patients, and the authors did not provide data to calculate a similar relative risk for nonsmokers only. The authors reanalyzed their data for "never smoked" women (Koo et al. 1985) and reported a relative risk of 1.75 for squamous cell carcinoma and 1.44 for large-cell undifferentiated carcinoma. Small numbers make histologic specific risks unstable, but the magnitude of the effect appears considerable: the attributable risk calculations indicate that 72.3% of lung cancer cases in nonsmoking Hong Kong women are causally linked to passive smoking. Wynder and Goodman (1983) reviewed some of the then available studies on passive smoking, pointed out their weaknesses, and discussed some pathophysiologic mechanisms which might favor peripheral (predominantly adenocarcinomas) as opposed to hilar (squamous and small-cell) carcinomas.

Kabat and Wynder (1984) presented a preliminary study of passive inhalation of tobacco smoke by a subset of nonsmoking lung cancer patients and controls extracted from an ongoing case-control study of tobacco-related cancers in selected hospitals from New York, Alabama, Illinois, Pennsylvania, and California. No excessive risk was found in passive smokers except for more frequent exposure among male cases in the work environment. Two weaknesses of this study are that the project was not designed to address the passive smoking issue, which accounts for the preliminary nature of the data, and the ill-defined population base resulting from a nonrandom selection of hospitals in six states.

A study of lung cancer, including 29 adenocarcinomas in nonsmoking women, has been reported from Los Angeles County. It includes 12 cases of bronchioalveolar cell carcinoma. No elevated risk was observed for parental smoking (RR = 0.6) and slightly elevated relative risks were observed for passive exposure from spouses (RR = 1.3) and work (1.3). The risk increased with the number of years of exposure to passive smoking from spouses and at work, but results were not statistically significant (Wu 1985).

A study of 792 patients with lung cancer in West Germany included 39 nonsmoking women (Knoth et al. 1983); 61% of whom lived with a smoker, triple the expected number based on the smoking habits of men in their respective age brackets.

A cohort of Rotterdam civil servants followed for up to 25 years failed to show an increase in mortality rates (all cancers) associated with passive smoking (Vandenbroucke et al. 1984). This finding is not unexpected since the contribution of lung cancer to general mortality in Holland is very small.

Gillis et al. (1984) reported on a cohort of 16,171 Scottish subjects followed for approximately 12 years. The lung cancer death rate for those reporting exposure to environmental tobacco smoke at the time of entry into the study was 13/10.000 compared to 4/10.000 for those not reporting such exposure.

A recent analysis of three population-based, case-control studies of lung cancer in New Jersey, Texas, and Louisiana (N. Dalager, in prep.) found a relative risk of 1.5 for nonsmokers living with a spouse who smoked. There was a significant linear trend with increasing exposure. The increase in risk was restricted to squamous and small-cell carcinomas.

Garfinkel et al. (1985) recently conducted a case-control study of lung cancer in women admitted to four hospitals in New Jersey and one in Ohio. A total of 134 cases in nonsmokers was ascertained. The odds ratio for women whose husbands smoked at home was 1.31 with a positive linear trend and odds ratio of 2.11 for women whose husbands smoked 20 or more cigarettes per day at home.

Hirayama (1984) reported on the interaction between passive smoking and nutritional factors in his cohort of Japanese nonsmoking women. It appears that consuming yellow-green vegetables daily reduces the lung cancer risk by approximately 30% relative to nondaily consumers of the same vegetables.

Most of the abovementioned studies are directed to lung cancer risk. Increase in risk for tumors of other sites has been reported in a few studies. Neutel and Buck (1971) reported a modest increase in childhood cancer in the offspring of mothers who smoke during pregnancy. Hirayama (1983) reported increased risk for nasal cancer and brain tumors. Preston-Martin et al. (1982) reported a risk of 1.5 for brain tumors in children who lived with a smoker. Sandler et al. (1985) reported on cancers of all sites diagnosed in persons of 15-59 years of age at the North Carolina Memorial Hospital. The controls were "friends" of the cases or, if such were not available, obtained by a telephone survey of a sample of the population. She reported an overall odds ratio of 1.6 associated with spouse smoking, with significant increases for cancers of the breast (1.8), cervix (1.8), and endocrine organs (3.2). Only two cases of lung cancer were found in her series. When exposure to tobacco smoke in childhood and adulthood was present, the overall risk increased to 2.7. If three or more household exposures were recorded, significant increases in risk were reported for smoking-related cancers (OR : 3.8), breast (3.3), cervix (3.4), and lymphoma-leukemia (6.8). A Canadian-based study of 33 women with cervical cancer, only ten of whom were nonsmokers, reported a dose-related increase in the risk of cervical cancer associated with the husband's smoking history but did not report a separate analysis for nonsmoking women (Brown et al. 1982).

Biologic Plausibility

Some laboratory evidence points to a possible role of passive smoking in carcinogenesis. A strong indication is derived from the chemistry of cigarette smoke which has consistently shown that the concentration of toxic and carcinogenic substances is much higher in sidestream (SS) than in mainstream (MS) smoke, as shown in Table 2. Of special concern are some nitrosamines which are 50 times more concentrated in sidestream smoke (Weiss 1983). This is especially relevant in the light of the possible role of nicotine-derived nitrosamines (Hoffmann and Hecht 1985) and the fact that passive smokers have considerable concentrations of cotinine in their blood and urine (Wald et al. 1984). The issue becomes more important in the light of solid evidence that newborn babies accumulate these metabolites from their smoking mothers (Greenberg et al. .1984). Experimental evidence shows the capacity of nasal, pulmonary, and hepatic tissues of near-term fetuses to enzymatically activate nicotine-derived nitrosamines to alkylating species which bind covalently to macromolecules (Castonguay et al. 1984).

OUTSTANDING ISSUES

Confounding by Active Smoking

Critics of the published work on passive smoking and cancer maintain that the reported effects may reflect the fact that some supposed nonsmokers are really hidden or closet smokers who deny their habit for sociocultural reasons. This bias may explain why the published relative risks for passive smokers are unreasonably high, incongruent with the dose estimated on the basis of theoretical models combined with measurements of inhaled constituents of cigarette smoke. Repace and Lowrey (1980) estimate that an office worker exposed to moderate smoking inhales the equivalent of five cigarettes per day whereas a musician working in a night club and having a chain smoker for a roommate inhales the equivalent of 27 cigarettes per day. Critics of this work have scaled down those estimates to 0.2 and one cigarette per day, respectively (Lee 1982; Vutuc 1984) and pointed out that risks of such low exposure are unmeasurable.

The problems of such estimates are well recognized not only because of the mathematical calculations but most importantly because of the uncertainties about how accurately they represent the real-life situations. Each environment differs in its impact on passive smoking. The most consistent epidemiologic associations have been obtained with exposure at home, mostly from the spouse's smoking. Wald et al. (1984) have shown that nonsmokers married to smokers not only have increased urinary cotinine excretion but also have higher exposure to smoke outside the home.

Extrapolation to passive smoking effects from active smoking experience ignores the fact that the active smoker also inhales sidestream smoke and, therefore, his risk reflects the effects of mainstream and sidestream smoke. Considering the higher concentration of toxins and carcinogens in sidestream smoke, a steeper dose-effect curve for this type of smoke should be expected. Another problem with the dose estimations is that the exposure to sidestream smoke probably occurs for many more years than mainstream smoke, in some cases even in the prenatal period.

Table 2
Selected Constituents of Cigarette Smoke Ratio of Constituents in Sidestream Smoke to Mainstream Smoke

Gas phase constituents	MS	SS/MS ratio	Particulate phase constituents	MS	SS/MS ratio
Carbon dioxide	20–60 mg	8.1	Tar	1–40 mg	1.3
Carbon monoxide	10–20 mg	2.5	Water	1–4 mg	2.4
Methane	1.3 mg	3.1	Toluene	108 μg	5.6
Acetylene	27 μg	0.8	Phenol	20–150 μg	2.6
Ammonia	80 μg	73.0	Methylnaphthalene	2.2 μg	28.0
Hydrogen cyanide	430 μg	0.25	Pyrene	50–200 μg	3.6
Methylfuran	20 μg	3.4	Benzo[a]pyrene	20–40 μg	3.4
Acetonitrile	120 μg	3.9	Aniline	360 mg	30.0
Pyridine	32 μg	10.0	Nicotine	1.0–2.5 mg	2.7
Dimethylnitrosamine	10–65 μg	52.0	2-Naphthylamine	2 mg	39.0

Reprinted, with permission, from Weiss et al. (1983).
SS, sidestream smoke; MS, mainstream smoke

Validation of Smoking Status

The problems of validation of passive smoking inhalation have been well-outlined by community surveys such as the one reported by Friedman et al. (1983) based on questionnaires received from 37,881 nonsmokers and exsmokers. In this survey, 63% reported some exposure to tobacco smoke, especially at younger ages (78.2% at ages 20-30). These data highlight the fact that the great majority of the population is subjected to other people's smoke. The same survey showed that 47% of women married to smokers reported zero exposure at home even though their spouses were not light smokers (76% of them smoked more than ten cigarettes per day). The data originated in supposedly healthy persons who took health examinations and are probably more health conscious; therefore, it should not be uncritically extrapolated to the general population, but it does point out the difficulties in classifying passive smokers on the basis of questionnaires. In that study the correlation between history of passive smoking and levels of thiocyanate and carbon monoxide in the blood was very poor. Johnson and Letzel (1984) have proposed systems to classify the different categories of passive smokers and quantify their exposure. They have shown that arbitrary rules for this quantification may give widely different results, which may explain why previous attempts in this direction have not been fruitful.

Techniques to measure nicotine and its metabolites in blood and serum have overcome the lack of specificity of other constituents of tobacco smoke. They discriminate clearly active from passive smokers (Wald and Ritchie 1984) and correlate well with the reported magnitude of passive exposure. The problem of validation of exposure years before the interview has not been solved, but the development of techniques to measure cotinine incorporation in hair extends the validation attempts backward over a longer, though limited, time period (Haley and Hoffmann 1985).

Low-dose Effect

There is consensus that the effect of passive smoking falls in the low-dose range in the incidence curve. This low dose makes the detection of such effect harder for several reasons. One such reason is the possibility that any effect detected may be due to confounders. This possibility becomes more tenable by the finding of the Friedman et al. (1983) survey. They reported that subjects more frequently exposed to passive smoking were also more frequent users of marijuana and alcohol and were more exposed to occupational hazards.

Histologic Types of Lung Cancer

Criticisms in this area have varied from theoretical expectations of the proportion of histologic types to questions about the validity of diagnoses. The Trichopoulos study (1981) supposedly excluded adenocarcinomas but included some cases without pathologic confirmation and did not carry out a review of pathology slides. The Hirayama study (1981) did not have histologic data available. The relatively high proportion of adenocarcinomas reported for females and for nonsmokers has led some critics to expect the passive smoking effect to be mostly for adenocarcinomas. Kabat and Wynder (1984) have postulated that since sidestream smoke mostly represents the gas-phase of the smoke, peripheral adenocarcinomas should be expected. In population-based, case-control studies of Hong Kong (Koo 1983) and the United States (N. Dalager, in prep.), however, the effects have been mostly in squamous cell carcinoma. Adenocarcinoma frequently includes bronchioalveolar carcinomas, which has not been associated with smoking. This issue clearly requires bigger and better samples to be resolved. If the effect applies predominantly or exclusively to some histologic types, inclusion of other types only dilutes the already barely detectable effect.

EPILOGUE

At the present time it cannot be categorically affirmed or denied that passive smoking is a cause of cancer in humans. The evidence now available, however, is suggestive of a low-dose effect in the causation of cancers of the lung, nasal cavity, and brain. The main support for this position is the consistency of the findings in diverse populations of Greece, Japan, Germany, and the United States, and the biologic plausibility provided by laboratory findings. Reports of the absence of association are fewer and have more serious shortcomings than reports of positive association.

The magnitude of the excess of cancer, if any, attributable to passive smoking is debatable. The discrepancy between reported relative risks (up to three for women with heavy smoking husbands) and calculations based on equivalents of the number of cigarettes smoked "actively" (1-7 per day) may indicate bias in study designs, but may also call for the examination of alternative pathogenetic mechanisms. Of particular importance in this regard is the fact that passive smoking may be present since childhood or even since prenatal life. Transplacental exposure to carcinogens experimentally increases the carcinogenic response of the offspring to postnatal exposure to the same or to a different carcinogen (Napalkov 1971; Vesselinovitch 1971). Mutagens in tobacco smoke could act as initiators whose effects would only be expressed by means of a later carcinogenic challenge.

The model of pulmonary carcinogenesis by tobacco smoke proposed by Doll and Peto (1978) postulates that the duration of exposure is the most important component of the equation, as shown by the proposed formula for the annual incidence in the age range 40-79. Incidence = $0.273 \times 10^{-12} \cdot (\text{cigarettes/day} + 6)^2 \cdot (\text{age} - 22.5)^{4.5}$. It is well known that fetal and infantile tissues require fewer doses for carcinogenic response. These considerations allow speculations for an important role of passive smoking in human carcinogenesis and should stimulate further scientific work. The biases of the reported studies can be overcome for the most part by larger samples, improved questionnaires, and the proper utilization of validation methods.

ACKNOWLEDGMENT

This work was supported by grant R01-CA40095 from the National Cancer Institute, NIH, USPHS.

REFERENCES

Brown, D., L. Pereira, and J.B. Garner. 1982. Cancer of the cervix and the smoking husband. *Can. Fam. Physician* 28: 499.
Castonguay, A., H. Tjälve, N. Trushin, and S.S. Hecht. 1984. Perinatal metabolism of the tobacco-specific carcinogen 4-(methylnitrosamino)-(3-pyridyl)-1-butanone in C57BL mice. *J. Natl. Cancer Inst.* 72: 1117.
Correa, P., L.W. Pickle, E. Fontham, Y. Lin, and W. Haenszel. 1983. Passive smoking and lung cancer. *Lancet* 2: 595.
Doll, R. and R. Peto. 1978. Cigarette smoking and bronchial carcinoma: Dose and time relationships among regular smokers and life-long non-smokers. *J. Epidemiol. Community Health* 32: 303.
Friedman, G.D., D. Petitti, and R. Bawol. 1983. Prevalence and correlates of passive smoking. *Am. J. Public Health* 73: 401.
Garfinkel, L. 1981. Time trends in lung cancer mortality in nonsmokers and a note on passive smoking. *J. Natl. Cancer Inst.* 66: 1061.
———. 1985. Involuntary smoking and lung cancer. A case-control study. *J. Natl. Cancer Inst.* (in press).
Gillis, C.R., D.J. Hole, V. Hawthorne, and P. Boyle. 1984. The effect of environmental tobacco smoke in two urban communities in the west of Scotland. *Eur. J. Respir. Dis.* (Suppl. 133) 65: 121.
Greenberg, R.A., N.J. Haley, R.A. Etzel, and F.A. Lode. 1984. Measuring the exposure of infants to tobacco smoke. *N. Engl. J. Med.* 310: 1075.
Haley, N.J. and D. Hoffmann. 1985. Analysis of nicotine and cotinine in hair to determine cigarette smoker status. *Clin. Chem.* (in press).
Hammond, E.C. and I.J. Selikoff. 1981. Passive smoking and lung cancer with comments on two new papers. *Environ. Res.* 24: 444.
Heller, W.D. 1983. Lung cancer and passive smoking. *Lancet* 2: 1309.
Hirayama, T. 1981. Non-smoking wives of heavy smokers have a higher risk of lung cancer: A study from Japan. *Br. Med. J.* 282: 183.
———. 1983. Passive smoking and lung cancer: Consistency of association. *Lancet* 2: 1425.
———. 1984. Lung cancer in Japan: Effects of nutrition and passive smoking. In *Lung cancer: Causes and prevention* (eds. M. Mizell and P. Correa), p. 175. Verlag Chemie, Florida.

Ho, J.H.C., C.L. Chan, K.K. Man, W.H. Lau, and G.K.H. Au. 1982. Characteristic features of cancer in Hong Kong. In *Cancer prevention in developing countries* (ed. K. Aoki), p. 33. Japan Scientific Society Press, Japan.

Hoffmann, D. and S.S. Hecht. 1985. Nicotine-derived N-nitrosamines and tobacco-related cancer: Current status and future directions. *Cancer Res.* **45**: 935.

Johnson, L.C. and H. Letzel. 1984. Measuring passive smoking: Methods, problems and perspectives. *Prev. Med.* **13**: 705.

Kabat, G.C. and E.L. Wynder. 1984. Lung cancer in nonsmokers. *Cancer* **53**: 1214.

Knoth, A., H. Bohn, and F. Schmidt. 1983. Passive smoking as a causal factor of bronchial carcinoma in female non-smokers. *Medizinische Klinik* **78**: 66.

Koo, L.C., J.H.C. Ho, and D. Saw. 1983. Active and passive smoking among female lung cancer patients and controls in Hong Kong. *J. Exp. Clin. Res.* **4**: 367.

Koo, L.C., J.H.C. Ho, N. Lee. 1985. An analysis of some risk factors for lung cancer in Hong Kong. *Int. J. Cancer* **35**: 149.

Lee, P.N. 1982. Passive smoking. *Food Chem. Toxicol.* **20**: 223.

McLennan, R., J. DaCosta, N.E. Derg, C.H. Law, Y.K. Ng, and K. Shanmugaratnam. 1977. Risk factor for lung cancer in Singapore Chinese, a population with high female incidence rates. *Int. J. Cancer* **20**: 854.

Miller, G.H. 1978. The Pennsylvania study on passive smoking. *J. Breath. Ill. Lung Assn.* **41**: 5.

Napalkov, N.E. 1971. Some general considerations on the problem of transplacental carcinogenesis. In *Transplacental carcinogenesis, International Agency for Research on Cancer, Publ. No. 4* (ed. L. Tomatis and U. Mohr), p. 1. IARC, Lyon, France.

Neutel, C.I. and C. Buck. 1971. Effect of smoking during pregnancy on the risk of cancer in children. *J. Natl. Cancer Inst.* **47**: 59.

Preston-Martin, S., M.C. Yu, B. Benton, and B.I. Henderson. 1982. N-Nitroso compounds and childhood brain tumors. *Cancer Res.* **42**: 5240.

Repace, J.L. 1984. Consistency of research data on passive smoking and lung cancer. *Lancet* **i**: 506.

Repace, J.L. and A.H. Lowrey. 1980. Indoor air pollution, tobacco smoke, and public health. *Science* **208**: 464.

Sandler, D.P., R.B. Everson, and A.J. Wilcox. 1985. Passive smoking and adulthood cancer risk. *Am. J. Epidemiol.* **121**: 37.

Trichopoulos, D., A. Kalandidi, L. Sparros, and B. McMahon. 1981. Lung cancer and passive smoking. *Int. J. Cancer* **27**: 1.

———. 1983. Lung cancer and passive smoking: Conclusion of Greek study. *Lancet* **ii**: 677.

Vandenbroucke, J.P., J.H.H. Verheesen, A. DeBruin, and B.J. Mauritz. 1984. Active and passive smoking in married couples: Results of 25-year follow-up. *Br. Med. J.* **288**: 1801.

Vesselinovitch, S.P. 1971. Comparative studies of perinatal carcinogenesis. In *International Agency for Research on Cancer Publ. No. 4. Transplacental carcinogenesis* (ed. L. Tomatis and U. Mohr), p. 14. Lyon, France.

Vutuc, C. 1984. Quantitative aspects of passive smoking and lung cancer. *Prev. Med.* **13**: 698.

Wald, N. and C. Ritchie. 1984. Validation of studies on lung cancer in non-smokers married to smokers. *Lancet* i: 1067.

Wald, N., J. Boreham, A. Bailey, C. Ritchie, J. Haddow, and G. Knight. 1984. Urinary cotinine as a marker of breathing other people's tobacco smoke. *Lancet* i: 230.

Weiss, S.T., I.B. Tager, M. Schenker, and F. Speizer. 1983. The health effects of involuntary smoking. *Am. Rev. Respir. Dis.* **128**: 933.

Wu, A.H., B.E. Henderson, M.C. Pike, and M.C. Yu. 1985. Smoking and other risk factors for lung cancer in women. *J. Natl. Cancer Inst.* **74**: 747.

Wynder, E.L. and M.T. Goodman. 1983. Smoking and lung cancer: Some unresolved issues. *Epidemiol. Rev.* **5**: 177.

COMMENTS

STELLMAN: Some of Dr. Correa's data were taken from a new study by Larry Garfinkel and Oscar Auerbach on passive smoking. I would like to show you some data from that study to illustrate some important concepts. Passive smoking must bear a weak association to lung cancer. The association is difficult to detect, certainly not with the great assurance that we have for active smoking. The problem that we have, really, is that, given the quality of information that is available to work with and the sensitivity of the statistical methods, the signal-to-noise ratio is very low. In Garfinkel's case-control study, they searched the records of four hospitals in order to find women who had lung cancer and who were also nonsmokers. From an 11-year period of record-searching, they found records of 1175 women who had "microscopic" proof of lung cancer according to the hospital records. Out of these 1175 women, the hospital records said that 892 were smokers, or about 76%; those cases were discarded as this was a study of nonsmokers. That left 283 women who, according to the hospital charts were either nonsmokers or whose smoking status was not stated, but who had microscopic proof of lung cancer. Then Auerbach took all the slide material for these people and reread them. He found, in his judgment, that 36 of these 283 were not lung cancer, at least there was no microscopic proof. He disagreed with that diagnosis. In this original screening, they excluded cytological diagnosis or clinical diagnosis, leaving only cases for which there was some genuine pathological evidence. All of the remaining 247 women, or their next-of-kin, were reinterviewed by interviewers who worked for the American Cancer Society: 113 of these turned out to be smokers. That left 134, or 47.3%, who were genuine nonsmokers with microscopic proof of lung cancer. Those are the data that I want to present; the study will appear soon in the *Journal of the National Cancer Institute*. But I think it's important to see that the opportunity for potential misclassification is immense. In this type of a study, where we're pursuing endpoints that are very difficult to track down, it is exceptionally important to verify and reverify what the outcomes, as well as the exposures are. Even then, there is still some uncertainty because in a retrospective study like this, dating back over 11 years, many of these women were dead at the time that the records were abstracted; and for those, the interviews are with next-of-kin, or proxy interviews. But in that case some of those interviews might not be as reliable as if they had been with the original subjects.

CORREA: Of these 134, for how many was the smoking status not stated and how many were reported as nonsmokers? Do you know?

STELLMAN: I can't recall.

TANNENBAUM: I'm not sure what point you're trying to make.

STELLMAN: This is a central point in epidemiology. You've seen slide after slide showing cases and controls, exposed to this, that, or the other thing. But just because an exposure is indicated, and a relative risk is computed, doesn't always mean the underlying data are correct.

TANNENBAUM: You're saying there are errors in misclassification.

STELLMAN: Absolutely. Some of the passive smoking studies which have been published might have a great deal of misclassification bias, in exposure and outcome.

CORREA: Several of them, including those of Hong Kong and the United States had histologic confirmation. The misclassification about passive and active smokers may be there.

TANNENBAUM: I think that the point about the difference in the chemistry of sidestream and mainstream smoke is the most critical point, because—Dietrich [Hoffmann] can correct me if I'm wrong—but in undiluted sidestream smoke you really have an excess of nitrogen-containing components compared with mainstream smoke. In mainstream smoke you therefore have a relatively high proportion of the hydrocarbons. So that if the hydrocarbons are causing lung cancer, then one may speculate that if the aromatic amines and the N-nitrosamines cause other types of cancer, such as bladder cancer, one should see these types of cancer more in passive smokers than lung cancer; with the sidestream smoke they inhale relatively more of these N-containing compounds than they inhale aromatic hydrocarbons. So, looking at lung cancer may be looking at the wrong thing. Maybe what we ought to be looking at is bladder cancer for nonsmokers. Now the problem is, of course, that the relative risk is much smaller, and so the chances of finding it, I think, are much weaker. But I was very impressed with how big the relative risks are for cervical cancer, and there we don't have the faintest idea of what's involved.

If the nitrogen compounds are involved, maybe that ought to be looked at more carefully. I don't know if I'm making myself clear. It's a very confusing subject. But let me just finish by saying that in the study we've been doing with aminobiphenyl, we have found a wide variation of aminobiphenyl in the blood of nonsmokers, and Nancy [Haley] has run cotinine for us. We have found—we haven't analyzed the data yet—but some of those people who are nonsmokers had cotinine in their urine so they are passive smokers to some extent. I don't know to what extent you can judge the exposure to cigarette smoke in any quantitative sense by the amount of cotinine. Could you help me on that?

HOFFMANN: In general, exposure of nonsmokers to tobacco smoke is small. Thus, it may not be possible to assign by epidemiological studies alone, a significant risk factor for lung or other types of cancer to nonsmokers who are environmentally exposed to constituents of tobacco smoke. However, knowledge of the nature of mainstream smoke and sidestream smoke and the relative uptake of such agents and the dose-and-effect relationships in carcinogenesis have led to the conclusion that passive smoke exposure entails some risk for lung cancer and, possibly, for other types of cancers, especially for bladder cancer as just discussed by Steve Tannenbaum. His ongoing studies with aromatic amines, as presented at this conference, should help us to assess the risk of passive smoking with regard to bladder cancer and the possible risk of other cancers associated with the exposure to aromatic amines.

TANNENBAUM: Can you estimate the amount of exposure to cigarette smoke?

HOFFMANN: Yes, you can differentiate between a passive smoker and an active smoker. That you can do.

TANNENBAUM: But for a passive smoker you cannot say anything about the amount of exposure.

HALEY: We will not convert cotinine levels in body fluids of passive smokers to cigarette equivalents absorbed. Based upon the differences in chemical composition of mainstream smoke and sidestream smoke as well as variation in biological half-life of cotinine in smokers and nonsmokers, such conversions seem inappropriate.

WINKELSTEIN: I tend to agree with Dietrich's [Hoffmann] point of view. Despite the problems of finding out how much people smoke, it can be done reliably and has been, and if you can measure the cotinine levels in their fluids, it seems to me that you can combine these observations into some kind of an index of exposure for each individual in the study.

HALEY: There are several factors which must be taken into account. Our data with infants make me cautious in defining cigarette equivalents. We are only measuring one compound present in sidestream smoke and one of its metabolites. As we know, the relative ratios of different smoke components in sidestream or mainstream smoke are not constant for all constituents. In addition, we must ask how the nicotine we measure is being absorbed. Is it inhaled or swallowed? Is it in room air or adherent to the multitude of things children put in their mouths? We must use caution in equating body cotinine to inhalation of X number of cigarettes.

CORREA: But the problem with your argument is that all the available indices, such as cotinine and carbon dioxide, refer to exposure within the last few weeks. So it's no good to quantitate. If the patient is saying that he smoked two packs a day 5 years ago, there's no way that the available tests will reflect that.

HARRIS: I'd like to comment about Steve's [Tannenbaum] statement, in which he said that hydrocarbons are responsible for lung cancer. I don't think we know that. I would also like to ask Dr. Haley if you study a group of individuals who are active smokers, and are smoking 1-5 cigarettes a day, and you study another group of samples who you absolutely know are not smoking but are passive smokers, can you unequivocally identify the active smokers from the passive smokers?

HALEY: We can identify the five cigarette per day smoker. The one cigarette per day smoker who does not inhale will be difficult to separate from passive smokers.

HARRIS: Is there an ongoing, blinded, epidemiological study?

HALEY: An international investigation of passive smoking is currently being conducted. It is a laboratory blinded study.

HARRIS: I think that will be a very important study.

STELLMAN: I have another problem that's really been troubling me about passive smokers, particularly with one or two studies. As far as I know, every active cigarette smoker is also a passive smoker; and, therefore, we pretty much know about all of the sites that are related to tobacco smoke, even cervical cancer. I think that there are some cancer sites which if we were going to find out about, we would know about now, like breast cancer and endocrine cancer. I cannot, for the life of me, rationalize how those two cancer sites popped up in some studies of passive smoking when not a single active smoking study has ever identified them. Can you explain it?

CORREA: There are two points here. One is that the active smoker is also a passive smoker. So I think that all those calculations that have been done so far are reflecting the combination of active and passive smoking. I don't think we have calculations for passive smoking alone, which would be probably, I guess, be more carcinogenic. The finding of risk for breast cancer I also find difficult to explain, but I am not ready to throw it out. First, because some tobacco metabolites are present in biologic fluids, like breast secretions; and second, as Dr. Haley has shown, the active smoker seems to be able to metabolize or get rid of the cotinine more easily than the passive smoker. This may indicate enzyme induction by the active smoker. Nancy [Haley] may want to speculate on that a little bit more. The issue is not just sidestream versus mainstream; it may be that if you are an active smoker, you induce enzymes to deal with carcinogenic metabolites more efficiently than if you are not.

HALEY: It is indicated that because of differences in enzyme induction with active smokers, toxic and carcinogenic agents may have different half-life times in smokers and passive smokers. We have also considered that women only passively exposed might not have the early menopause associated with smoking. However, Sandler and Everson have data suggesting that passively exposed women also have an earlier age of menopause.

CORREA: Which brings into focus the question of endocrine interaction.

CONNEY: It is important to reemphasize that although active cigarette smokers have increased levels of the cytochrome P-450 enzymes, passive smokers have little or no increase in the levels of these enzymes. Accordingly, it is likely that active smokers, but not passive smokers, will have an enhanced metabolism of certain steroid hormones that play a role in the carcinogenic process.

HOFFMANN: Until recently, nothing was known about an increased risk for nasal cancer in active smokers. When Hirayama found an increased risk for nasal cancer in women who were married to heavy smokers, this appeared surprising until 6 months later when NCI published a large field study showing that cigarette smokers have a higher risk of nasal cancer. I would just like to make the point that we should not reject off-hand the possibility of a specific type of cancer risk in nonsmokers because this aspect has not been studied in active smokers.

TANNENBAUM: I'm confused then because data were presented showing that smokers had a higher risk for breast cancer.

WINKELSTEIN: In the Cederlof study there is an elevated relative risk for breast cancer among smokers. However, the data are purely descriptive and unaccompanied by biological explanation or epidemiological comment.

TANNENBAUM: What's the consensus?

WINKELSTEIN: The consensus is that cigarette smoking is not related to breast cancer.

Smokeless Tobacco and Oral/Pharynx Cancer: The Role of Cofactors

DEBORAH M. WINN*
Biostatistics Branch, DCE, E&B
National Cancer Institute
Bethesda, Maryland 20892

OVERVIEW

Epidemiologic and experimental evidence suggests that the use of smokeless tobacco is an important risk factor for cancers of the oral cavity. In our study in North Carolina, white women with oral and pharynx cancer were four times more likely to use oral snuff than controls. Among women with cancer in the cheek and gums, the risks rose to nearly 50-fold for long-term use. This paper describes the role of cofactors in modifying the oral cancer risks associated with the use of smokeless tobacco in the North Carolina study population. Relative risks are similar for blacks and whites when factors such as the anatomic site of cancer are taken into account. Neither a usual adult diet high in fruits and vegetables, nor smoking and alcohol drinking influenced the magnitude of the association between smokeless tobacco use and oral cancer. However, the risk of snuff-induced oral cancer was enhanced in the presence of poor condition of gums and teeth. Squamous cell carcinomas were the predominant cancer type reported regardless of the tobacco habits of the cases. Future research on smokeless tobacco and cancer risks should emphasize quantitation of cancer risks by years of use and amount used, research on chewing tobacco specifically, estimation of the risks of smokeless tobacco use among persons who have quit the smokeless tobacco habit, and interactions between other potential oral cancer risk factors and smokeless tobacco. It will also be important to assess the natural history of the potentially precancerous oral lesions that sometimes occur after initiation of a smokeless tobacco habit and whether smokeless tobacco use is related to other forms of cancer in addition to oral and pharynx cancer.

INTRODUCTION

To evaluate reasons for the high mortality rate for oral and pharynx cancer among white women in the Southeastern United States (Mason et al. 1975), we compared the use of tobacco and other characteristics in a group of women in North Carolina with mouth and throat cancer to that in a comparison group of women without

---
Present address: National Center for Health Statistics, Room 2-58, 3700 East-West Highway, Hyattsville, Maryland 20782.

these cancers. Our results (Winn et al. 1981a) showed that among white women oral snuff use was associated with a fourfold increased risk of oral and pharynx cancer. Risks were far higher for women with cancers in the cheek and gum where the tobacco was routinely placed, reaching close to 50-fold for 50 or more years of use. Snuff, powdered or ground tobacco taken by mouth, is one of several related forms of smokeless tobacco.

Alcohol drinkers who smoke increase their risk of oral cancer beyond that expected based on the sum of the individual effects of the two habits (Rothman and Keller 1972). In India persons who both smoke and chew tobacco (usually mixed with other ingredients such as areca nut or betel leaf) have exceptionally high risks for cancers of the oral cavity, pharynx, larynx, and esophagus (Jayant et al. 1977). Since these findings point to the importance of multiple factors in oral cancer etiology, further assessment of the North Carolina study population determined whether the risk of oral cancer associated with the use of smokeless tobacco varies with the presence of cofactors, such as race, alcohol drinking, and diet. If persons with a particular combination of habits or characteristics seem highly susceptible to the impact of smokeless tobacco, then targeting of preventive programs to groups at unusually high risk may be appropriate. We also examined the histologic characteristics of the cancers occurring in tobacco users to understand the nature of the disease process.

Briefly, cases were women hospitalized with or dying from cancers of the oral cavity or pharynx in North Carolina between 1975 and 1978. Histologic data were abstracted from the "pathologic diagnosis" section of the pathology report on each case in the hospital sample. Two female controls per case were sought from the same source as the case, matched on age, race, and geographic areas of residence. Tobacco information and other data were collected from the women themselves or from the next-of-kin of deceased or incompetent study subjects; interviews were completed with 91% of 255 cases and 82% of the 502 controls. Relative risks (RR) were estimated by the odds ratio (Mantel and Haenszel 1959). Confidence intervals were calculated using the procedure of Gart (1971).

RESULTS

Figure 1 shows that snuff use was strongly related to cancer of the gum and buccal mucosa (where the tobacco typically is placed) regardless of respondent type (self versus next-of-kin), with white cases more than 15 times more likely to use snuff than controls; the lower bounds of the 95% confidence intervals were 3.4 for self respondents and 2.4 for next-of-kin interviews. (Only four blacks in the study had developed gum and buccal mucosal cancer.) The figure also shows the racial similarities in the magnitude of the association between snuff and cancer in other parts of the mouth and pharynx; from the interviews conducted with the study subjects ("self" interviews), relative risks were 5.6 for whites (95% confidence interval

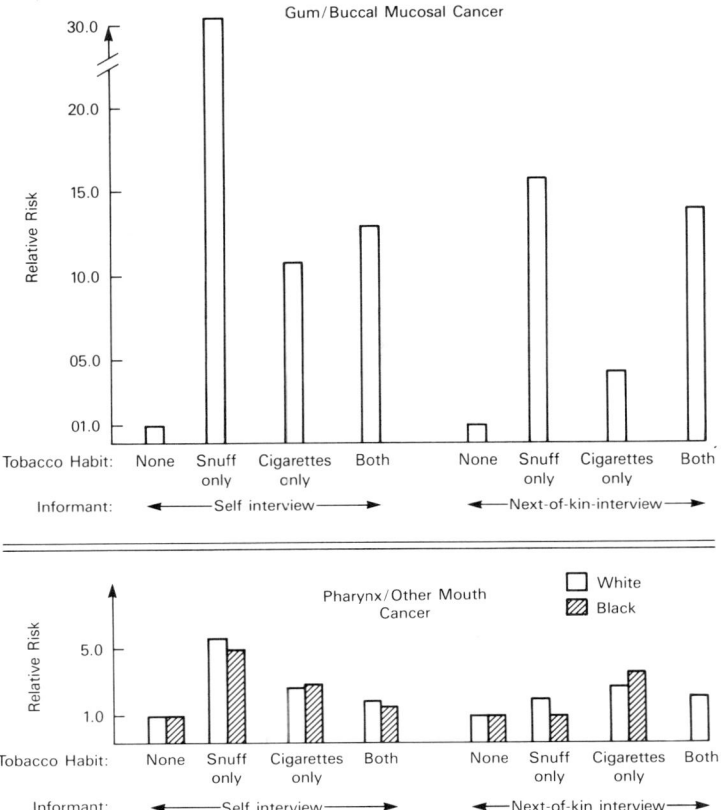

Figure 1
Relative risks of gum/buccal mucosal cancer and of other mouth and pharynx cancer by type of tobacco habit, race, and informant

1.3-24.3) and 5.0 for blacks (95% confidence interval 0.4-135.6). The relative risks of both gum/buccal mucosa and pharynx/other mouth cancer associated with snuff use tended to be higher when estimated from interviews conducted with the women themselves than from interviews with next-of-kin.

The average age at diagnosis or death of women with gum and buccal mucosal cancer was 69 compared with 65 for cancer in other parts of the mouth. Also, white women were generally older than black women; only a quarter of the 36 black cases in the hospital sample were over age 65 when the cancer was diagnosed, whereas more than half of the whites were over 65 at diagnosis. Gum and buccal mucosal cancer also accounted for a smaller proportion of the black (11%) than the white cases (24%) diagnosed in hospital. The proportion of snuff users among the cases in the two races were similar, however (47% of the black cases versus 46% of the whites). Three of the four black cases with gum/buccal mucosal cancer used snuff.

Other potential cofactors, in addition to race, were also examined. A usual adult diet high in fruits and vegetables was associated with a reduced oral cancer risk in this population, with high consumers (21 or more portions per week) at approximately one-half the risk of low consumers of fruits and vegetables (less than 11 portions per week) (Winn et al. 1984). However, no consistent variation in the snuff-associated relative risks is evident by the amount of fruits and vegetables consumed; oral cancer cases with a low dietary intake of fruits and vegetables were 4.6 times more likely to use snuff than controls, while relative risks for moderate and high intake of fruits and vegetables were 2.5 and 4.3, respectively.

Table 1 shows relative risks of oral and pharyngeal cancer associated with various combinations of snuff dipping, alcohol drinking, and cigarette smoking. Smokeless tobacco users who smoked cigarettes and/or drank alcohol were not at higher risk than women who only took snuff. However, snuff dippers who consumed alcohol usually drank very little; only 14% had as much as 2 oz of alcohol per day. Also, women who dipped snuff and smoked on average used snuff for fewer years (33) than women who only used snuff (47). Women with both habits also smoked fewer cigarettes per day, 15 versus 21, than those who only smoked.

Usual lifelong oral hygiene and dentition status, as reported by the respondent, were modifiers of the relative risks of smokeless tobacco as shown in Table 2 (Winn et al. 1981b; Blot et al. 1983). Although the relative risk associated with snuff use did not differ significantly among the levels of each type of health index, the magnitude of the association between smokeless tobacco and cancer increased with increasingly poorer dental status as measured by the general condition of the teeth

Table 1
Relative Risks for Oral and Pharynx Cancer by Type of Tobacco and Alcohol

Tobacco and alcohol use	Cases	Controls	RR	95% Confidence interval
No tobacco and alcohol habits	37	136	1.0	—
Snuff dipper only	81	78	3.8	2.3–6.3
Snuff and cigarettes only	6	6	3.7	1.0–13.9
Snuff and alcohol only	10	26	1.4	0.6–3.4
All three habits	10	13	2.8	1.0–7.6
Cigarettes only	19	48	1.5	0.7–2.9
Alcohol only	4	30	0.5	0.1–1.6
Cigarettes and alcohol	60	68	3.2	1.9–5.5

Reprinted from Winn et al. (1984)

Table 2
Association Between Smokeless Tobacco Use and Oral/Pharynx Cancer by Dental Characteristics

Dental characteristic	Cases using snuff[a]	RR[b]	95% Confidence interval
Teeth lost			
None	9	1.8	0.4–7.0
1–9	14	2.2	0.8–6.0
>= 10	75	3.7	2.0–6.9
Condition of teeth			
Excellent	6	1.3	0.2–6.6
Good	31	2.9	1.3–6.7
Fair	22	4.9	1.8–14.0
Poor	46	5.7	2.4–13.6
Condition of gums			
Excellent	2	0.8	0.1–7.5
Good	57	3.8	2.0–7.1
Fair	22	3.6	1.3–10.3
Poor	21	4.3	1.1–18.1
Ever had gum disease			
No gum disease	80	3.2	1.9–5.2
Gum disease	20	6.4	1.7–26.4
Ever used mouthwash regularly			
No	45	4.4	2.1–9.2
Yes	46	3.5	1.6–7.3
Years since started wearing dentures			
No dentures	38	2.7	1.3–5.5
0–10	21	14.6	1.7–321.1
11–30	23	3.3	1.2–9.2
>= 31	7	1.6	0.4–6.4

[a]Includes smokeless tobacco users who smoke
[b]Referent = nonusers of tobacco

and by tooth loss. The health of the gums also made an impact on the relative risks associated with smokeless tobacco, but the trends were less clear. In women whose category of gum condition was less than excellent, the snuff-associated relative risks remained at about 4; however, the presence of gum disease doubled the relative risk due to snuff. Snuff use was most strongly associated with oral and pharynx cancer (RR = 14.6) in those who started wearing dentures in the previous 10 years. One final indicator of oral hygiene, i.e., mouthwash use, also made a significant impact on smokeless tobacco-associated relative risks, with users having lower relative risks than nonusers.

Squamous cell carcinoma accounted for 83% of the 141 cancers reported in cases in the hospital sample. (Histologic type was poorly documented in cases ascertained through death certificates.) Eight women, 6% of the sample, had verrucous carcinomas. All but one of the verrucous carcinomas occurred in the smokeless tobacco users, accounting for 9% of the 53 snuff dippers and 14% of the 14 snuff users who also smoked. Well-differentiated squamous cell carcinomas also occurred more frequently in the smokeless tobacco users, accounting for 42% of all the cancers in the snuff users, but only 25% of the 50 cases who only smoked and one-quarter of the 24 nonusers of tobacco. In the total study population, far more of the snuff dippers (31%) with cancer reported that they had had leukoplakia or white patches in the mouth than did nonusers of tobacco (10%) or smokers (9%).

Finally, an alternative method of statistical analysis (a conditional logistic analysis) (Lubin 1981), taking into account the matching of individual cases and controls, yields results similar to those presented previously by stratified logistic modeling (Prentice 1976). Table 3 shows crude and adjusted relative risks, via the conditional matched regression analysis, for snuff use. The relative risk for white women nonsmokers actually rose from 4.2 to 5.2 when the matching was taken into account.

DISCUSSION

Our earlier research (Winn et al. 1981a) indicated that the high death rates from oral cancer among Southern women could be accounted for by the snuff dipping

Table 3
Comparison of Results for Snuff Dipping and Cigarette Smoking[a]

Race	Smoker	Snuff dipper	RR from simple analysis[b]	RR from conditional logistic regression[c]
White	No	No	1.0 (R)	1.0 (R)
		Yes	4.2	5.2
	Yes	No	2.9	3.1
		Yes	3.3	3.5
Black	No	No	1.0 (R)	1.0 (R)
		Yes	1.5	1.4
	Yes	No	2.6	5.5
		Yes	3.0	3.2

[a] Data from the North Carolina oral cancer study.
[b] Data from Winn et al. (1981a).
[c] For potential confounders included in model, see Winn et al. (1981a). Separate models for blacks and whites. Industry variables in model for whites only, since few blacks had jobs in these industries.
R = referent

habits of the women in the area. These findings from the North Carolina study population are consistent with other evidence concerning the cancer risks associated with smokeless tobacco. Numerous case-control and cohort studies have shown that smokeless tobacco is related to an increased risk of oral cancer (Connolly et al. 1986); this includes other research conducted in the southern United States (Vogler et al. 1962; Westbrook et al. 1980) as well as in other areas of the United States (Wynder et al. 1957a) and in Scandinavia (Wynder et al. 1957b). Risks associated with chewing tobacco are less well documented than for snuff. In addition to our report, at least one other study has shown a dose-response effect: that increasing usage of smokeless tobacco is associated with increasing risks of gum/mouth cancer (Williams and Horm 1977). The cancers occurring in smokeless tobacco users are often described as arising exactly where the tobacco was routinely placed (Landy and White 1961; McGuirt 1983), lending further reinforcement to an interpretation of a causal association between unsmoked tobacco and oral cancers. Epidemiologic research on related habits outside of the United States is also supportive of an important role of smokeless tobacco in cancer etiology. In India and other parts of Asia and the Pacific Islands, the oral use of mixtures which usually contain unsmoked tobacco as a chief component is a major contributor to the extremely high oral cancer rates in these areas (World Health Organization 1984). Experimental studies have shown that N-nitrosamines are present in smokeless tobacco in high amounts (Hoffmann and Hecht 1985) and two of these substances N-nitrosonornicotine (NNN) and 4-(methylnitrosamino)-1-(3-pyridyl)-1-butanone (NNK), are strong animal carcinogens even at low doses (Hoffmann and Hecht 1985).

An understanding of the link between smokeless tobacco and cancer is important because of the increasing popularity of smokeless tobacco in America, especially by youth. In surveys in the 1980s of school populations, an estimated 8-36% of boys were smokeless tobacco users (Connolly et al. 1986). An early age at initiation of the habit is common; in one study 11% of boys age 8-9 were users of smokeless tobacco (Hunter et al. 1980). One-third of the women in the North Carolina study who used snuff started the habit by age 10. In the North Carolina study women with oral cancer who used snuff took on average 9.7 g per day, which is lower than the 11.9 g (Gritz et al. 1981) and 15.9 g (Squires et al. 1984) reported as usual daily intake by college men in two small studies. It has been estimated that a snuff user taking 1 g of tobacco per day for 30 years would have had a lifetime total of about 0.5 mg/kg of NNK (Hecht et al. 1983). The North Carolina women with oral cancer had a median lifetime intake of NNK of 6.2 mg/kg (calculated by assuming that their "usual adult" daily intake was the same over all the years that the product was used). This level of NNK is nearly as high as the 9 mg/kg (12 mg) given in a single dose to hamsters, which yielded tumors above the level of the controls and is above the extrapolated minimum tumor-generating dose of certain other nitrosamines known to produce tumors in laboratory animals (Hoffmann et al. 1984).

In the North Carolina study next-of-kin served as the respondent when the study subject was deceased or physically unable to respond. Relative risks were generally higher for interviews done with the women themselves than for interviews with next-of-kin. Proxy interviews are a crucial element in many epidemiologic studies of chronic diseases with a high mortality rate, and next-of-kin generally give valid interview responses to broadly defined questions, including smoking. The results of the "self" interviews indicated that blacks and whites with other mouth and pharynx cancer were similar in their relative risks for snuff and cigarette smoking. Too few black women had developed gum or buccal/mucosal cancer to permit analysis by tobacco habit. The deficit of black women with cancer of this site is due in part to the much younger age distribution of the blacks compared to the whites. Cancer incidence data in the United States also shows that patients with gum and buccal mucosal cancer have a higher median age at diagnosis than women with cancer in any other oral or pharynx site except the lip (Young et al. 1981).

Snuff dippers who also smoked or consumed alcohol did not have greater relative risks than women who only dipped snuff, since in the North Carolina study population, smokeless tobacco use was negatively correlated with drinking alcohol and smoking. An understanding of potential interactions, not readily evaluable in our study, would be important for several reasons. If the new generation of smokeless tobacco users, boys and young men, is found to be more likely to adopt a smoking habit concurrently with or after quitting smokeless tobacco use due to habituation to nicotine, the result will be an expanded pool of persons with multiple habits. Moreover, alcohol appears to increase the permeability of the oral mucosa of the pig to N-nitrosonornicotine (Hall et al. 1985), one of the animal carcinogens present in smokeless tobacco, which suggests a potential mechanism for an enhanced effect of two habits. Finally, in India it has been reported that persons who both smoke bidis (local cigarettes) and chew tobacco with other ingredients have many times the risk of mouth cancer than expected on the basis of the individual habits alone (Jayant et al. 1977).

We did find that snuff was more strongly associated with oral cancer among those with the poorest dental status and according to some indices, gum status and dentures. Deteriorating oral status may be a consequence of the use of smokeless tobacco, especially since some of the indicators of poor oral status were not associated with cancer risk in nonusers of tobacco. Alternatively, it may be possible that the nitrosamine level is increased in persons whose oral bacteria level is high due to poor oral hygiene or gum and teeth problems. This question needs considerably more research.

A usual adult diet high in fruit and vegetables had been shown in this study population to be significantly more common in controls than cases (Winn et al. 1984), suggesting a protective effect due possibly to beta-carotene and/or vitamin C. However, this dietary factor had no impact on the relationship between smokeless tobacco and cancer.

Verrucous carcinomas, which have distinctive histologic features, have been described in case reports of smokeless tobacco users (Sorger and Myrden 1960; Fonts et al. 1969). In the present study, relatively few women had verrucous carcinoma mentioned on the pathology report, but these carcinomas only occurred in the tobacco users. Although verrucous carcinoma may be commonly underdiagnosed (Kraus and Perez-Mesa 1966), our finding is consistent with that described in a large North Carolina hospital (Wynder et al. 1957a) where only four of 57 oral cancer patients with a smokeless tobacco habit had histologically verified verrucous carcinoma. In our study the overwhelming proportion of smokeless tobacco users had squamous cell carcinomas, which in the United States is the most common form of cancer occurring in the oral cavity and pharynx (Young et al. 1981).

We found that women with oral cancer who had a snuff habit reported leukoplakia more frequently than women with other or no habits. Leukoplakia has been reported in other studies of oral cancer patients with a smokeless tobacco habit (Wynder et al. 1957a; Vogler et al. 1960). Cancer transformation rates between 3-17% in populations of patients with leukoplakia (Silverman et al. 1984) suggest that this condition may be a premalignant lesion for oral cancer. Leukoplakia can develop in smokeless tobacco users according to one small study of college athletes (Christen et al. 1979), and other oral lesions have been reported in surveys of youth after only a few years of smokeless tobacco use (Greer and Poulson 1983). More research is needed to understand which lesions are the most problematic in terms of ultimate oral cancer risk, especially in view of reports that carcinoma is more frequently present in leukoplakias with a nodular, multicolored appearance than in other leukoplakias (Axell et al. 1984).

Future research studies should also evaluate whether the cessation of a smokeless tobacco habit results in a reduced level of cancer risk. It is unknown whether the risk of oral cancer is lower in quitters of smokeless tobacco, but even former smokeless tobacco users retained an increased risk of pancreatic cancer in a recent cohort study (Heuch et al. 1983). These findings concerning smokeless tobacco and cancer of the pancreas in humans and evidence of metabolic activation of tobacco-specific nitrosamines in a variety of human organs (Castonguay et al. 1983) suggest the need for more research on the effects of smokeless tobacco on tissues distant from the mouth.

SUMMARY

Our findings from the North Carolina study indicate: (1) Similarities in snuff-associated relative risks in blacks and whites and a lack of modification of snuff-associated risks by a usual diet high in fruits and vegetables, smoking, or alcohol intake. (2) That the association between smokeless tobacco and oral cancer may be exacerbated by poor dentition and certain gum conditions. (3) That squamous cell carcinomas are by far the most common cancer associated with smokeless tobacco use. Verrucous carcinoma was more common among tobacco users (of smokeless and smoking products), but accounted for only 6% of oral/pharynx cancers in women in the study. (4) The amount of snuff usually used per day by the women with oral cancer was less than that reported in two recent studies of college men. These women had an estimated lifetime dose of NNK, a carcinogen found in smokeless tobacco, of roughly 6.2 mg/kg. (5) Our findings are consistent with other epidemiologic studies which show in totality that smokeless tobaccos are potent oral cancer risk factors. (6) High rates of smokeless tobacco use in young persons have made it important to understand the health risks associated with smokeless tobacco. (7) Future research should emphasize quantification of the magnitude of risk associated with chewing tobacco, identifying high-risk premalignant lesions, risks associated with cancers in anatomic sites outside of the mouth and throat, systematic studies of the histologic forms associated with cancer in smokeless tobacco users, risks in former smokeless tobacco users, and the role of cofactors involved in modifying the risks of smokeless tobacco use.

ACKNOWLEDGMENTS

The author thanks Dr. William J. Blot of the National Cancer Institute for his insightful comments and discussions during the writing of this manuscript.

REFERENCES

Axell, T., P. Holmstrup, I.R.H. Kramer, J.J. Pindborg, and M. Shear (eds.). 1984. International seminar on oral leukoplakia and associated lesions, related to tobacco habits. *Community. Dent. Oral Epidemiol.* 12: 146.

Blot, W.J., D.M. Winn, and J.F. Fraumeni, Jr. 1983. Oral cancer and mouthwash. *J. Natl. Cancer Inst.* 70: 251.

Castonguay, A., G.D. Stoner, H.A. Schut, and S.S. Hecht. 1983. Metabolism of tobacco-specific N-nitrosamines by cultured human tissues. *Proc. Natl. Acad. Sci. U.S.A.* 80: 6694.

Christen, A.G., R.K. McDaniel, and J.E. Doran. 1979. Snuff dipping and tobacco chewing in a group of Texas college athletes. *Tex. Dent. J.* 97: 6.

Connolly, G.N., D.M. Winn, S.S. Hecht, J.E. Henningfield, B. Walker, and D. Hoffmann. 1986. The reemergence of smokeless tobacco. *N. Engl. J. Med.* 314: 1020.

Fonts, E.A., R.H. Greenlaw, B.F. Rush, and S. Rovin. 1969. Verrucous squamous cell carcinoma of the oral cavity. *Cancer* 23: 152.

Gart, J.J. 1971. The comparison of proportions: Review of significance tests, confidence intervals, and adjustments for stratification. *Rev. I. I. Sta.* 39: 148.

Greer, R.O. and T.C. Poulson. 1983. Oral tissue alterations associated with the use of smokeless tobacco by teenagers. *Oral Surg.* 56: 275.

Gritz, E.R., V. Baer-Weiss, N.L. Benowitz, H. Van Vunakis, and M.E. Jarvik. 1981. Plasma nicotine and cotinine concentration in habitual smokeless tobacco users. *Clin. Pharmacol. Ther.* **30**: 201.

Hall, B.K., P. Cox, C.A. Squier, and C. Lesch. 1985. Effects of tobacco derivatives and low concentrations of ethanol on oral mucosa. *J. Dent. Res.* **64**: 279.

Hecht, S.S., J. Adams, S. Numoto, and D. Hoffmann. 1983. Induction of respiratory tract tumors in Syrian golden hamsters by a single dose of 4-4-(methylnitrosamino)-1-(3-pyridyl)-1-butanone (NNK) and the effect of smoke inhalation. *Carcinogenesis* **4**: 1287.

Heuch, I., G. Kvale, B.K. Jacobsen, and E. Bjelke. 1983. Use of alcohol, tobacco, and coffee, and the risk of pancreatic cancer. *Br. J. Cancer* **48**: 637.

Hoffmann, D. and S.S. Hecht. 1985. Nicotine-derived N-nitrosamines and tobacco-related cancer: Current status and future directions. *Cancer Res.* **45**: 935.

Hoffmann, D., K.D. Brunneman, J.D. Adams, and S.S. Hecht. 1984. Formation and analysis of N-nitrosoamines in tobacco products and their endogenous formation in consumers. In *N-nitroso compounds: Occurrence, biological effects and relevance to human cancer* (ed. I.K. O'Neill, R.C. Von Borstel, C.T. Miller, J. Long, and H. Bartsch), IARC Scientific Publications no. 57, p. 743. Oxford University Press, Oxford.

Hunter, S.M., L.S. Webber, and G.S. Berenson. 1980. Cigarette smoking and tobacco usage behavior in children and adolescents: Bogalusa Heart Study. *Prev. Med.* **9**: 701.

Jayant, K., V. Balakrishnan, L.D. Sanghvi, and D.J. Jussawalla. 1977. Quantification of the role of smoking and tobacco chewing in oral, pharyngeal, and esophageal cancers. *Br. J. Cancer* **35**: 232.

Kraus, F.T. and C. Perez-Mesa. 1966. Verrucous carcinoma: Clinical and pathologic study of 105 cases involving the oral cavity, larynx, and genitalia. *Cancer* **19**: 26.

Landy, J.J. and H.J. White. 1961. Buccogingival carcinoma of snuff dippers. *Am. Surg.* **26**: 442.

Lubin, J.H. 1981. A computer program for the analysis of matched case-control studies. *Comput. Biomed. Res.* **14**: 38.

Mantel, N. and W. Haenszel. 1969. Statistical aspects of the analysis of data from retrospective studies of disease. *J. Natl. Cancer Inst.* **22**: 719.

Mason, T.J., F.W. McKay, R. Hoover, W.J. Blot, and J.F. Fraumeni, Jr. 1975. *Atlas of cancer mortality for U.S. counties 1950-1969*, DHEW Publ. (NIH) 75-780. U.S. Government Printing Office, Washington, D.C.

McGuirt, W.F. 1983. Snuff dipper's carcinoma. *Arch. Otolaryngol.* **109**: 757.

Prentice, R. 1976. Use of the logistic model in retrospective studies. *Biometrics* **32**: 599.

Rothman, K.J. and A.Z. Keller. 1972. The effect of joint exposure to alcohol and tobacco on the risk of cancer of the mouth and pharynx. *J. Chronic Dis.* **25**: 711.

Silverman, S., M. Gorsky, and F. Lozada. 1984. Oral leukoplakia and malignant transformation. *Cancer* **53**: 563.

Sorger, K. and J.A. Myrden. 1960. Verrucous carcinoma of the buccal mucosa in tobacco chewers. *Can. Med. Assoc. J.* **83**: 1413.

Squires, W.G., T.A. Brandon, S. Zinkgraf, D. Bonds, G.H. Jartung, T. Murray, A.S. Jackson, and R.R. Millar. 1984. Hemodynamic effects of oral smokeless tobacco in dogs and young adults. *Prev. Med.* **13**: 195.

Vogler, W.R., J.W. Lloyd, and B.K. Milmore. 1962. A retrospective study of etiological factors in cancer of the mouth, pharynx, and larynx. *Cancer* **15**: 246.

Westbrook, K.C., J.Y. Sven, J.M. Hawkins, and D.C. McKinney. 1980. Snuff dipper's carcinoma: Fact or fiction? In *Prevention and detection of cancer, part II. Detection* (ed. H.E. Nieburgg). vol. 2, p. 1367. Marcel Dekker, New York.

Williams, R.R. and J.W. Horm. 1977. Association of cancer sites with tobacco and alcohol consumption and socioeconomic status of patients: Interview study from the Third National Cancer survey. *J. Natl. Cancer Inst.* **58**: 525.

Winn, D.M., W.J. Blot, C.M. Shy, L.W. Pickle, A. Toledo, and J.F. Fraumeni, Jr. 1981a. Snuff dipping and oral cancer among women in the Southern United States. *N. Engl. J. Med.* **304**: 745.

Winn, D.M., W.J. Blot, and J.F. Fraumeni, Jr. 1981b. Snuff dipping and cancer. *N. Engl. J. Med.* **305**: 230.

Winn, D.M., R.G. Ziegler, L.W. Pickle, G. Gridley, W.J. Blot, and R.N. Hoover. 1984. Diet in the etiology of oral and pharynx cancer among women in the Southern United States. *Cancer Res.* **44**: 1216.

World Health Organization. 1984. Control of oral cancer in developing countries. *Bull. W.H.O.* **62**: 817.

Wynder, E.L., I.J. Bross, and R.M. Feldman. 1957a. A study of the etiological factors in cancer of the mouth. *Cancer* **10**: 1300.

Wynder, E.L., S. Hultberg, F. Jacobsson, and I.J. Bross. 1957b. Environmental factors in cancer of the upper alimentary tract. *Cancer* **10**: 1300.

Young, J.L., C.L. Percy, and A.J. Asire. 1981. *Surveillance, epidemiology and end results: Incidence and mortality data, 1973-1977.* Monogr. 57, NIH Publ. 81-2330. U.S. Government Printing Office, Washington, D.C.

COMMENTS

STELLMAN: Is it possible that another explanation for the dentition response that we see in many studies of mouth cancer is that people with mouth cancer tend, as you have already shown, to have poor diet and this is a manifestation of just a very poor diet, an effect, rather than a cause?

WINN: That's possible. I would think that if diet and oral hygiene interact, you'd probably see it most easily in studies outside the United States—maybe in a developing country where there is a wider range of dietary intakes and oral care than in the United States.

YOAKUM: Has there been any examination of the microflora to test for the presence of relevant bacteria and viruses such as herpes type I?

WINN: Not that I am aware of. You mean in terms of swabbing the mouth and seeing what is growing there?

YOAKUM: Yes, find out what's growing there. Something different or all the same?

WINN: There's been no research that I know of.

HARRIS: I have two questions. Is there any evidence that the age of starting to use snuff has an influence on the risk?

WINN: I looked at that and I saw almost no difference between cases and controls in the median age at which use of the product started. However, three-quarters of the women using smokeless tobacco started before adulthood and so are concentrated in a relatively small number of years of onset.

HARRIS: The second question relates to offspring of women using snuff. Is there any effect on birth weight, or anything else that's been affected?

WINN: There has been one study in India on tobacco-chewing women. The chewers were more likely to have stillbirths, a lower birth rate, and a greater proportion of male births than the women in the comparison group. This has not been studied in the United States.

HARRIS: So these questions about birth weight relate to carbon monoxide; and a study of tobacco smokers, as opposed to smokeless tobacco, might sort out its importance.

WINN: Actually, doing a study of nonusers of tobacco, smokeless tobacco users, and smokers might be a useful way of sorting out some of the health effects related to smoking from those related to using noncombusted tobacco.

HOFFMANN: I want to comment that it was Spiegelhalder from Heidelberg who found nitrate in the saliva of nonsmokers. But you have to realize that the average intake of snuff per day is about 10 g, meaning that the snuff dippers' oral cavity is exposed to an additional 100-200 mg of nitrate daily. Some of this is reduced to nitrite. Thus, in the saliva of a nonsmoker or nonchewer, you wouldn't expect much nitrate relative to tobacco consumers.

TANNENBAUM: No. The hypothesis in the Spiegelhalder study was that people who had poor oral hygiene would have more nitrite.

HOFFMANN: Yes, but when there is no nitrate to reduce.

TANNENBAUM: There is plenty of nitrate. Saliva has a lot of nitrate. You could be right.

HOFFMANN: We were amazed at the difference in nitrate of nonusers and users.

TANNENBAUM: You could be right. That's the only study I know in which oral hygiene has been looked at.

HOFFMANN: Deborah [Winn], you presented information about two teenagers and we do know of at least four cases of young men with cancer of the oral cavity all of whom used snuff and died very early. So we may assume that snuff is a potent carcinogen. Disregarding very few occupations, I do not know of any other environmental agent which induces cancer so rapidly so early in life except perhaps the polycyclic aromatic hydrocarbons in the soot that Percival Pott held accountable for the scrotal cancer of young boys who worked as chimney sweeps in 18th century England. If I were the government, I would make a registry for cancer of the oral cavity in these young people. I thought that should be done because it is of major concern. Snuff-dipping in young people is a new and steadily increasing habit. Should we wait, as in the case of cigarette smoking and lung cancer, to have an epidemic of cancer, or should we clearly delineate the risk factors now and intervene? I believe a national cancer registry of such cases must be the first step.

WINN: I think that would be a good idea. Young oral cancer patients who used smokeless tobacco are being identified through an informal network of physicians and others at the moment; however, no systematic or exhaustive effort is being made to find these patients.

ENZELL: Was the snuff used by these women dry snuff or wet snuff?

WINN: Mostly dry. Almost exclusively dry snuff.

ENZELL: So it's different from what people have usually consumed in earlier studies.

WINN: In most of the studies done in women in the South, probably most of the snuff used is of the dry type. But in the case reports or studies in men or in other parts of the United States, other forms of smokeless tobacco are likely to be involved. Although not quite as many studies have been done in these areas as in the South, positive associations between smokeless tobacco use and oral cancer have been reported in Minnesota and New York.

ENZELL: But isn't that a very minor portion of the market?

WINN: Yes. Dry snuff is now a minor portion of the U.S. market.

ENZELL: I'm just trying to see the difference between the results that I am aware of and the results that you have arrived at. My feeling is that there might be quite different effects of the two products.

WINN: It's possible that there are variations in risk. From an epidemiological point of view, there are very high relative risks associated with snuff use in studies from the southeastern United States. Reported or estimated relative risks in parts of the United States where moist snuff is likely to be used are not consistently as high. Nevertheless, positive associations have been observed in both places; and nitrosamines are isolatable from all of these various forms of smokeless tobacco.

HOFFMANN: Nitrosamines are higher in the moist snuff than in the dry snuff.

ENZELL: Yes, but you focus on nitrosamines. I'm not saying that. Are you convinced that these are the only carcinogens? I mean, it seems that this is putting magic into the word, nitrosamine.

HOFFMANN: The tobacco-specific nitrosamines are by far the highest concentration of carcinogens in snuff.

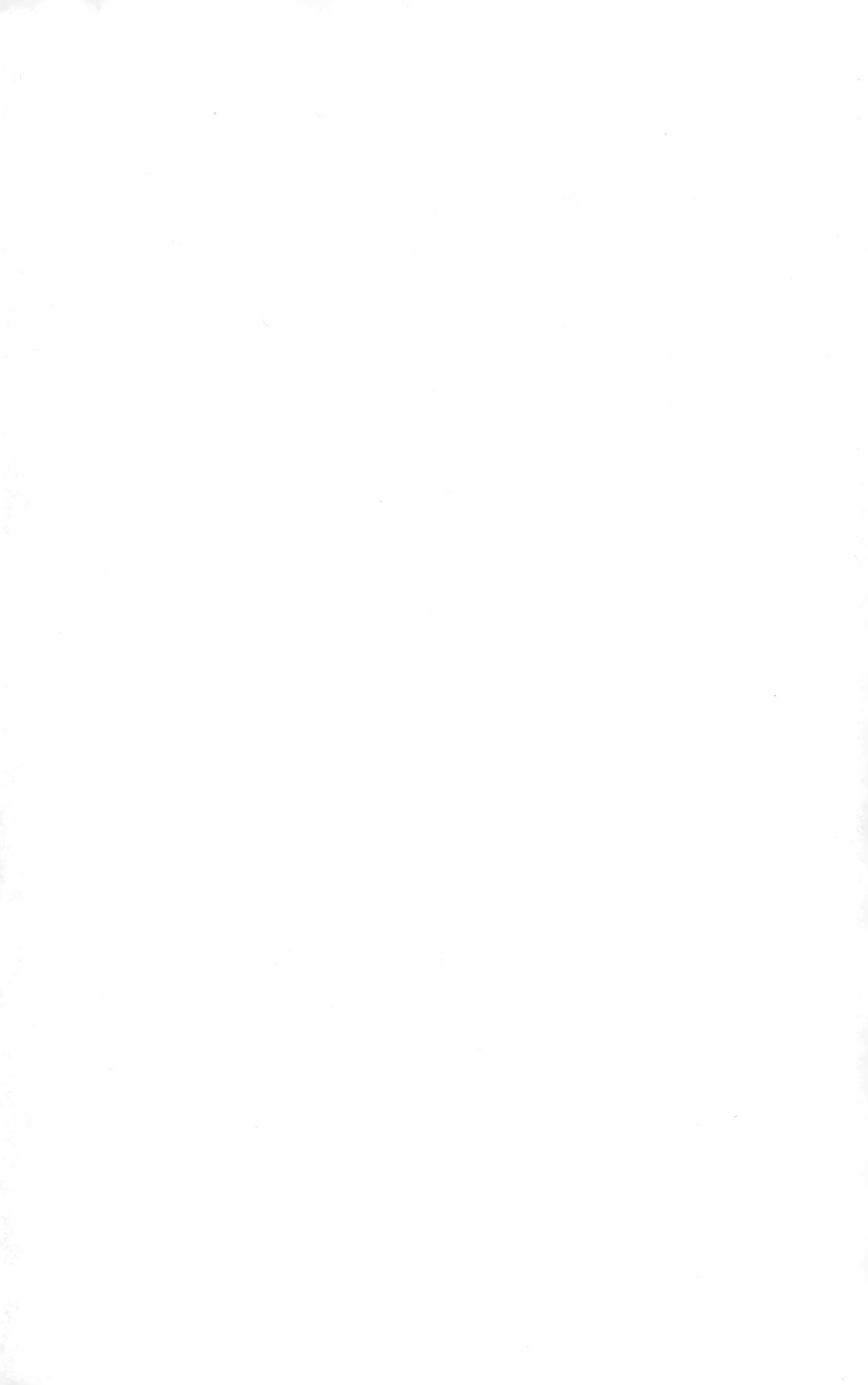

Interactions between Smoking and Other Exposures: Occupation and Diet

STEVEN D. STELLMAN
American Cancer Society
New York, New York 10001

INTRODUCTION

There are two important reasons for investigating the relationship between tobacco smoking and other factors in the causation of illness. In the first place, smoking is causally related to a very large number of diseases, including those which cause the majority of deaths in our society. Many of these diseases, particularly cancers of the lung and other sites, also have environmental causes in addition to smoking. Many of these environmental factors increase the quantitative risk of diseases by amounts similar to or often less than the risks associated with smoking; yet many people exposed to these factors also smoke, so that it is often a major methodological problem in epidemiological studies to disentangle the effects due to smoking from those due to other exposures.

The second reason for pursuing smoking-environment interactions is that some substances, notably asbestos, increase the risk of smoking-related disease far above the amount expected if smoking and asbestos exerted their effects independently. This effect, often called synergism, has profound implications for predicting future numbers of cases of diseases (Selikoff 1981), as well as for developing strategies for prevention.

Most multiple-factor studies have centered around cigarette smoking and occupational exposures. The literature on this subject is now sufficiently abundant that the 1986 Surgeon-General's report on smoking and health is devoted exclusively to occupation. Among the topics treated at length in that report are general workplace interactions, chronic lung disease, and cancer. Among the exposures considered are petrochemicals, aromatic amines, pesticides, asbestos, radon daughters, and cotton dust.

Rather than attempt to cover these topics which have already been reviewed in great depth in that report, in detail, this paper will be confined to presenting a superficial summary of the interaction problem, with some interesting illustrations from studies of both occupation and nutrition in relation to smoking and cancer. I will mention some of the problems encountered in trying to analyze these situations epidemiologically and present some new American Cancer Society data which may help us as we proceed to investigate the interrelationships between smoking and other exposures.

The 1979 Surgeon-General's report lists six ways in which cigarette smoking can interact with the occupational environment to increase risk of illness or injury (U.S. Dept. Health, Education, and Welfare 1979).

(1) A working environment may facilitate body absorption of the toxic components of cigarette smoke.
(2) Cigarette smoking can transform workplace chemicals into more toxic substances.
(3) A worker can be doubly exposed to the toxic constituents of tobacco smoke and to the same constituents in the workplace.
(4) The health effects from environmental exposure can be concurrent with similar health effects from smoking.
(5) The synergistic effects of all agents can pose a grave health problem to workers.
(6) Accidents can be caused by smoking in the industrial environment.

During the past few years, an elaborate—and sometimes controversial—mathematical formalism has been developed for describing and quantifying such interactions, particularly as they apply to measuring the contributions to total risk of disease due to individual exposures (Walker and Rothman 1972; Rothman 1976, 1981; Saracci 1977, 1980; Rothman et al. 1978; Walter and Holford 1981). Formal definitions have been proposed for causal types of concepts, such as interaction and synergy. The main difficulty in this area has not been lack of good statistical ideas so much as lack of good data. As will be shown below, the basic environmental dosage measurements, which are hard enough to obtain reliably for a single exposure, become very tenuous when applied two at a time. Nevertheless, there are now available a number of useful examples to illustrate the wide range of interactions between these various exposures and smoking.

To simplify the discussion and focus attention on the factors themselves, I will present data from a number of multiple-factor studies in terms of two simple models: additive and multiplicative. The numerical aspects of these models are presented in Table 1, in terms applicable to studies in which either relative risks or

Table 1

Comparison of Additive and Multiplicative Models for Two Simultaneous Exposures

Exposure	Relative risk	Rate
Neither	1.0	I_o
Smoking	s	sI_o
Additional factor	a	aI_o
Both		
Additive model	(s + a − 1)	$(s - a - 1) I_o$
Multiplicative model	sa	saI_o

absolute rates are available. If s is the relative risk conferred by smoking in the absence of the second exposure, and a is the relative risk due to the second exposure in the absence of smoking, then according to the additive model the relative risk among persons exposed to both should be $s + a - 1$, whereas according to the multiplicative model it should be sa. Extension to multiple levels of exposure is straightforward. The key to developing both models is that risks due to any combination of exposures must always be measured relative to a common reference point.

SMOKING AND OCCUPATION

Figure 1 shows the relative risk for lung cancer in relation to both smoking and shipyard work according to the data of Blot and Fraumeni (1981) combined across four studies. Smoking apart, it is assumed that the excess lung cancer risk among shipyard workers is due mainly to exposure to asbestos, although other contributory factors are certainly possible. Except for former smokers, the relative risk (RR) among shipyard workers is higher at each level of smoking, compared to the

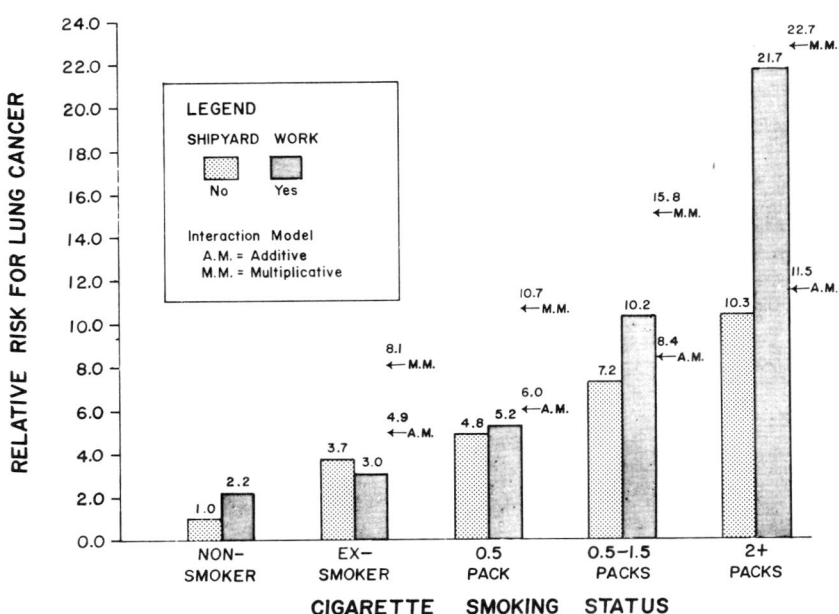

Figure 1
Relative risk for lung cancer according to number of cigarettes smoked per day and whether or not subject worked in a shipyard. Data from four case-control studies combined. Data from Blot and Fraumeni (1981).

RR among nonshipyard workers. At the level of 0.5 to 1.5 packs per day, the actual RR among shipyard workers is higher than the additive model predicts, but less than the multiplicative model, whereas among the heaviest smokers, it is nearly the same as the multiplicative model. Table 2 shows the lung cancer death rates determined by Hammond et al. (1979) among asbestos insulation workers according to whether or not they smoked and according to the source of information on cause of death (death certificate versus best evidence). In either case, the actual rate among those exposed to both asbestos and cigarette smoking is well above the additive model, and, in the case of death certificate ascertainment, is nearly multiplicative (601.6 observed versus 633.6 predicted).

Stellman and Garfinkel (1984) recently reported on the mortality experience of 10,322 men employed in woodworking industries and followed up for 12 years in an American Cancer Society study. Figure 2 shows the standardized mortality ratio (SMR) for lung cancer, according to smoking habit and usual employment as nonwoodworker, woodworker, or in the carpenter-joiner subgroup. The mortality rates for woodworkers in general and for the carpenters among them were higher than in the nonwoodworkers only among smokers of 20 or more cigarettes per day. Figure 3 shows the analogous SMR pattern for bladder cancer, with similar findings. In the case of lung cancer, the risks of smoking and woodworking seem to be additive, but with bladder cancer they are more nearly multiplicative.

Whether or not exposure to ionizing radiation in the form of radon daughters, particularly through underground mining, increases lung cancer risk multiplicatively has yet to be resolved. Relative risks for lung cancer among smoking Swedish underground miners of iron ore, computed by Damber and Larsson (1985), shown in Table 3, agree well with those predicted with a multiplicative model. On the other

Table 2

Comparison of Observed Cancer Death Rates with Predictions of Additive and Multiplicative Models

Exposure	Lung cancer death rate	
	Best evidence	Death certificate
Neither	11.3	11.3
Smoking	122.6	122.6
Asbestos	80.2	58.4
Both		
Actual	693.8	601.6
Predicted		
Additive model	191.5	169.7
Multiplicative model	870.1	633.6

Based on data from Hammond et al. (1979)

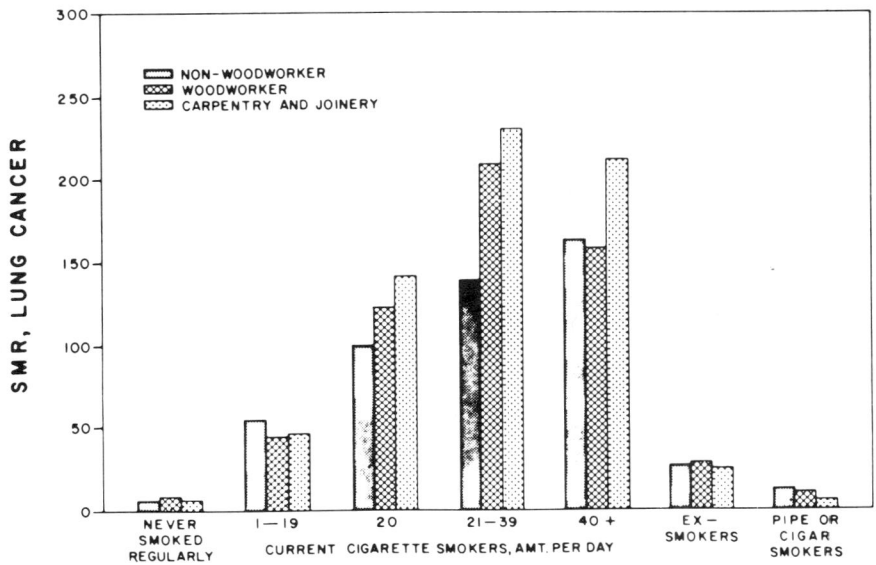

Figure 2
Standardized mortality ratios (*SMR*) for lung cancer by occupation (woodworker or not) and smoking habits. All categories are relative to nonwoodworkers who were current smokers of 20 cigarettes per day (= 100). Reprinted, with permission, from Stellman and Garfinkel (1984).

hand, several other studies (Edling 1982; Radford and St Clair Renard 1984) show risks that are additive.

Hirayama (1981) has reported age-standardized death rates from all cancer, lung cancer, and stomach cancer (Table 4) among material metal workers, in the context of a very large prospective study of the general population in Japan. According to his data, the actual rates for all cancers and for stomach cancer are considerably above those predicted by either model, whereas the lung cancer rate is consistent with an additive model.

In a case-control study in an industrialized area of Northern Italy, Pastorino et al. (1984) computed relative risks for lung cancer in relation to smoking and employment in occupations in which exposures to known carcinogens are likely. Such exposures included asbestos, polycyclic aromatic hydrocarbons, chromium, nickel, and arsenic compounds, bis-chloromethyl ether, chloromethyl methyl ether, and vinyl chloride. Subjects were classified as not exposed (−), or as definitely or potentially exposed (+,?). Figure 4 shows the relative risks. For the heaviest smokers, the RR was 20, which is higher than that predicted by an additive model (12.5) but less than a multiplicative model (27.5).

Table 3
Comparison of Observed Cancer Death Rates with Predictions of Additive and Multiplicative Models

Exposure	Relative risk for lung cancer
Neither	1.0
Smoking	7.4
Underground mining	5.5
Both	
Actual	40.6
Predicted	
Additive model	11.9
Multiplicative model	40.7

Based on data from Damber and Larsson (1985)

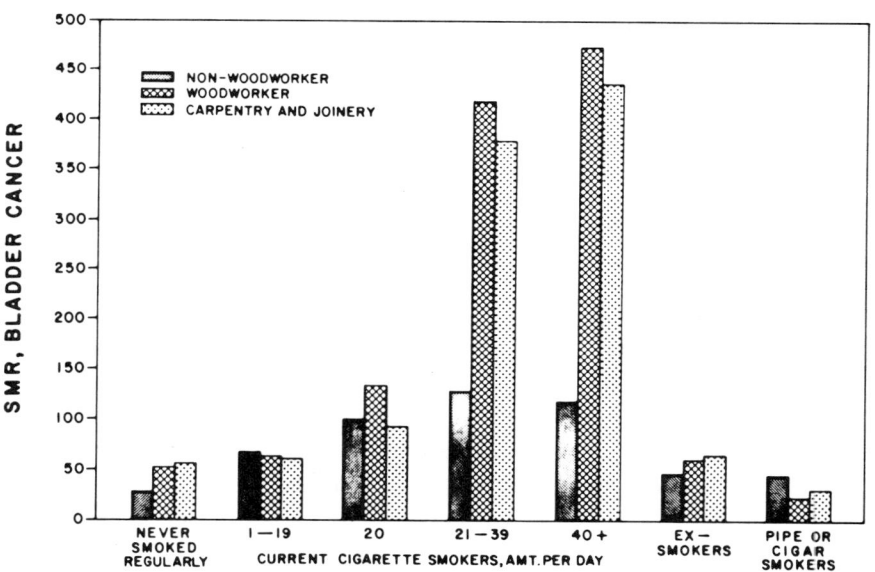

Figure 3
Standardized mortality ratios (*SMR*) for bladder cancer by occupation (woodworker or not) and smoking habits. All categories are relative to nonwoodworkers who were current smokers of 20 cigarettes per day (= 100). Reprinted, with permission, from Stellman and Garfinkel (1984).

Table 4
Comparison of Observed Cancer Death Rates with Predictions of Additive and Multiplicative Models

Exposure	Age-standardized death rate per 100,000 from:		
	All cancers	Lung cancer	Stomach cancer
Neither[a]	304.3	20.7	136.5
Daily smoking	495.9	85.5	200.7
Material metal workers	305.1	62.5	180.8
Both			
Actual	851.7	142.1	400.3
Predicted			
Additive model	496.8	127.3	244.3
Multiplicative model	497.5	258.2	264.9

[a] Approximated by total study population nonsmokers
Based on data from Hirayama (1981)

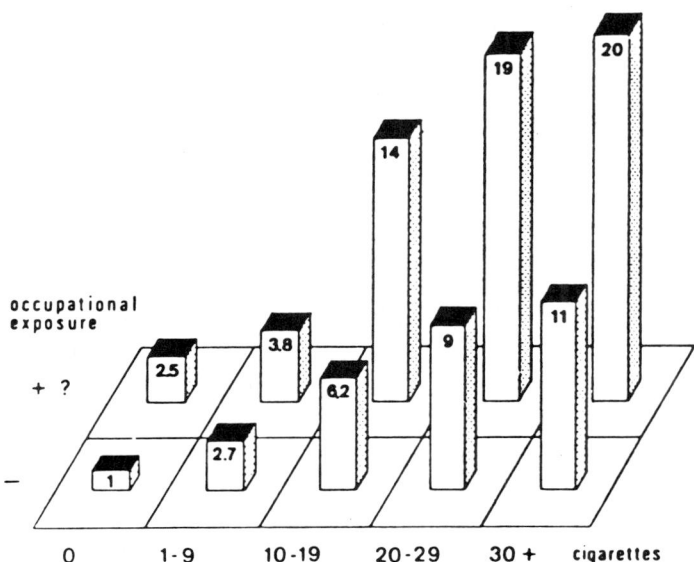

Figure 4
Relative risk for lung cancer by definite (+) or possible (?) occupational exposure to industrial carcinogens, according to number of cigarettes smoked per day. Reprinted, with permission, from Pastorino et al. (1984).

SMOKING AND DIET

In addition to interactions between smoking and occupation, the interactions with alcohol consumption have been studied extensively. The recent surge of interest in nutritional aspects of carcinogenesis has also led to a realization that the same principles may also apply. In studies of diet and lung cancer, for example, it is essential to take smoking habits into account, so as not to mistakenly report an apparent diet-lung cancer effect that might actually be due to confounding by smoking.

Alcohol plays an etiologic role in cancers of the mouth, larynx, oral cavity, and esophagus (Wynder and Stellman 1977, 1979). It has been widely stated that alcohol is not a carcinogen by itself but that it promotes the carcinogenic effects of tobacco smoke. However, it has always been difficult to settle this point, because of the cultural nature of heavy drinking: It is very rare to find a heavy drinker who is not also a smoker. Consequently, the error bounds for estimates of RR in heavy drinkers in the absence of smoking are usually too large to permit drawing firm conclusions about the carcinogenicity of alcohol alone.

Further difficulties in estimating the relative risks of alcohol accurately arise from uncertainties in assigning dosages. Some heavy drinkers consume similar quantities of alcohol each day, as with cigarette smoking; but others drink in binges, spaced by short or long periods of time. The epidemiologist must consequently make drastic assumptions about exposure in order to aggregate sufficient numbers of cases into a small enough number of categories for useful analysis.

Figure 5 shows a reasonable way in which such categorization has been done (Mashberg et al. 1981). Here, drinking has been classified according to the number of "whisky equivalents" (we) consumed per day, as a way of normalizing beer, wine, and spirit consumption on the same scale. An interesting feature of this case-control study of oral squamous carcinoma is the use as a reference group of "minimal" smokers and "minimal" drinkers, rather than nonsmoking nondrinkers. This distinction was necessary because of the high prevalence of both smoking and drinking in the entire study population. Among "minimal" smokers, the RR rose with the number of we per day. At each higher level of smoking, the RR among heavier drinkers was higher than among "minimal" drinkers, but the relationships are not consistent. Table 5 shows the interaction models at the highest levels of smoking and drinking. The RR (104.7) is somewhat between the additive (30.2) and multiplicative (185.6) models.

An alternative classification scheme for alcohol consumption was proposed by Olsen et al. (1985) in a case-control study of cancer of the larynx. Figure 6 shows smoking- and alcohol-specific RRs, at levels of 0-100, 101-200, 201-300, and 301+ g of alcohol per week. As in the preceding study, the reference levels of both alcohol and tobacco usage were not restricted to total abstainers.

A number of investigators have recently begun to examine the interaction between smoking and specific food item consumption. Table 6 shows the SMR for

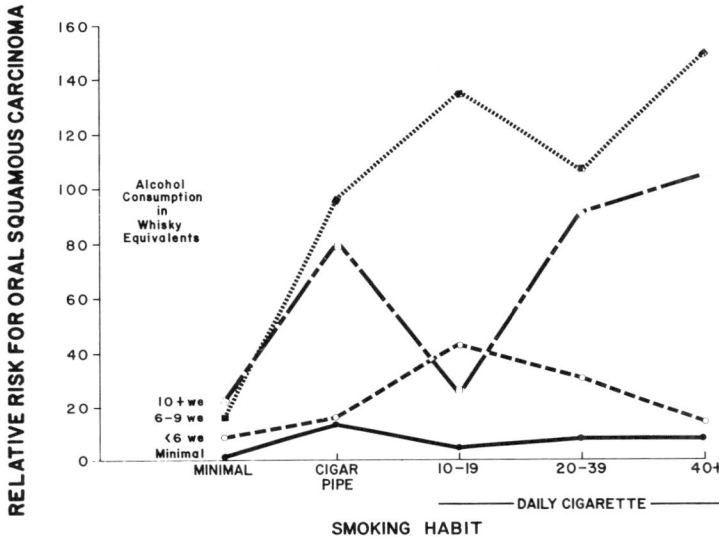

Figure 5
Relative risk for oral squamous carcinoma, according to number of cigarettes smoked per day and number of "whisky equivalents" consumed per day. Reference group consists of "minimal" drinkers and smokers, rather than nondrinkers and nonsmokers. (*we*) Whisky equivalents. Data from Mashberg et al. (1981).

Table 5
Comparison of Relative Risks with Predictions of Additive and Multiplicative Models

Exposure	Relative risk for oral squamous carcinoma
"Minimal" smoking and drinking	1.0
Smoking 40 or more cigarettes per day	8.0
Drinking 10 or more whisky equivalents per day	23.2
Both	
Actual	104.7
Predicted	
Additive model	30.2
Multiplicative model	185.6

Based on data from Mashberg et al. (1981)

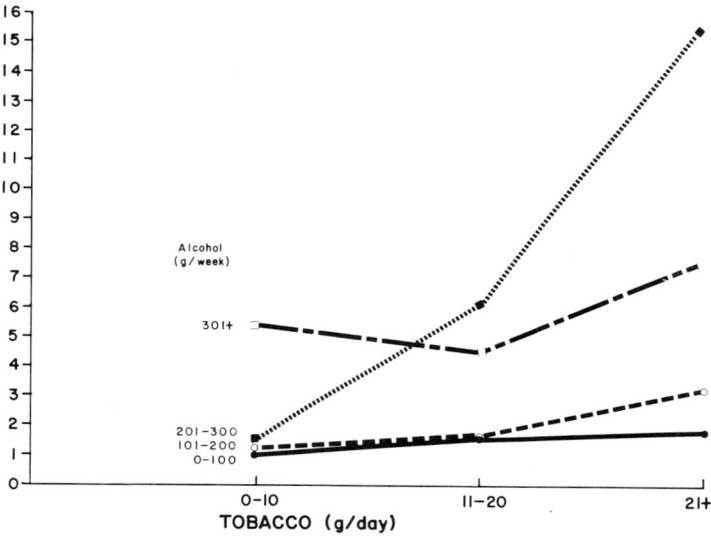

Figure 6
Age- and sex-adjusted relative risk for larynx cancer according to number of cigarettes smoked per day and number of g of alcohol consumed per week. Data from Olsen et al. (1985).

Table 6
Comparison of Observed Cancer Death Rates with Predictions of Additive and Multiplicative Models

Exposure	Age-standardized death rate per 100,000 from lung cancer	
	Males	Females
Neither	14.5	11.7
Daily smoking	66.3	19.0
Avoidance of green-yellow vegetables	32.4	16.7
Both		
Actual	79.5	33.9
Predicted		
Additive model	84.1	24.0
Multiplicative model	147.8	27.1

Based on data from Hirayama (1979)

lung cancer in both men and women in Hirayama's large-scale prospective study (Hirayama 1979) in relation to smoking and *avoidance* of green-yellow vegetables, which was considered to be the risk factor of interest. The observed RR for men was close to the additive, whereas for women the observed RR exceeded both the additive and multiplicative models.

The relationship between consumption of fruit and fruit juice was examined by Wang and Hammond (1985) using data from the American Cancer Society's 12-year follow-up study. Figure 7 shows the relative risk for lung cancer according to the number of days per week that fruit or fruit juice was consumed, with additional information on the regular use of vitamin supplements. The left half of the figure refers to all subjects while the analysis in the right half is restricted to current smokers of one pack or more per day. Lack of consumption of fruit or fruit juice was seen to be a powerful risk factor for lung cancer in both groups. To examine the interaction between fruit consumption and smoking, however, it was necessary to recompute the RRs in relation to a common reference group. Figure 8 shows the result of this recalculation. Heavy smokers who consumed little or no fruit or juice

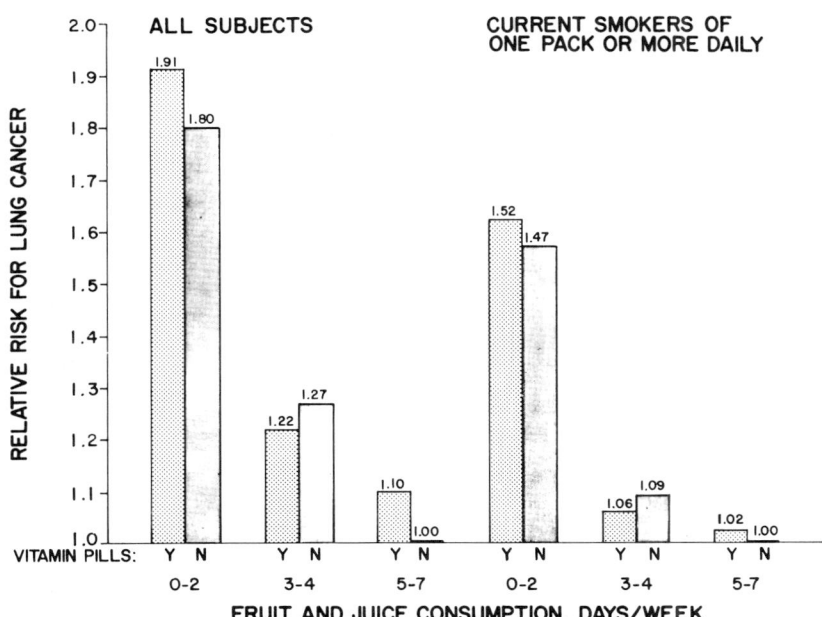

Figure 7
Relative risk for lung cancer among nearly 500,000 men surveyed by American Cancer Society and followed up 1960-1966, according to number of times per week subjects consumed fruits or fruit juices, and whether or not subjects took regular vitamin supplements. Data from Wang and Hammond (1985).

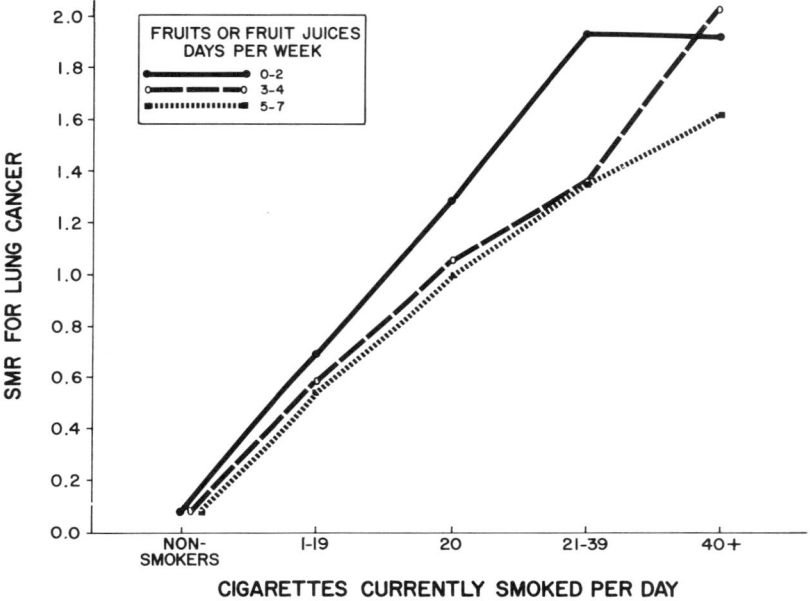

Figure 8
Standardized mortality ratio for lung cancer among the same subjects as in Figure 7, according to number of cigarettes smoked per day (current smokers only) and the number of times per week subjects consumed fruits or fruit juices. The reference group is men who smoked 20 cigarettes per day and who consumed fruits or juice 3-4 times per week.

had RRs higher than those of frequent consumers. The joint risk was slightly greater than either additive or multiplicative, which in fact were equal to each other because the relative risk in nonsmokers was independent of the second factor (fruit and juice consumption).

DISCUSSION

Table 7 compares the predictions from additive and multiplicative models in a number of the examples cited above. In four of the studies cited, including two of asbestos-exposed workers, the multiplicative model seemed to predict the effect of joint exposure. In one study (avoidance of green-yellow vegetables, females only), the additive model appeared best. In two studies, the observed RR lay in between the two models, and in two others the prediction far exceeded even the multiplicative model.

It is important not to take such findings too literally. This type of analysis is fairly new and is fraught with many methodological pitfalls. The most serious

Table 7
Additive Versus Multiplicative Models in Studies of Smoking, Other Exposures, and Cancer

Exposures		Outcome	Observed	Predicted A.M.	Predicted M.M.	References
Smoking	Other					
Ever smoked	Asbestos insulator	Lung cancer mortality	601.6	169.7	633.6	Hammond et al. (1979)
Smoked 2+ packs/day	Shipyard worker	Lung cancer RR	21.7	11.5	22.7	Blot and Fraumeni (1981)
Ever smoked	Underground miner	Lung cancer RR	40.6	11.9	40.7	Damber and Larsson (1985)
Daily smoker	Material metal worker	Cancer mortality	851.7	496.8	497.5	Hirayama (1981)
		Lung cancer mortality	142.1	127.3	258.2	Hirayama (1981)
		Stomach cancer mortality	400.3	244.3	264.9	Hirayama (1981)
Smoked 30+ cigarettes per day	Occupational exposure to likely carcinogens	Lung cancer RR	20.0	12.5	27.5	Pastorino et al. (1984)
Smoked 40+ cigarettes per day	Drank 10+ whisky equivalents/day	Oral cancer RR	104.7	30.2	185.6	Mashberg et al. (1981)
Daily smoker	Lack of green-yellow vegetables	Lung cancer mortality, male	79.5	84.1	147.8	Hirayama (1979)
		Lung cancer mortality, female	33.9	24.0	27.1	Hirayama (1979)
Smoked 40+ cigarettes	Fruit or juice 0–2 times/week	Lung cancer RR	24.0	20.3	20.3	American Cancer Society (unpubl.)

A.M., additive model; M.M., multiplicative model

problem is classification of exposure. Figure 9 shows the distribution of smoking and alcohol consumption in mouth cancer cases and controls reported by Wynder and Stellman (1977). These exposures are highly correlated so that while any large study can be expected to observe statistically useful numbers of nondrinking nonsmokers and heavy-drinking heavy smokers the number of heavy-drinking nonsmokers will invariably be very small (and subjects falling into that category by self-report possibly unreliable), making it difficult to estimate the parameter a in Table 1. Misclassification of just a few subjects can lead to a large bias in a, as well as in the predictions of the models. In such cases it is prudent to rely on qualitative examination of smoking- and second-factor specific rates or risks, as in the figures, and not put too much weight on models.

On the other hand, in such clear-cut cases as asbestos where there is no doubt as to the synergistic effect (Frank 1979), such information is of tremendous public health importance and is vital for establishing prevention strategies.

The most challenging task of all is to collect the needed data in the first place. Table 8 shows the number of epidemiologic studies of tobacco-related diseases that

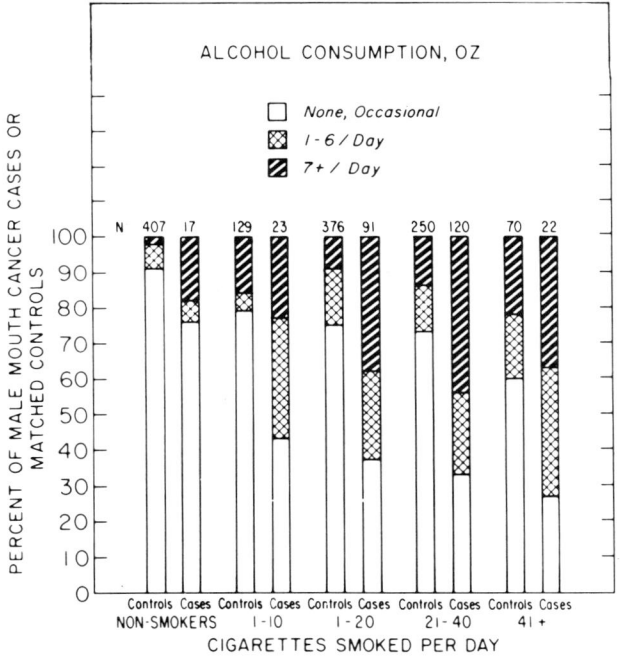

Figure 9
Correlation of alcohol and tobacco consumption among male mouth cancer cases and controls. Reprinted, with permission, from Wynder and Stellman (1977).

Table 8
Smoking Information in 32 Original Articles in Volume 26 of the *Journal of Occupational Medicine* (1984) on Epidemiology of Tobacco-related Diseases

Subject matter	Number of studies	Number with smoking data
Respiratory effects, including pulmonary function and radiographic testing	12	8
All cause SMR	5	0
Lung cancer	2	2
Coronary artery disease	1	1
Reproductive outcomes	3	1
Sleep	1	1
Reviews of studies which included tobacco-related outcomes	2	1
Surveillance and corporate medical programs	6	2
Total	32	16

were published in a recent volume (1984) of the *Journal of Occupational Medicine* according to whether or not smoking information was also collected. Smoking data was available in only 16 of 32 such articles. These omissions were not necessarily the fault of the authors since many studies were based upon historical sources in which no smoking data were present. Nevertheless, one obviously cannot study interactions between occupation and smoking data unless one has the smoking data first. Without such data, one cannot tell for certain to what extent smoking has influenced the results.

Similar remarks may be made concerning dietary studies. Figure 10 shows the distribution of smoking habits among men who scored high, medium, and low on scales which measured the frequency of consumption of foods high in vitamins A and C. Data were collected in 1982 by the American Cancer Society as part of a follow-up study of over 1.2 million men and women. Men who scored low on the vitamin scale were twice as likely to smoke cigarettes as men who scored high. It is clear that any analysis of lung cancer mortality (or any other outcome which is thought to be related to vitamin A or C intake) must simultaneously control for cigarette smoking.

REFERENCES

Blot, W.J. and J.F. Fraumeni. 1981. Cancer among shipyard workers. In *Banbury report 9: Quantification of occupational cancer* (ed. R. Peto and M. Schneiderman), p. 37. Cold Spring Harbor Laboratory, Cold Spring Harbor, New York.

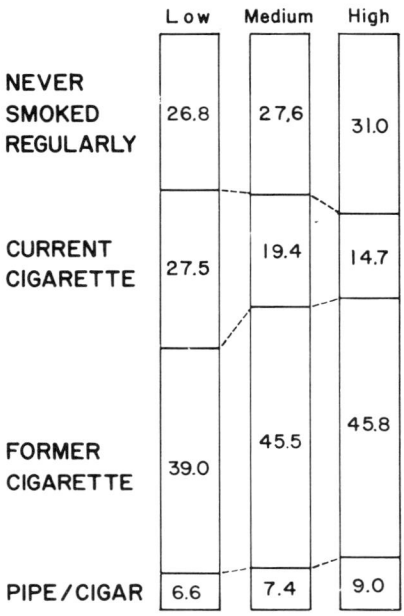

Figure 10
Distribution of smoking habits, adjusted for age among men surveyed in 1982 American Cancer Society follow-up study, according to whether they scored high, medium, or low on a scale which measures frequency of consumption of foods rich in vitamins A. and C.

Damber, L. and L.-G. Larsson. 1985. Underground mining, smoking, and lung cancer: A case-control study in the iron ore municipalities in Northern Sweden. *J. Natl. Cancer Inst.* **74**: 1207.

Edling, C. 1982. Lung cancer and smoking in a group of iron ore miners. *Am. J. Ind. Med.* **3**: 191.

Frank, A.L. 1979. Public health significance of smoking-asbestos interactions. *Ann. N.Y. Acad. Sci.* **330**: 791.

Hammond, E.C., I.J. Selikoff, and H. Seidman. 1979. Asbestos exposure, cigarette smoking and death rates. *Ann. N.Y. Acad. Sci.* **330**: 473.

Hirayama, T. 1979. Diet and cancer. *Nutr. Cancer* **1**: 67.

――――. 1981. Proportion of cancer attributable to occupation obtained from a census, population-based, large cohort study in Japan. In *Banbury report 9: Quantification of occupational cancer* (ed. R. Peto and M. Schneiderman), p. 631. Cold Spring Harbor Laboratory, Cold Spring Harbor, New York.

Mashberg, A., L. Garfinkel, and S. Harris. 1981. Alcohol as a primary risk factor in oral squamous carcinoma. *CA:A Cancer Journal for Clinicians* **31**: 146.

Olsen, J., S. Sabreo, and U. Fasting. 1985. Interaction of alcohol and tobacco as risk factors in cancer of the laryngeal region. *J. Epidemiol. Community Health* **39**: 165.

Pastorino, U., F. Berrino, A. Gervasio, V. Pesenti, E. Riboli, and P. Crosignani. 1984. Proportion of lung cancers due to occupational exposure. *Int. J. Cancer* **33**: 231.

Radford, E.P. and K.G. St Clair Renard. 1984. Lung cancer in Swedish iron miners exposed to low doses of radon daughters. *N. Engl. J. Med.* **310**: 1485.

Rothman, K.J. 1976. Causes. *Am. J. Epidemiol.* **104**: 587.

——. 1981. Occam's razor pares the choice among statistical models. *Am. J. Epidemiol.* **108**: 347.

Rothman, K.J., S. Greenland, and A.M. Walker. 1978. Concepts of interaction. *Am. J. Epidemiol.* **112**: 467.

Saracci, R. 1977. Asbestos and lung cancer: An analysis of the epidemiological evidence on the asbestos-smoking interaction. *Int. J. Cancer* **20**: 323.

——. 1980. Interaction and synergism. *Am. J. Epidemiol.* **112**: 465.

Selikoff, I.J. 1981. Constraints in estimating occupational contributions to current cancer mortality in the United States. In *Banbury report 9: Quantification of occupational cancer* (ed. R. Peto and M. Schneiderman), p. 3. Cold Spring Harbor Laboratory, Cold Spring Harbor, New York.

Stellman, S.D. and L. Garfinkel. 1984. Cancer mortality among woodworkers. *Am. J. Ind. Med.* **5**: 343.

——. 1986. Smoking habits and tar levels in a new American Cancer Society prospective study of 1,200,000 men and women. *J. Natl. Cancer Inst.* **76**: 1057.

U.S. Department of Health, Education, and Welfare. 1979. *Smoking and health: A report of the Surgeon General.* U.S. Department of Health, Education, and Welfare, Public Health Service, Office of the Assistant Secretary for Health, Office on Smoking and Health, DHEW Publication No. (PHS)-79-50066.

Walker, A.M. and K.J. Rothman. 1972. Models of varying parametric form in case-referent studies. *Am. J. Epidemiol.* **115**: 129.

Walter, S.D. and T.R. Holford. 1981. Additive, multiplicative, and other models for disease risks. *Am. J. Epidemiol.* **108**: 341.

Wang, L.-D. and E.C. Hammond. 1985. Lung cancer, fruit, green salad, and vitamin pills. *Chin. Med. J.* **98**: 206.

Wynder, E.L. and S.D. Stellman. 1977. Comparative epidemiology of tobacco-related cancers. *Cancer Res.* **37**: 4608.

——. 1979. Impact of long-term filter cigarette usage on lung and larynx cancer risk. A case-control study. *J. Natl. Cancer Inst.* **62**: 471.

COMMENTS

TANNENBAUM: Jeff Harris has published a paper showing different ways of analyzing the cigarette smoking data. I'm sure you're familiar with it. He showed that the cancers which appear at an earlier age as a result of risks, don't show up as dramatically when you use age standardization. When you just say what the relative risk is to cigarette smoking, you do not show that the deaths may also be occurring at an earlier age.

STELLMAN: That's right. That's a problem, caused by our practice of age standardization. When we do our initial runs we always analyze mortality by 5-year cohorts. But this generates stacks and stacks of paper, and we must have a way of summarizing the age-specific rates. Unless there are major obvious differences between the rates in different cohorts, we generally feel that combining them is a reasonable way of reducing the data; but obviously it can obscure data as well.

WINKELSTEIN: I think, generally speaking, that epidemiologists feel that environmental associations get weaker as age goes up. This is a sort of general rule. Probably the reason is that people get sick in more ways as they get older; so there are more factors at work. Some specific factors are likely to show a lower association.

TANNENBAUM: A paper was just published this year from Walter Willett, showing that even the consumption of green and yellow vegetables made a difference, even above age 65.

WINKELSTEIN: It may, but if you look at the Framingham data, for example, look at smoking in coronary disease, there's no association shown in people who entered the study after the age of 45—in the cohort study.

TANNENBAUM: You may be right. There may be some factors that may not make so much of a difference. For other factors it may make a difference. Actually, maybe that's part of the problem when you're dealing with two variables each of which may have an associated risk. I guess one of the problems is that your model assumes that dose and time are contemporaneous.

STELLMAN: For cohort studies like the ones that we do, that is usually true. But in case-control studies, that is not often true; and for most industrial cohort studies it is not true either.

TANNENBAUM: No, but when you showed your analysis of whether it was an arithmetic or a multiplicative model, there were several different exposure models which you could have used. I mean, where you have the two variables: A occurred before B; A occurring at the same time as B; A occurring after B.

STELLMAN: This is such an idealistic simplification of a terribly complex situation that it's almost embarrassing to present it that way.

TANNENBAUM: No, it's interesting. It's an interesting start. Let's take a specific case: wood workers and smoking. Is the number of years that they worked as wood workers overlapped with the number of years that they smoked?

STELLMAN: Yes.

CORREA: I think that the point that you are making is the sequence. If you have a promoter, it will show an effect only if it is present after an initiator and not if it is present before that factor.

STELLMAN: For most of the examples that I presented, these exposures were contemporaneous for many years. So it's not like a two-stage skin painting experiment. In the United States, people in the generation we studied started smoking around the age of 20, and they smoked the rest of their lives. They died around 60 and 70. So we have 40 years of smoking, and we have at least 30 years of the same occupation.

TANNENBAUM: So it is mostly that model, is what you're saying?

STELLMAN: That is correct.

HOFFMANN: Do you have data, or are there too few cases on nasal cancer in wood workers and their smoking habits?

STELLMAN: Yes, there are data, but too few cases to analyze. The expected number of nasal cancers was 0.03, and the observed number was 2. So, the relative risk was very large, but the confidence limits were very wide.

WINKELSTEIN: I think that the point that Steve [Stellman] made is a very important one. Epidemiologists must begin to look at the joint action of factors, rather than spending so much of their efforts on trying to separate out all of the actions.

Concluding Remarks

CURTIS C. HARRIS* AND DIETRICH HOFFMANN†
*Laboratory of Human Carcinogenesis
National Cancer Institute
Bethesda, Maryland 20892
†Naylor Dana Institute for Disease Prevention
American Health Foundation
Valhalla, New York 10595

Recent advances in biotechnology have provided us with the tools to answer long-standing and nagging questions in biomedical research. Tobacco carcinogenesis is one of the areas to which these new techniques and knowledge of the fundamental mechanisms of cell and molecular biology are being applied.

In the first session of the conference, Laboratory-Epidemiology Studies, which was chaired by Dietrich Hoffmann, the speakers discussed (1) the uptake by smokers of tobacco components; (2) the effects of tobacco smoking on endogenous formation of N-nitroso compounds, including carcinogenic N-nitrosamines; (3) the use of macromolecular adducts as indicators of biologically effective doses of tobacco smoke components; and (4) DNA adducts, micronuclei and urinary mutagens as indicators of the genotoxicity of tobacco smoke.

Nancy Haley discussed the uptake of tobacco smoke components. Cotinine, a major metabolite of nicotine, can be used as a sensitive and specific semiquantitative measure of both active and passive exposure to tobacco smoke. Haley also reviewed the data on this subject, including those showing that smokers, who use cigarettes with low nicotine yields compensate by smoking a greater number of cigarettes. Because the capacity to enzymatically metabolize nicotine to cotinine varies among individuals and because cotinine is only one of several metabolites, the quantitative assessment of tobacco smoke exposure depends on the development of methods to measure the complete spectrum of nicotine metabolites, including nicotine-N'-oxides and nicotine dioxides.

Polycyclic aromatic hydrocarbons (PAH) are one of the chemical classes of tobacco smoke components of which the carcinogenic properties have been extensively studied in laboratory animals. PAH, formed by incomplete combustion of tobacco and many other organic materials, also may be associated with increased risk of lung cancer in humans. George Becher described a high-pressure liquid chromatographic method for determining PAH and their metabolites in urine. Extracts from urine of tobacco smokers show significantly higher levels of PAH than do urine specimens from nonsmokers. Becher emphasized that environmental monitoring of PAH may exaggerate exposure levels if the bioavailability of PAH absorbed to airborne particles is not considered. For example, particles must be small enough to be inhaled, and the elution of PAH in the lung may vary depending on the type of carrier particle.

Three participants discussed the effects of tobacco smoking on the endogenous formation of *N*-nitroso compounds, including carcinogenic *N*-nitrosamines. Allan Conney reported substantial day-to-day and person-to-person differences in the urinary excretion of *N*-nitrosodimethylamine (NDMA), a carcinogen, and *N*-nitrosoproline (NPRO), which is not carcinogenic, in healthy volunteers who ate their usual diets. Urinary excretion of NDMA increased approximately 45-100% in individuals who smoked tobacco and consumed alcoholic beverages on a daily basis. Conney speculated that this increase may be related to the presence of substantial concentrations of NDMA and nitrosating gases in tobacco smoke, and he suggested that alcohol may inhibit the metabolism of NDMA. Interestingly, he also reported a correlation between atmospheric concentrations of NO_2 and urinary excretion of NDMA, but not of NPRO. Helmut Bartsch described the NPRO test he and his coworkers recently developed for assessing endogenous nitrosation. Endogenous synthesis of *N*-nitroso compounds occurs at a higher rate in tobacco smokers, chewers of tobacco and betel quid, and snuff dippers. Tobacco smokers may be exposed to milligram quantities of nitrogen oxides, which are nitrosating agents, and nicotine and other nitrosatable amines. The concentration of thiocyanate is increased to millimolar levels in tobacco smokers and its potent catalytic action may further enhance endogenous nitrosation. Aldehydes in tobacco smoke (e.g., formaldehyde and acetaldehyde) endogenously react with L-cysteine, followed by nitrosation to form *N*-nitrosothiazolidine-4-carboxylic acid and *N*-nitroso-2-methylthiazolidine-4-carboxylic acid. Dietary supplementation with ascorbic acid may reduce urinary excretion of these compounds. Like Conney, Bartsch found large interindividual variations in the urinary excretion of *N*-nitroso compounds. For unknown reasons, ascorbic acid may decrease, increase, or have no effect on endogenous nitrosation in different individuals using various tobacco products. This variation in response requires further study before a protective effect of ascorbic acid can be assumed. Gerhard Scherer presented the results of two preliminary experiments in which endogenous formation of NPRO increased in tobacco smokers in the first but not in the second experiment. He speculated that urinary nitrate levels may not have been sufficiently high to increase NPRO formation in the second study.

Preliminary investigations, discussed at the conference by Stephen Hecht and presented in this volume by Karam El-Bayoumy, indicate that cigarette smokers excrete aromatic amines such as aniline and o-toluidine in the urine, but further studies on dietary confounders and interpersonal variation of such data are needed.

Steve Tannenbaum described a promising approach for determining internal doses of the activated metabolites of chemical procarcinogens found in tobacco smoke. He is investigating hemoglobin adducts of tobacco-related aromatic amines. Because hemoglobin has a lifetime of about 120 days in humans and the adducts are not believed to be repaired, hemoglobin adducts represent the accumulated level of exposure. 4-Aminobiphenyl, a carcinogen in humans and one of the aromatic amines found in tobacco smoke, was selected for study. A range of 20-100 ng of 4-aminobiphenyl was found in tobacco smoke from one pack of cigarettes; on the basis of the hemoglobin adduct data, an intake of 15-35 ng per pack of cigarettes was estimated. Therefore, this approach may be useful as an internal dosimeter of exposure to certain carcinogens found in tobacco smoke.

In addition to hemoglobin adducts, the formation of adducts between reactive chemicals and DNA may be used as an internal indicator of tobacco smoke exposure. DNA is a macromolecular target that may be important in the carcinogenicity of tobacco smoke. Kurt Randerath described the results of a ^{32}P-postlabeling nucleotide chromatography assay developed in his laboratory. ^{32}P-Fingerprints of presumed DNA adducts induced in mouse skin by topical exposure to cigarette smoke condensate showed several adducts. Although the precise structures of the presumed DNA adducts are not known, it is likely that they are derivatives of aromatic or large unsaturated chemicals. The presumed adducts appear to be unrelated to those formed by the following aromatic chemicals found in tobacco smoke: benzo[a]pyrene, benz[a]anthracene, dibenz[a,h]anthracene, pyrene, chrysene, fluoranthene, benzo[g,h,i]perylene, 4-aminobiphenyl, 2-naphthylamine, and nicotine-derived tobacco-specific N-nitrosamines. ^{32}P-Fingerprints from placental and bronchial DNA revealed putative DNA adducts in tobacco smokers that were not found in DNA from nonsmokers.

Micronuclei are formed from chromosome and chromatid fragments caused by clastogenic events, including exposure to DNA-damaging carcinogens. Hans Stich and Miriam Rosin presented data indicating an elevated frequency of micronucleated cells in the oral cavities of tobacco chewers. Beta-carotene administration (180 mg/week) for 10 weeks reduced the frequency of micronucleated cells in the oral mucosa of snuff dippers. Pelayo Correa described the use of the micronucleus test to examine exfoliated epithelial cells from several tissue sites (i.e., bronchus, oral cavity, bladder, and uterine cervix) associated with tobacco smoke carcinogenesis. Increases in the frequencies of micronucleated cells were found in all four tissue types from tobacco smokers. Nonsmokers married to smokers did not have elevated levels of micronucleated cells, indicating that the micronucleus test is not sensitive enough to detect the genotoxic effects of passive smoking.

Edmond LaVoie presented data comparing the mutagenicity in a *Salmonella typhimurium* assay of urine from smokers and nonsmokers who ate either a typical western diet (high meat and fat content) or a vegan diet. Smokers' urine had higher levels of mutagenic activity. Surprisingly, the vegan diet was associated with higher levels of urinary mutagenicity than was the typical western diet. The effect of diet was sufficiently pronounced to confound uncontrolled studies comparing urinary mutagenicity in smokers and nonsmokers.

New aspects of tobacco carcinogenesis were the topic of Session 2, which was chaired by Peter Magee. Speakers discussed (1) the analysis of synthetic and natural additives to tobacco products, (2) perinatal metabolism of N-nitrosamines in laboratory animals, (3) carcinogens found in smokeless tobacco, and (4) molecular interactions between aldehydes found in tobacco smoke and macromolecules in the respiratory epithelium.

Clove-containing cigarettes have become increasingly popular in the United States, especially among adolescents, and have been associated with acute illnesses including hemoptysis, pulmonary edema, and bronchospasm. Marcus Wise described the chemical analysis of these cigarettes. By combining gas chromatography and mass spectrometry, the smoke was determined to be chemically similar to conventional tobacco smoke except that it also contained clove oil components (e.g., 15 mg of eugenol per cigarette). Other clove oil constituents detected were eugenol acetate, beta-caryophyllene, alpha-humulene, and caryophyllene epoxide. The toxicity, including carcinogenicity of these individual constituents has not yet been adequately tested.

The aroma of tobacco smoke is influenced by aging and various curing processes. Curt Enzell described the complex chemical reactions and products formed. Isoprenoids are the most important tobacco aroma constituents. Several hundred of these isoprenoids have been identified and they undergo singlet oxygen reactions, epoxidations, and rearrangements during the postharvest processes. The pathobiological effects of these and other odoriferous agents are unknown.

Maternal tobacco smoking may have toxic effects on the fetus, including growth retardation, spontaneous abortion, and neonatal death. Hans Tjälve discussed the transplacental disposition and metabolism in laboratory animals of N-nitrosamines found in tobacco and its smoke. Whole-body autoradiograms clearly showed the disposition in fetal tissues of the tobacco-specific N-nitrosamines, 4-(methylnitrosamino)-1-(3-pyridyl)-1-butanone (NNK) and N'-nitrosonornicotine, and another N-nitrosamine found in tobacco smoke, N-nitrosodiethylamine. The sites of N-nitrosodiethylamine disposition correlated with the tissue sites of tumor formation. The tobacco-specific N-nitrosamines have not as yet been tested for transplacental carcinogenicity.

The use of smokeless tobacco has been increasing. Klaus Brunnemann discussed the carcinogens found in this form of tobacco. Tobacco-specific, nicotine-derived N-nitrosamines are present in concentrations ranging from 8 ppb to 339,000 ppb in smokeless tobacco products and in tobacco and betel nut mixtures obtained from different countries. In addition, areca alkaloids in the betel nut can be nitrosated to form areca-specific N-nitrosamines, including methylnitrosaminopropionitrile, a potent carcinogen in laboratory animals. Low concentrations of benzo[a]pyrene and polonium-210 also have been found in smokeless tobacco products. Finally, musk ambrette, one of the synthetic additives introduced into some tobacco products, is mutagenic in *S. typhimurium*, a finding that once again points to our lack of information concerning the possible hazards of such tobacco additives.

Aldehydes, including formaldehyde, acetaldehyde, and acrolein, are present at high concentrations in tobacco smoke and may contribute to its carcinogenicity.

Formaldehyde and acetaldehyde each have been shown to cause respiratory tract cancer in experimental animals. Henry Heck described studies designed to elucidate the interactions between these aldehydes and cellular macromolecules found in the rat nasal mucosa. DNA-protein cross-links were formed by either formaldehyde or acetaldehyde exposure but were not detected in studies with acrolein. However, acrolein markedly depleted glutathione concentrations and increased the number of DNA-protein cross-links induced by formaldehyde. Therefore, the effects of interactions between various aldehydes and between aldehydes and other constituents of tobacco smoke will require further investigation.

Session 3, Biochemical, Cellular, and Molecular Studies on Human Tissues and Cells, was chaired by Allan Conney. The speakers discussed a variety of subjects, including metabolism of chemical carcinogens, DNA repair, formation of DNA adducts, and transformation of human epithelial cells in vitro.

Ismail Parsa described an in vitro model system of adult human pancreas carcinogenesis using N-nitroso compounds. The tobacco-specific N-nitrosamine, NNK, when administered twice a week at 20 μg/ml, was reported to cause in vitro transformation of pancreatic epithelial cells. The DNA adduct O^6-methylguanine was also detected by immunocytochemistry in some of the nuclei of the carcinogen-exposed cells.

Stephen Hecht also discussed tobacco-specific N-nitrosamines. NNK was found to be a more potent carcinogen in the rat than the more ubiquitous N-nitrosodimethylamine, even though the latter compound is a more efficient DNA methylating agent than is NNK. Hecht also described sensitive immunocytochemical methods for detecting DNA damage and hemoglobin adducts caused by N-nitrosamines.

Herman Autrup reviewed the metabolic pathways of carcinogenic polycylic aromatic hydrocarbons in cultured human tissues. Oral mucosa and lung and bladder epithelia all have the enzymes required to metabolically activate these carcinogens, which are found primarily in the particulate phase of tobacco smoke. Wide interindividual variations in formation of DNA adducts were found.

Roland Grafstrom presented the second paper concerning aldehydes. He discussed the effects on cultured human bronchial epithelial and fibroblastic cells of aldehydes found in tobacco smoke. Formaldehyde and acrolein each caused DNA damage and mutations and inhibited DNA repair processes. Grafstrom speculated that these aldehydes might have cocarcinogenic activities.

Anthony Pegg discussed the DNA repair enzyme, O^6-alkylguanine-DNA-alkyltransferase, and factors affecting its activity. This enzyme restores the structure of DNA in a single step. Rodents generally have five- to tenfold lower repair activity than do humans. In addition, intertissue and interindividual differences in repair activity have been found.

Curtis Harris described the transfection of oncogenes associated with human lung cancer into normal human bronchial epithelial cells in vitro. In this model system, the v-Ha-*ras* oncogene caused a cascade of events leading to the development of malignant cells that formed invasive and metastatic carcinomas when xenotransplanted into athymic nude mice.

Fred Beland discussed the metabolic activation of aromatic amines. He emphasized the role of specific enzymatic pathways, including oxidation by prostaglandin *H* synthase, *N*-oxidation, and acetylation, which are responsible for the metabolism of this group of chemicals. Urinary pH and genetic factors also influence the pharmacokinetics of aromatic amines.

Session 4, New Associations of Tobacco Use and Cancer, was chaired by Warren Winkelstein, who also discussed the association between tobacco smoking and carcinoma of the uterine cervix. This association has been found in 15 of 18 cohort and case-control studies. The relative risk in these studies has been as high as 12.7, and positive dose-response relationships have been found in some of them.

Pelayo Correa discussed the passive smoking-cancer issue. In his review, he concluded that the available evidence suggests a low-dose effect in the causation of respiratory tract cancers. The magnitude of this increase of lung cancer cannot be precisely defined. The possibly increased susceptibility of fetuses and children was also discussed.

The use of smokeless tobacco is considered to be an important risk factor for oral cancer. Deborah Winn described the possible influence of cofactors. In a study of North Carolina women, cases with oral and pharyngeal cancer were four times more likely than controls to have used oral snuff. Relative risks were similar for blacks and whites. Poor condition of gums and teeth enhanced the risk of oral cancer. However, neither a high intake of fruits and vegetables, nor tobacco smoking and consumption of alcoholic beverages, altered the magnitude of the relative risk between smokeless tobacco and oral-pharyngeal cancer.

In the final presentation of this session, Steven Stellman reviewed the data concerning interactions between smoking and other factors such as occupation and diet. He discussed the methodological difficulties associated with such studies. Emphasis was placed on analysis of synergistic interactive effects, for example, the effect of smoking coupled with occupational exposure to certain hazardous agents, such as asbestos. The difficulties frequently encountered in such studies include problems of classification and sample size, which Stellman illustrated by comparing the results of several studies in which the interactive effects of smoking and alcoholic beverage consumption were investigated. Finally, he pointed out that smoking data had not been collected in a large number of studies of tobacco-related diseases that were published in occupationally oriented journals.

It is hoped that the publication of the proceedings of this conference will stimulate new and collaborative research activities. We are convinced that the pursuit of such research activities will advance our understanding of tobacco carcinogenesis and this will hopefully hasten the day when we can ultimately prevent cancer diseases resulting from the widespread use of tobacco.

Name Index

Aagaard, J., 315, *323*
Aaronson, S.A., *312*
Aasen, A.J., 176
Abbots, J., *xii*, 95, 227
Abel, E.L., 13, *16*
Abernethy, D.J., 216, *225*
Adamkiewicz, J., *256*
Adams, J.B., *338*
Adams, J.D., *17, 18, 58, 133, 145, 192,*
    199, 204, *210, 211,* 233, *242, 371*
Adlkofer, F., **137-148**
Aeschbacher, H.U., 122, 126, *132*
Agrawal, H.P., *95*
Ahmad, R.A., *322*
Alexander, L.T., *211*
Alitalo, K., 106, *107*
Althoff, J., *193*
Altman, N.H., *323*
Ambrosius, D., *84*
Ames, B.N., 86, *94,* 121, 123, 131, *132, 134,* 332
Amin, A., *268*
Amstad, P., *282,* **299-314**
Anderson, I., 151, *159*
Andjelkovich, D.A., *226*
Angus, D., *132*
Anson, J.F., *323*
Appelman, L.M., 216, 224, *225, 228*
Archer, G., *310*
Archer, M.C., *30, 58, 145*
Arenholt, D., *267*
Aristizabal, N., *118*
Arjungi, K.N., 205, *209*
Arlauskas, A., *132*
Armitage, P., 302, *309*
Armstrong, R.N., *269*
Arndt, R., *177*
Aronow, W.S.A., 8, *16*
Ashby, J., *94,* 208, *209*
Ashoor, S.H., *133*
Ashton, H., 3, 4, *16*
Asire, A.J., *372*
Au, G.K.H., *354*
Auerbach, O., 8, *17*
Aune, T., *292*
Austin, D.J., *177,* 329, 330, 331, 333, *337, 338*
Autrup, H., *242,* **259-271,** 260, 261, 262, 263, 264, 265, 266, *266, 267, 268, 269,* 270, 271, *282, 310, 311,* 401
Avitts, T.A., **85-98,** *94,* 95
Axell, T., 369, *370*
Axelrad, C.M., *17, 18, 133*

Babiuk, C., 216, *226*
Baccetti, S., *133*
Baer-Weiss, V., *371*
Bailey, A., *355*
Baird, W.M., 266, *269*
Baker, R., 122
Balakrishnan, V., *371*
Bamborschke, S., 288, *292*
Barfold, N.M., *323*
Barham-Hall, D., *322*
Barrett, L.A., *242*
Barrie, M.D., *226*
Barrow, C.S., 216, *226*
Bartholomew, J.C., *269*
Bartley, J.C., *269*
Bartsch, H., 21, 29, *30,* **45-61,** 45, 46, 47, 48, 51, 54, *57,* 58, *59,* 60, 61, 71, 73, 97, 136, 137, 144, *145, 146,* 194, **197-213,** *210, 211,* 287, 288, *292,* 325, 398
Basu, D., *43*
Basrur, P.K., *226*
Battey, J., *310, 311*
Bawol, R., *353*
Beauchamp, R.O., Jr., 216, *226*
Becher, G., **33-44,** 34, 35, 36, 38, 39, 40, *42, 43,* 44, *397*
Beckett, M.A., 299, *311*
Bedell, M.A., *293, 294*
Bedenko, V., *268*
Beland, F.A., 72, 73, 74, 98, 135, 136, 212, 229, 256, **315-326,** *322, 323, 324,* 324, 325, *326,* 402
Belich, J.M., 233, *242*
Ben, T., *312*
Benestad, C., *42*
Benigno, B.E., *338*
Benowitz, N.L., 4, *16, 371*
Benton, B., *18, 193, 354*
Benyajati, C., 224, *226*
Berenson, G.S., *371*
Bereziat, J.-C., *59*
Berggren, M., *310,* 331, 333, *337*
Berrino, F., *393*
Bertness, V., *310*
Bhide, S.V., 46, *57, 58,* 205, *209,* 211, *212*
Bialer, M., 266, *267*
Billings, K.C., *293, 294*
Bird, R.P., 216, *226*
Bishop, J.M., *108*
Bjelke, E., *371*
Bjørseth, A., 34, 35, 36, *42*
Blakey, D.H., *107*

Blettner, M., *109*
Bloomfield, R.D., *242*
Blot, W.J., *60, 109, 212,* 364, *370,* 379, 389, *391*
Bock, F.G., xi, *xii,* 302, *309*
Bock, K.W., 316, *323*
Boger, E., *84*
Bogovski, P.A., 143, *145*
Bohm, B., *109*
Bohn, H., *354*
Bonds, D., *372*
Bonin, A., *132*
Bordelon, C.B., *95*
Boreham, J., *355*
Boreiko, C.J., 216, *225,* 227
Bos, R.P., 122, *132*
Botero, S., *118*
Boucheron, J.A., *294*
Bourgade, M.-C., *59*
Box, R.P., *134*
Boyd, M.R., 260, *267*
Boyland, E., 47, *57,* 209
Boyle, J.M., *256*
Boyle, P., *353*
Boyle, S., *30*
Brand, R., *338*
Brandon, T.A., *372*
Branton, P., *256*
Brasure, J., *337*
Brennand, J., *293*
Bresch, H., *193*
Bresnick, E., *267*
Bright, C.C., 6, *18*
Brinton, L.A., *337*
Brittebo, E.B., 190, *191,* 217, *226*
Brooks, B.J., *310, 311*
Bross, I.J., *109, 372*
Brown, D., 348, *353*
Brown, J.P., 131, *133*
Brown, K.D., 303, *309*
Bruce, W.R., *107,* 113, *118, 146*
Brugh, M., *267*
Brunnemann, K.D., *17, 18,* 29, *30,* 47, 51, 56, *58, 60,* 71, *109,* 118, *133,* 137, 143, 144, *145,* 146, *192,* **197-213**, 198, 199, *210, 211, 212,* 212, *371,* 400
Bryan, G.T., *324*
Bryant, M.S., **63-75,** *70, 256*
Bucci, T.J., *322*
Buck, C., 180, *193,* 343, 345, 348, *354*
Buck, R.D., 217, *227*
Buckley, J.D., *108,* 330, 331, 332, *337*
Buhler, D.R., *134*
Buiatti, E., *133*
Burgade, M.-C., *211*
Burton, H.R., 164, 166, *176*
Bush, L.P., *176*

Busser, R., *42, 337*
Bussman, C.J.M., *227*
Butt, K.M.H., *242*
Butterworth, B.E., *267*
Butts, W.C., 4, *16*
Byers, S.T., *337*

Caderni, G., *268*
Calmels, S., **45-61,** 56, *57*
Cao, E.-H., *294*
Carlini, E., 158, *160*
Carmella, S.G., **245-257**
Carney, D.N., *311*
Cartwright, R.A., *133,* 321, *322*
Casanova, M., **215-230,** *226*
Casanova-Schmitz, M., 217, 218, 219, 220, *226*
Case, R.A.M., 315, *322*
Cassale, V., *57*
Casto, B.C., 304, *309*
Castonguay, A., **179-195,** 181, 184, 186, 190, *191, 192,* 210, 233, *242, 255, 256,* 349, *353,* 369, *370*
Caton, J.E., *133*
Cederlof, R., 329, 331, *337*
Cefalo, R.C., *94*
Chadha, M.S., *209*
Chadjaeva, M.C., *109*
Chamrakulov, F.S., *109*
Chan, C.L., *354*
Chang, J.C.F., *226, 256*
Chang, S.K., 53, *58*
Chappuis, C., 122, 126, *132*
Charlet, J., *338*
Chart, I.S., *323*
Chatterjee, K., *109*
Cheeke, P.R., *134*
Chen, C.B., *226*
Chortyk, O.T., 83, *83*
Christen, A.G., 369, *370*
Christensen, B., *267*
Chu, F.S., *133*
Chu, K.C., *84*
Chung, F.-L., *192,* 242
Churg, J., *311*
Clarke, E.A., 330, 331, *337*
Clatterbuck, B.E., *294*
Clayson, D.B., *70*
Cleary, C.M., **233-244**
Coates, C., *17*
Cohen, B., *210*
Colburn, N., *312*
Cole, P., 315, *323*
Coleman, D.T., *134*
Colledge, A., 166, *176*
Connor, T.H., 77, *83*
Conney, A.H., 19, **21-32,** *30,* 31, 32, **44,**

[Conney, A.H.]
  72, 96, 195, 243, 257, 262, *267*,
  270, 284, 297, 340, 359, 398, 401
Connolly, G.N., 367, *370*
Connor, R.J., *242*
Connor, T.H., 126, *133*, 216, *226*
Conrad, M., *192*
Cooper, D.P., *293*
Coria, C.F., *338*
Correa, P., 8, *16*, 72, **113-119**, 119, 161, 325, 326, 339, 340, **343-360**, 344, 346, *353*, 356, 358, 359, 395, 399, 402
Corsico, C.D., *292*
Cotgreave, I.C., 275, *282*
Cowell, R.H., *337*
Cox, P., *371*
Craddock, V.M., 288, *292*
Crespi, M., *57*
Croisy, A., *58*, *210*
Crosignani, P., *393*
Cuello, C., *118*
Curren, R.D., *282*
Curtis, J.R., *109*
Curvall, M., *177*

DaCosta, J., *354*
Dahl, A.R., 217, *226*
Dahl, K., *30*
Damber, L., 380, 382, 389, *392*
Daniel, F.B., *269*
Dannan, G.A., *322*
Darroudi, F., *227*
Dauer, A.D., *160*
David, R.M., *226*
Davis, B.B., *324*
Davis, H.J., *338*
Davis, L.J., *309*
Day, R.S., 289, *292*, *294*
De Bruin, A., *354*
DeGaudemaris, R., *17*
Deichmann, W.B., *323*
Deilhaug, T., 288, *292*
DeLarco, J.E., *311*
DeMarini, D.M., 303, *309*
Demole, C., 170, *176*
Demole, E., 166, 170, *176*
Demple, B., 287, *292*
Derg, N.E., *354*
Descotes, G., *59*, *146*
De Serres, F.J., 86, *94*
Deshpande, V.A., 205, *210*
de Smet, P.A.G.M., 100, *107*
Deutsch, J., *43*
Devereux, T.R., 266, *267*
Dicker, P., *309*
Dietrich, P.S., 131, *133*

Diliberto, J.J., *267*
Di Paolo, J.A., 304, *309*
Djurić, Z., 320, *322*
Dolan, M.E., 289, 291, *292*, *293*, *294*
Dolara, P., 132, *133*, *268*
Doll, R., 33, 34, 41, *42*, *108*, 302, *309*, *337*, *338*, 352, *353*
Domoradzki, J., 289, *292*
Donahue, J., **77-84**
Donaldsen, B., 139, *146*
Donofrio, D.J., *227*
Dooley, K.L., 316, *322*, *323*
Doolittle, D.J., *267*
Doran, J.E., *370*
Downie, N.M., 223, *226*
Draper, H.H., *226*
Druckrey, H., 45, *58*
D'Souza, A.V., *211*
Duncan, A.M.V., *107*
Dünger, M., *84*
Dunn, B.P., *59*, *109*
Dunn, C.Y., *312*
Duque, E., 117, *118*
Dyroff, M.-C., *293*, *294*

Eadie, J.S., 190, *192*
Eastman, A., 266, *267*
Edling, C., 381, *392*
Eggset, G., *293*
Ehrenberg, L., *70*
Einbrodt, H.J., 41, *43*
Eisenstadt, E., *133*
Ekert, B., *269*
El-Bayoumy, K., **77-84**, *83*, 398
El-Gerzawi, S., *108*
Emminger, A., *193*
Emura, M., *192*
Eng, V.W.S., *109*
Enggist, P., 166, *176*
Enoch, H.G., *133*
Enzell, C.R., 73, 74, **163-178**, 163, 164, 166, 169, 170, 171, 172, *176*, *177*, 177, 178, 374, 375, 400
Epstein, S.S., *30*
Erickson, L.C., 289, 290, *294*
Ericson, L.C., *282*
Ernster, V.L., *95*, *227*, *338*
Essigmann, J.M., *293*
Esterbauer, H., *282*
Esteve, J., *60*
Etzel, R.A., 4, 13, *17*
Evans, A.E.J., 77, *84*
Evans, D., *310*
Everett, D.W., *84*
Everson, R.B., **85-98**, 92, 93, 94, *94*, 180, *192*, *269*, *354*
Ewig, L.C., *282*

Falck, H.L., *42*
Falk, H.L., *337*
Farber, E., 85, *94*, 225, *226*
Farishian, R.A., 190, *192*
Fasting, U., *393*
Feldman, R.M., *109*, *372*
Fergusson, D.M., 13, *17*
Feron, V.J., 216, 224, *225*, *226*, *228*
Fett, D., *146*
Feyerabend, C., *18*
Fiala, E.S., *83*, *84*
Fifer, E.K., *322*
Fischer, S.M., *269*
Fisenne, I., *210*
Fisher, T., 144, *146*
Flammang, T.J., 320, 321, *322*
Flander, L., *118*
Fleurdelys, B., *309*
Fogh, J., *311*
Foiles, P.G., 21, 205, *210*, 233, *242*, **245-257**, 247, *255*
Folsom, A.R., 6, *17*
Fontham, E., *16*, **113-119**, *353*
Fonts, E.A., 369, *370*
Foote, R.S., 288, *293*, *294*
Forichon, J., *57*
Fornace, A.J., Jr., *282*
Fouts, J.R., *267*
Fowler, K.W., *293*
Foye, C.A., **233-244**, *242*
Fraenkel-Conrat, H., *227*
Frank, A., *242*, *268*, 390, *392*
Fraumeni, J.F., Jr., *58*, *60*, *109*, *212*, *370*, *371*, 379, 389, *391*
Frazelle, J.H., *225*
Fredeick, C.B., *323*
Freisen, M., **45-61**, *58*, *59*, *145*, *210*, *211*
Friberg, I., *337*
Friedman, G.D., 351, *353*
Friend, N., *118*
Fujiki, H., *309*
Fujimori, T., *176*
Furlong, J.W., *267*
Furth, M.E., 306, *309*
Furuya, K., *242*

Gabrielson, E.W., *282*, *312*
Gaffney, B.L., 291, *293*
Gangolli, S.D., *193*
Gardner, J.W., *118*, *337*
Garfinkel, L., 8, *17*, 345, 346, 348, *353*, 380, 381, 382, *393*
Garland, W.A., **21-32**, 21, 22, *30*
Garner, J.B., *353*
Garner, R.C., 65, *70*, 122, *133*
Garren, L., *59*
Garro, A.J., *133*

Gart, J., 362, *370*
Garven, L., *211*
Gazdar, A.F., *310*, *311*
Gelbart, S.M., 122, *133*
Gelboin, H.V., *43*, 94, *95*, *242*
Genoble, L., *210*
Genta, V., *268*
George, D., *108*
German, J., 101, 107, *108*
Gervasio, A., *393*
Gibson, J.E., *227*
Giercksky, K.-E., *293*
Gillies, P.A., 4, *17*
Gillis, C.R., 345, 348, *353*
Gillum, R., *17*
Gilman, A.G., 308, *309*
Gjika, H.B., *18*, *133*
Glashan, R.W., *322*
Glowinski, I.B., 65, *70*
Goldberg, M.T., 106, *107*
Goldberg, T., *118*
Goldfarb, M., *311*
Goldmacher, V.S., 216, *226*
Goldsmith, R., 131, *134*, 315, *324*
Goodman, M.T., 347, *355*
Gore, C.W., *323*
Gori, G.B., xi, *xii*
Gorsky, M., *371*
Gothoskar, S.V., 205, *209*, *211*
Gounot, A.-M., *57*
Grace, M., *324*, *338*
Grafström, R.C., 229, 230, *242*, *267*, 271, **273-285**, 276, 277, 278, 279, 280, 282, *282*, 283, 284, 285, 288, *293*, *310*, 313, 339, *401*
Graham, F.L., 306, *309*
Graham, S., *337*
Gralla, E.J., *227*
Grasso, P., 83, *83*, *256*
Gray, R., *256*
Green, C.L., 291, *293*
Green, H., 299, *309*
Green, L.C., 66, *70*, 252, *256*
Greenberg, E.R., 331, 333, 334, *337*
Greenberg, R.A., 4, *17*, 349, *353*
Greenland, S., *393*
Greenlaw, S., *393*
Greenlaw, R.H., *370*
Greer, R.O., 369, *370*
Gridley, G., *109*, *372*
Griest, W., *159*
Grimmer, G., 33, *42*
Gritz, E.R., 367, *371*
Gross, E.A., *227*, *228*
Grover, P.L., *268*
Grunberger, D., 254, *256*
Grygiel, J.J., *267*
Guengerich, F.P., 381, *322*

Guenther, E., 152, *159*
Guerin, M.R., **151-162**, 153, *159*
Gupta, R.C., 85, 86, 87, 88, *94, 95*
Guynn, R.W., 219, *227*

Hackett, P., *160*
Haddow, J., *355*
Hadley, W.M., 217, *226*
Haenszel, W., *353*, 362, *371*
Haenzel, W., *16, 118*
Haglund, R.E., *95*
Hague, B.F., Jr., *190*
Haley, N.J., **3-19**, 3, 4, 6, *17, 18*, 18, 19, 73, 98, *118*, 124, *133, 145*, 161, 195, *211*, 270, *338*, 341, 351, *353*, 357, 358, 359, 397
Hall, B.K., 368, *371*
Hallstrom, I., *70*
Hamada, H., *18*
Hamilton, J.L., *176*
Hammond, E.C., *311*, 346, *353*, 380, 387, 389, *392, 393*
Hammons, G.J., 316, 317, *322*
Hannan, M.A., *133*
Harley, N.H., 206, *210*
Harrington, G.W., *58*
Harris, C.C., xi-xii, 18, 19, 31, *42*, 44, 74, 75, 161, 213, 230, 241, *242*, 257, 260, 261, 262, 263, 264, 265, *267, 268, 269*, **273-285**, 274, 279, *282, 283, 293*, 295, **299-314**, 299, *309, 310, 311, 312*, 312, 313, 314, 324, 373, **397-402**, 401
Harris, R.W.C., 330, 331, *337*
Harris, S., *393*
Hartige, P., *58*, 131, *133*
Harvey, R.G., 35, *42*
Hatch, G., *269*
Haugen, A., 34, *42, 268, 282, 292*, 304, *309, 310*
Hautefeuille, A.A., *211*
Hauwert, P.C.M., *134*
Hawkins, J.M., *372*
Hawthorne, V., *353*
Hearn, W.L., *146*
Heath, R.W., 223, *226*
Hebertson, R.M., *118, 337*
Hecht, S.S., *17*, 21, 29, *30, 42*, 46, 55, 56, *58*, 60, 61, **77-84**, 78, *83*, 88, *95*, 147, 161, 177, **179-195**, 190, *191, 192*, 205, *210*, 216, *226*, 229, 233, *242*, 243, **245-257**, 245, 246, 247, 251, 254, 255, *256*, 256, 257, 260, *268, 269*, 284, 285, 287, *293, 309*, 324, 349, *353, 354*, 367, *370, 371*, 398, 401
Heck, H. d'A., **215-230**, 218, *226*, 227,
[Heck, H. d'A.]
228, 228, 229, 230, 284, 285, 401
Heddle, J.A., 106, *107*
Hein, D.W., 320, *324*
Hellberg, D., *118*
Heller, W.D., 343, *353*
Hemminki, K., 85, *95*
Henderson, A.R., 288, *292*
Henderson, B.E., *18, 193, 355*
Henderson, B.I., *354*
Henderson, G., *160*
Henderson, P.Th., *132, 134*
Henningfield, J.E., *370*
Hennings, H., *312*
Herbosa, E.G., *211*
Herz, W., 172, *177*
Heuch, I., 369, *371*
Higgins, C., 153, *159*
Higgins, E., *322*
Hilfrisch, J., *192*
Hill, G.B., 331, 333, *338*
Hill, P., 3, 4, *17*
Hirata, Y., *18*
Hirayama, T., 8, *17, 59*, 329, 331, *337*, 343, 345, 346, 348, 351, *353*, 381, 383, 386, 387, 382, *392*
Hirs, A., 151, *159*
Hirsch, J.M., 204, 205, *210*
Ho, J.H.C., *18*, 346, *354*
Hodgson, R.M., 260, *268, 269*
Hoffman, N.D., *338*
Hoffmann, D., xi-xii, **3-19**, 3, 6, 8, *17, 18*, 21, 29, *30*, 31, 32, 41, *42*, 43, 45, 46, 47, 51, 55, 56, *58, 60*, 60, 64, 65, 70, *70*, 71, 72, 74, 75, **77-84**, 77, 82, 83, *83, 84*, 88, *95*, 109, 110, *118*, **121-136**, 125, *133, 134*, 137, 143, 144, *145*, 146, 147, 148, 153, 158, *160*, 160, 162, 178, 180, 181, *192*, 194, **197-213**, 198, 199, 204, 205, 206, *210, 211, 212*, 212, 213, *226*, **233-244**, 233, *242*, 244, **245-257**, 245, 246, 255, *256*, 259, *268, 269*, 270, 274, 279, *283*, 287, *293*, 302, *309, 311*, 315, *323*, 341, 349, 351, *353, 354*, 357, 358, 367, *371*, 374, 375, 395, **397-402**, 397
Hoffmann, I., *323*
Hole, D.J., *353*
Holford, T.R., 378, *393*
Hollis, G.F., *310*
Holly, E., 117, *118*
Holmstrup, P., *370*
Holowaschenko, H., *30*
Homburger, F., *84*
Honda, M., *133*
Hoover, R.N., *58, 109, 133*, 315, *323, 371, 372*

Hopkins, R., 3, *18*
Horm, J.W., 329, 330, 331, 332, *338*, 367, 372
Hornby, A.P., *109*
Horowitz, A.D., 303, *309*
Horwood, L.T., *17*
Hosker, M.E., *322*
Hosomi, J., *268*
Howard, P.C., *322*
Howard, P.H., *43*
Hrubec, Z., *337*
Hsu, I.-C., 265, *268*, 269
Hubert, P., *84*
Huh, N., *256*
Hultberg, S., *372*
Hunter, S.M., 367, *371*

Ide, F., 265, *268*
Iitaka, Y., *134*
Iqbal, Z.M., 29, *30*
Irvin, T.R., *95*
Isaac, P.F., 4, *18*
Ishikawa, T., *268*
Ishmael, J., *323*
Issenberg, P., *30*
Ittah, Y., 260, *268*
Iwaoka, W.T., 131, *133*

Jackson, A.S., *372*
Jackson, F., *242*
Jacob, P., *16*
Jacobs, D., *17*
Jacobsen, B.K., *371*
Jacobsson, F., *372*
Jacobsson, M., *292*
Jaffe, R.L., 122, *133*
Jartung, G.H., *372*
Jarvik, M.E., *371*
Jarvis, M., 12, *18*, 144, *145*
Jayant, K., 362, 368, *371*
Jeffrey, A.M., 262, *267*, *268*, *309*
Jeger, O., *176*
Jenkins, R., *160*
Jennette, K.W., *268*
Jensen, O.M., *60*
Johansson, S.L., *210*
Johnson, K.K., *338*
Johnson, L.C., 351, *354*
Johnson, W.H., *177*
Jones, R.A., *293*
Jones, R.T., *16*, *242*
Joubert, L., *17*
Junker, N., *177*
Jurd, L., 131, *133*
Jussawalla, D., 205, *210*, *371*

Kabat, G.C., 8, *18*, 344, 347, 351, *354*
Kadlubar, F.F., **315-326**, 316, 317, 318, 319, 320, 321, *322*, *323*, *324*
Kahn, M.A., *322*
Kalandidi, A., *354*
Kalinowski, A.E., *323*
Kaminsky, L.S., *322*
Kanapilli, G.M., *43*
Kaneko, M., *282*, *310*
Kann, J.M., *145*
Kantor, A.F., 55, *58*, *133*
Karlsson, K., *177*
Karran, P., 289, 290, *293*
Kasperbauer, M.J., 164, *176*
Kato, K., *176*
Kaufman, D.G., *242*, 260, *268*
Kawachi, T., *133*, *134*
Kawamura, H., 229, 308, *310*
Keith, C.H., *227*
Keller, A.Z., 362, *371*
Kelly, R.E., *70*
Kelsey, W., *312*
Kenward, B., *338*
Kerley, S.A., *160*
Kerns, W.D., 216, *227*
Kidd, J.G., 335, *338*
Kieler, J., *267*
Kiese, M., 65, *70*
Kinesbury, E.W., *269*
King, M.-C., *338*
Kirkman, H., 88, *95*
Kirsch, I.R., *310*
Kirstein, U., *256*, *294*
Kitano, N., *18*
Kleihues, P., *292*, *294*
Klein, E., 106, *108*
Klein, G., 106, *108*
Kligerman, A.D., *226*
Knight, G., *355*
Knoth, A., 344, 347, *354*
Kodama, H., 166, *176*
Kodama, M., *282*, *310*
Koeman, J.H., *134*
Kohn, K.W., 276, *282*
Koivula, T., *227*
Koivusalo, M., 217, 218, *227*, *228*
Konieczny, M., 35, *42*
Koo, L.C., 8, *18*, 344, 346, 347, 351, 352, *354*
Korba, B.E., *282*, *311*, *312*
Kornychuk, H., **21-32**
Kostenbauder, H.B., *267*
Kasuge, T., *134*
Kotin, E., 332, *337*
Kotin, P., 34, *42*
Kozam, G., 158, *159*
Kramer, I.R.H., *370*

Name Index

Kraus, F.T., 369, *371*
Kreyberg, L., 329, *337*
Kristmundsdotir, F., *17*
Krokan, H., 275, *282*, 292
Krone, C.A., 131, *133*
Krumperman, P.H., *134*
Kruysse, A., *226*
Kuehneman, M., *16*
Kuenzig, W., **21-32**
Kuroki, T., 260, *268*
Kusmierek, J.T., 287, *294*
Kuvshinov, J.P., *109*
Kvale, G., *371*

LaBaume, L.B., 219, *227*
Ladd, K.F., 29, *30*, 47, *58*, 137, 143, 144, *145*
Lagerwey, W.J., *134*
Lake, B.G., *193*
Lam, C.-W., **215-230**, 218, 219, 221, 223, 224, *226*, 227
Lama, C., *311*
Lambert, R., *57*
Land, H., 305, *310*
Land, P.D., *146*
Landy, J.J., 367, *371*
Langenbach, R., 265, *268*
Langley, D., *133*
Langone, J., 4, *18*, 124, *133*
Larsson, B., 190, *192*
Larsson, L.-G., 380, 382, 389, *392*
Laszlo, J., *xii*, 95, 227
Lau, W.H., *354*
Laval, F., 288, *293*
Laval, J., 288, *293*
LaVeck, M., *282*, 300, *310*
LaVoie, E., **121-136**, *134*, 134, 135, 136, 147, 161, 162, 260, *268*, *269*, 399
Law, C.H., *354*
Layde, P., *338*
Lechner, J.F., 260, 262, *268*, 273, 275, 276, *282*, *283*, **299-314**, 299, 300, 304, 306, 308, *309*, *310*, *311*
Lee, M.-S., *323*
Lee, N., *18*, *354*
Lee, P.N., 349, *354*
Lee, R.E., *118*, *338*
Leeman, L., *311*
Lefkowitz, M., *243*
Legator, M.S., *83*, *133*
Leijdekkers, Ch.-M., *134*
Lentz, J.C., *242*
Lesch, C., *371*
Letzel, H., 351, *354*
Leuchtenberger, C., 303, *310*
Leuchtenberger, R., *310*

Levin, L.I., 330, *338*
Levin, W., *268*, *269*
Levine, R.J., *227*
Lewis, J.D., 190, *192*
Lichti, U., *312*
Liehr, J.G., 88, *95*
Lijinsky, W., 206, *210*
Lilienblum, W., 316, *323*
Lin, Y., *16*, **113-119**, *256*, *353*
Lindahl, T., 287, *292*, *293*
Lindamood, C., 288, *293*
Lindsay-Smith, V., *133*
Lloyd, A.G., *193*
Lloyd, J.W., *372*
Loda, F.A., *17*
Lodovici, M., 265, *268*
Loeb, L.A., xi, *xii*, 88, 216, *227*
Loechler, E.L., *293*
Löfberg, B., **179-195**, 187, 189, *192*
Lombardo, C., *134*
Longnecker, D.S., *243*
Lorich, U., *337*
Lower, G.M., Jr., *324*
Lowrey, A.H., 349, *354*
Lozada, F., *37*
Lu, S.H., 51, *58*, *256*
Lubin, J.H., 366, *371*
Luepker, R., *17*
Lundin, F.E., Jr., 299, *310*, *338*
Lyon, J.L., 117, *118*, 330, 331, *337*

Maach, C.A., *338*
Mabrouk, A.F., 83, *84*
McBride, O.W., *310*
McCann, J., *132*
McCarthy, T., 287, *293*
McClendon, I.A., *310*
McCormick, J.J., *292*
McCullough, B., *133*
McDaniel, R.K., *370*
McDonald, D.B., *322*
McDowell, E., *242*
MacGregor, J.T., 131, *133*
McGuirt, W.F., *371*
McKay, F.W., *371*
McKenna, M.J., 216, *227*
McKinney, D.C., *372*
McLennan, R., 346, *354*
Maclure, M., **63-75**
McMahon, B., *354*
McNulty, M.J., *226*
McPherson, K., *337*, *338*
Maercklein, P.B., 300, 308, *311*
Magee, P.N., 60, 72, 97, 146, 147, 162, 180, *192*, 194, 228, 243, 257, 296, 313, 399

Maher, V.M., *292*
Mahon, G.A.T., *59*
Malan-Shibley, L., *312*
Malaveille, C., **45-61**, *210*, *211*
Maly, E., 41, *43*
Mantel, N., *324*, 362, *371*
Mao, Y., *324*, *338*
Margison, G.P., 287, *292*, *293*
Marky, L.A., *293*
Marquardt, H., 4, *17*
Marsh, W.H., *242*
Marshall, J.R., 331, 333, *337*
Marshall, M.V., 126, *133*
Martin, C.N., *70*
Martin, J., *228*
Martin, M.V., *322*
Martin, P.M.D., 331, 333, *338*
Martinez, D., 41, *43*
Maru, G.B., *292*
Masada, Y., 152, *159*, 315, *323*
Mashberg, A., 384, 385, 389, *393*
Mason, T.J., 361, *371*
Mass, M.J., 260, *268*
Masui, T., **299-314**, 300, 306, 308, *310*
Matiakin, E.G., *109*
Matney, T.S., *226*
Matsukura, S., 12, *18*
Mattern, M.R., 292, *294*
Mauritz, B.J., *354*
Maxwell, J.C., 198, *210*
Mazzoli, S., *133*
Meeuwissen, C.A.J.M., *134*
Melick, W.F., 64, *70*
Melikian, A.A., 260, *269*
Menon, M.M., *211*
Merabishvili, V.M., *108*
Mergens, W.J., *30*
Meyer, S.A., *294*
Michels, S., 41, *43*
Michelson, J., *59*
Milievskaya, I.L., *108*
Millar, R.R., *372*
Miller, D.W., *324*
Miller, E.C., 85, *95*, 260, *269*, *323*
Miller, G.H., 343, 344, *354*
Miller, J.A., 85, *95*, *323*
Miller, R.H., **85-98**
Milmore, B.K., *372*
Minaire, Y., *57*
Minchin, R.F., *267*
Minna, J.D., *310*, *311*
Minski, M.J., *193*
Mirvish, S.S., 29, *30*
Mitchum, R.K., *323*
Mitelman, F., 100, *108*
Mitra, S., 288, *293*, *294*
Mizuno, T., *310*

Mohammad, A., 218, *227*
Mohr, U., 180, 181, 187, 191, *192*, *193*
Moldeus, P., *282*, 303, *310*
Mommsen, S., 315, 320, 321, *323*
Montesano, R., 21, 29, *30*, 45, *57*, *192*, 256, 287, 288, *292*
Mookherjee, B.D., *177*
Moolgavkar, S.H., 315, *323*
Moore, R.E., *309*
Morgan, D.L., 279, *283*, 299, 308, *311*
Morgan, K.T., 225, *226*, *227*, *228*
Morgan, R.W., *337*
Morimoto, K., 290, *292*, *293*
Moser, C.E., Jr., *283*, *311*
Moss, R.A., 6, *18*
Mossman, B.T., *267*
Mould, A.J., *133*
Muir, C.S., *108*
Mulder, G.J., *323*
Muller, B., *176*
Munakata, K., *268*
Muñoz, N., *57*
Murray, T., *372*
Myers, G., *269*
Myrden, J.A., 369, *371*
Myrnes, B., *292*, *293*

Nagao, M., 131, *133*
Nagarajrao, D., *57*
Nagata, C., *282*, *310*
Naguib, S.M., 329, 330, 331, *338*
Nair, J., **45-61**, 49, 52, 53, 54, *57*, *58*, *59*, **197-213**, 198, 206, 207, 208, *210*, *211*
Nakajima, H., *18*
Nakano, H., 300, 305, *310*
Nakayama, A., *58*
Nakayama, J., 260, *269*
Nakayama, T., 276, *282*, 303, *310*
Napalkov, N.E., 352, *354*
Napalkov, N.P., 102, *108*
Naryka, J.J., *70*
Natarajan, A.T., 224, *227*
Nath, J., *134*
Nau, M.M., 305, *310*, *311*
Nehls, P., 247, *256*
Nesnow, S., 265, *268*
Neurath, G.B., 82, *84*
Neutel, C.I., 180, *193*, 343, 345, 348, *354*
Neville, C., *310*
Newan, M.J., *42*
Newman, A.M., *337*
Newmark, H.L., *30*, *58*, *107*, *109*, *118*, *145*
Newsome, J.R., *227*
Ng, Y.K., *354*
Nicholson, W.J., *133*

Nilsson, S., *118, 338*
Nishida, T., *177*
Nordfors, K., *177*
Norkus, E.P., **21-32**, *29*
Norman, V., *227*
Norstrand, K., *293*
Numoto, S., *371*

Obe, G., 216, *227*
O'Connor, P.J., *292*
Ohloff, G., 173, *176*
Ohmori, T., *226*
Okamoto, T., *134*
Okin, E., *309*
Olcott, H.S., *227*
Olsen, J., 384, 386, *393*
Olsson, P., *292*
Omenn, G.S., 94, *95*
Ong, T.M., *134*
Ohshima, H., **45-61**, 45, 46, 47, 48, 49, 50, 51, 54, 54, *57, 58, 59*, 137, 144, *145*, **197-213**, 198, *210, 211*
Onderdonk, J., *324*
O'Neill, I.K., *59, 211*
Ory, H., *338*
Osterman-Golkar, S., 64, *70*
Ozanne, C., *311*

Paches, A.I., 102, *108*
Paganuzzi, M., *134*
Pal, K., *268*
Palladino, G., 4, 6, *18*, 199, 204, *211*
Palmiri, C., *146*
Panigrahi, G.B., 208, *211*
Papageorge, A.G., *311*
Parada, L.F., *310*
Parida, B.B., *109*
Pariza, M.W., 131, *133*
Park, N.H., 205, *211*
Parke, D.V., 82, *84*
Parker, K., *18*
Parkes, H.G., 77, *84*
Parkin, D.M., *108*
Parorie, W.D., *211*
Parsa, I., 194, 195, **233-244**, 233, 234, 240, 241, *242, 243*, 243, 244, 401
Parshikova, S.M., *109*
Pastorino, U., 381, 383, 389, *393*
Patrianakos, C., 64, 65, 70, *70*, 77, 82, *84*, 315, *323*
Patterson, D.L., *227*
Patterson, E., *312*
Pavkov, K.L., *227*
Pearson, J.T., *322*
Pechacek, T., *17*

Pegg, A.E., 73, 74, 97, 98, 228, 243, 244, 254, *256*, 282, 283, 284, **287-297**, 287, 288, 289, 290, 291, *292, 293, 294*, 295, 296, 297, 312, 313
Pein, F.G., *84*
Pequignot, G., *60*
Percy, C.L., *372*
Pereira, L., *353*
Perez-Mesa, C., 369, *371*
Perin-Roussel, O., 260, *269*
Perry, W., *294*
Perucho, M., 300, 305, *310, 311*
Pesenti, V., *393*
Petitti, D., *353*
Peto, R., 32, *42*, 103, *108*, 254, *256*, 352, *353*
Petrakis, M.L., 332, *338*
Petrakis, N., *118*
Pettis, E.W., *310*
Phillips. D.H., 88, *95*
Phillips, J.C., 187, *193*
Pickle, L.W., *16, 60, 109*, 212, *353, 372*
Pignatelli, B., **45-61**, 53, *59*, 143, *145, 146*
Pike, M.C., *355*
Pillsbury, H.C., 6, *18*
Pindborg, J.J., *370*
Place, A.R., *226*
Poddubni, B.K., *109*
Poirier, M., 243, *269, 312*
Poljakov, B.P., *109*
Popp, J.A., *228*
Poulsen, T.C., 369, *370*
Poupko, J.M., 65, *70*, 319, *323*
Pour, P., *242*
Pratap, A.I., *209*
Prentice, R., 366, *371*
Preston-Martin, S., 8, *18*, 180, *193*, 348, *354*
Preussmann, R., 29, *30*, 45, *58, 192*, 246, *256*
Prokopczyk, B., **197-213**
Prue, D.M., 6, *18*
Purchase, I.F.H., 317, *323*
Puzrath, R.M., 122, *133*

Raafat, M., 101, *108*
Radford, E.P., *393*
Radok, P., *242*
Radomski, J.L., 317, *323*
Radomski, R.M., *70*, 144, *146*
Radomski, T., *70, 323*
Radtke, H.E., *70*
Ragan, D.L., 216, *227*
Rajewsky, M.F., *256, 294*
Ramazotti, V., *57*
Ranadive, K.J., 205, *209, 211*

Rand, M.J., 4, *18*
Randall, H.W., *228*
Randerath, E., **85-98**, 87, 88, 89, 91, *94, 95*, 98, 147, 297
Randerath, K., **85-98**, 85, 86, 87, 88, 93, *94, 95, 96,* 96, 97, 98, 147, 148, 294, 295, 399
Rao, A.R., 208, *211*
Rao, K.V.N., 191, *193*
Rathkamp, G., 83, *83*
Rautenstrauch, V., 172, *176*
Razzon, T., *134*
Recio, L., 122, *133*
Reddy, E.P., *312*
Reddy, J.K., *243*
Reddy, M.V., **85-98**, 85, 86, 88, 89, *94, 95*
Reid, D.J., *17*
Reid, W.W., 166, *176*
Repace, J.L., 346, 349, *354*
Repetto, M., 41, *43*
Reznik-Schuller, H., 190, *192, 193*
Rheinwald, J.G., 299, *311*
Rhim, J.S., *312*
Riboli, E., *393*
Rice, J.M., 180, *193*
Richards, B., *133*
Richardson, F.C., 291, *294*
Richter-Reichhelm, H.-B., *192*
Ristow, H., 216, *227*
Ritchie, C., 351, *355*
Rivenson, A., *83, 210, 211*, **245-257**
Rizio, D., 198, *211*
Robins, P., *292*
Rodriguez, E., **113-119**
Rodriguez, Q., *160*
Roeraade, J., *177*
Rogers, H.J., *322*
Rogers, W.R., **121-136**, 122, *133*
Rooma, M.A., *145*
Rosenberg, J., *16*
Rosi, D., *133*
Rosin, M.P., 100, 101, 102, 103, 106, 107, *108, 109,* 109, 110, 111, 113, 114, 117, *118*, 212, 299
Rothman, K.J., 103, *108*, 362, 371, 378, *393*
Rothstein, M., *58*
Rottenberg, V.I., *109*
Rous, P., 335, *338*
Rovin, S., *370*
Rowland, J., *43*
Rowley, J.D., 100, 106, *108*
Rozengurt, E., *309*
Rubio, F., **21-32**
Rush, B.F., *370*
Russel, R., *176*
Russell, M.A.H., 6, *18,* 144, *145*

Russfield, A.B., *84*

Sabreo, S., *393*
Sacks, S.T., *338*
Sadagopa Ramanujan, V.M., *83*
Saffhill, R., *256*
Sagle, N.A., *160*
Sailo, J., *109*
St Clair Renard, K.G., 381, *393*
Saladino, A.J., 276, *282, 311*
Salloojee, Y., *18*
Sams, J.P., *30*
San, R.H.C., 86, *96, 109*
Sandler, D.P., 344, 348, *354*
Sanger, B., *160*
Sanghvi, L.D., *371*
Santella, R.M., *70, 94, 323*
Santodonato, J., 40, *43*
Sapp, J.P., *211*
Saquem, S., *269*
Saracci, R., 378, *393*
Sarles, D., *119*
Sasson, I.M., 117, *118,* **121-136**, 122, *134,* 332, *338*
Sato, S., 131, *134*
Sausville, E., *310, 311*
Saw, D., *354*
Scalese, S., *134*
Scarpelli, D.G., *242*
Schachter, S., *18*
Schafer, P., *242, 309*
Schauenstein, E., *280*
Schechter, F., 151, 159, *160*
Schenck, K.M., *269*
Schenker, M., *355*
Scherer, G., **137-148**, 146, 398
Schmeltz, I., *42*, 77, *84, 268*
Schmid, W., *118*
Schmidt, F., *354*
Schneider, A., *310*
Scholtzhauer, W.S., 83, *83*
Schottenfeld, D., 103, *108*
Schreiber, O., *84*
Schuetzle, D., 83, *84*
Schulte-Elte, K.H., 172, *176*
Schurdak, M.E., 88, *95, 96*
Schut, H.A.J., *242, 370*
Schwab, M., 106, *108*
Scicchitano, D., *292, 293, 294*
Scolnick, E.M., *309, 311*
Scott, J.C., *210*
Scott, R.E., 300, 308, *311*
Scriban, R., *146*
Scudiero, D.A., 289, 290, *292, 294*
Seeley, T., *311*
Segerback, D., *70*

Seidman, H., *392*
Seino, Y., *133, 134*
Selikoff, I.J., *299*, 304, *311*, 346, *353*, 377, *392*,
Selkirk, J.K., *242*
Sell, A., 158, *160*
Sellajumar, A., *43*
Selvin, S., *338*
Sen, N.P., 139, *146*
Sepkovic, D.W., 4, 6, 8, *17, 18*
Seremet, T., *267*
Setlow, R.B., *294*
Shackney, S.E., *323*
Shah, A., *57*
Shamsuddin, A.M., *282, 310, 312*
Shanmugaratnam, K., *354*
Shannon, F.T., *17*
Shear, M., *370*
Shergalis, W.A., *58*
Shih, T.Y., 306, *311*
Shillitoe, E.J., *338*
Shimizu, K., *311*
Shirname, L.P., 208, *211*
Shivapurkar, N.M., 205, *209*
Shoyab, M., 303, *311*
Shudo, K., *134*
Shy, C.M., 60, *109*, 212, *372*
Siegel, M., *311*
Sieno, Y., *18*
Silverman, S., 369, *371*
Sim, P., *268*
Sinclair, N.M., *18*
Singer, B., 254, *256*, 287, *292, 294*
Singer, G.M., 216, *227*
Sipahimalani, A.T., 206, 207, *209, 211*
Sirtori, C., 122, *134*
Sjostedt, S., 331, 333, *337*
Sjunneskog, C., *293*
Skegg, D.C.G., *337*
Skipper, P.L., **63-75**, *70, 256*
Slaga, T.J., 265, *269, 312*
Sloneker, S.D., *267*
Smans, M., *108*
Smith, D.G., *337*
Smith, F.G., Jr., 190, *193*
Smith, H.S., *269*
Smolarek, T.A., 266, *269*
Sofer, W., *226*
Son, O.S., 82, *84*
Sontag, S.J., 122, *133*
Soreng, A.L., 106, *109*
Sorger, K., 369, *371*
Sousa, J., 122, *134*
Spandidos, D.A., 306, *311*
Sparks, D., *323*
Sparros, L., *359*
Speilgelhalder, B., 29, *30*

Speizer, F., *355*
Spielhoff, R., *193*
Spingarn, N.E., 131, *134*
Spiro, M., *269*
Spit, B.J., *226*
Sporn, M.B., *108, 310*
Squier, C.A., *371*
Squires, W.G., 367, *372*
Srivastava, S.K., *312*
Stampfer, M.R., 260, *269*
Stanish, W.M., *118, 337*
Starr, T.B., 217, 224, *226, 227, 228*
Stavric, B., 131, *134*
Stedman, R.L., *309*
Steinhagen, W.H., *226*
Stellman, S.D., 193, 213, 313, 325, 326, 330, 331, *338*, 339, 340, 355, 356, 358, 359, 372, **377-395**, 380, 381, 382, 382, 390, *393*, 394, 395, 402
Stenbäck, F., 34, 41, *43*
Stepney, T., *16*
Stevens, R.G., 315, *323*
Stewart, B.W., 246, *256*
Stich, H.F., 53, *59*, 86, *96*, **99-111**, 101, 102, 103, 104, 106, *108, 109*, 113, 114, 117, *118*, 208, *211*, 399
Stich, W., 104, *108, 109*
Stokes, P.E., *311*
Stoner, G.D., 261, 262, *267, 268, 269, 282, 309, 310, 370*
Stony, G.D., *242*
Stott, W.T., 216, *227*
Strickland, J.E., *310*
Styles, J.A., *209*
Sugimura, T., *59*, 131, *134, 309*
Sullivan, J.W., *58*
Sun, J.D., 34, *43*
Sundqvist, K., **273-285**
Sutton, A.L., *242*
Sven, J.Y., *372*
Swain, A.P., *309*
Swann, P.F., 56, *59*
Swanson, M., *337*
Swenberg, J.A., 190, *192*, **215-230**, 217, 221, 225, *227, 228*, 299, 292, *293, 294*
Swern, D., *58*

Tager, I.B., *355*
Takagi, M., *268*
Takeda, K., *134*
Taminato, T., *18*
Tannenbaum, S.R., 19, 31, 32, **63-75**, 70, 71, 72, 73, 74, 96, 109, 110, 119, 135, 144, *146*, 194, 212, 229, *256*, 271, 283, 284, 285, 296, 326, 340,

[Tannenbaum, S.R.]
  356, 357, 359, 360, 373, 393, 394, 395, 398
Taylor, B., *17*
Taylor, H.W., 206, *210*, 216, *227*
Telford, R., *16*
Terracini, B., *60*
Thakker, D.R., *268, 269*
Tharp, R., *192*
Theall, G., 260, *269*
Theiss, J.C., *226*
Theuws, J.L.G., *132, 134*
Thilander, H., 204, *210*
Thilly, W.G., *216, 226*
Thomaele, J., *256*
Thomas, D.B., 329, 330, 331, *338*
Thompson, J.W., *16*
Thurnham, D.I., *109*
Tilton, K.A., *17, 133*
Tjälve, H., **179-195**, 184, 187, 189, 190, 191, *192, 193*, 194, 195, 217, *226, 353,* 400
Todaro, G.J., *311*
Tokiwa, T., *310, 311*
Tokuhata, G.K., 329, 331, *338*
Toledo, A., *60, 212, 372*
Toledo, M.A., *109*
Toorchen, D., *192*
Topal, M.D., *192*
Trapeznikov, N.N., *109*
Trevathan, E., 330, 331, *338*
Trichopoulos, D., 343, 344, 351, *354*
Trivers, G.E., *42*
Trump, B.F., *242, 267, 282, 293,* **299-314**, *309, 310, 312*
Trushin, N., **179-195**, *192, 210, 242,* **245-257**, *255, 256, 353*
Tserkovny, G.F., *108*
Tso, T.C., 204, *210,* 211
Tsuda, M., 47, *59*
Tsuji, T., *134*
Tswi, K., *134*
Tucker, J.D., *134*
Turchi, A., *133*
Turesky, R.J., *70*
Turner, J.A., 172, *177*
Turnstall-Pedoe, H., *18*
Tuyns, A.J., 56, *59, 60*

Uchikashe, M., *18*
Ullberg, S., 181, *193*
Umbenhauer, D., 254, *256, 294*
Unruh, L.E., *323*
Uotila, L., 218, *227,* 228

Vahakangas, K., *42, 267*

Vahlne, A., *210*
Valerio, M.G., *312*
van Bladeren, P.J., 260, *269*
Vanderbroucke, J.P., 347, *354*
van der Eb, A.J., 306, *309*
van der Heijden, C.A., *228*
Van der Hoeven, J.C.M., 131, *134*
Van Dongen, C.G., *84*
Van Doorn, R., 122, *134*
Van Haaften, C., *242*
van Kesteren-van Leeuwen, A.C., *227*
Vanucci, V., *133*
Van Vunakis, H., *18, 133, 371*
Varmus, H.E., *108*
Verheesen, J.H.H., *354*
Vernier, R.L., 190, *193*
Vernster, V.L., *xii*
Vesey, C., *18*
Vesselinovitch, S.D., *191*
Vesselinovitch, S.P., 352, *354*
Vessey, M.P., *337*
Vial, Ch., *176*
Vigny, P., 260, *269*
Vinato, J.F., *177*
Vincent, P., *57*
Vineis, P., 56, *60*
Vitzthum, O.G., 83, *84*
Vogler, W.R., 367, 369, *372*
Vogt, C., *177*
Vohra, S.K., *58*
Volden, G., *293*
Volger, G., 99, *109*
von Hippel, P.H., 217, *228*
Voragen, A.G.J., *134*
Vutuc, C., 349, *354*
Vyas, K.P., *260*

Wagenaar-Zegers, M.A.P., *134*
Wagoner, J.K., *310*
Wahlberg, I., 164, 166, 168, 169, 170, 172, *176, 177*
Wahrendorf, J., *59*
Wakabayashi, K., 131, *134*
Wakefield, L.M., *310*
Wald, N., 349, 351, *355*
Waldstein, E.A., 288, *294*
Walker, A.M., 378, *393*
Walker, B., *370*
Walker, E.A., *145*
Walker, S.E., 47, *57*
Wallin, I., *177*
Walter, S.D., 378, *393*
Walters, C.L., *57*
Wang, C.Y., 316, *324*
Wang, L.-D., 387, *393*
Ward, J.B., Jr., *83, 133, 226*
Wargovich, J., 113, *118*

Wargovich, M.J., 106, *107, 109*
Warner, K.E., *xii, 95, 227*
Watson, A.P., 204, *211*
Weaver, J.A., *95*
Webber, L.S., *371*
Weber, A., 144, *146*
Weber, W.W., *70,* 320, *324*
Webster, L.A., *338*
Weeks, C.E., *269*
Weeks, M.O., *311*
Wefald, F.C., *267*
Weinberg, R.A., *310*
Weinstein, I.B., *268, 269, 309*
Weis, C.C., *322, 323, 324*
Weisburger, E.K., 78, *84, 323*
Weisburger, J.H., *84,* 131, *134*
Weiss, S.T., 346, 349, 350, *355*
Wenke, G., 46, *60,* 206, 207, *211, 212*
Werkhoff, P., *84*
West, D.W., *118, 337*
Westbrook, K.C., 367, *372*
Westra, J.G., *322*
White, H.J., 367, *371*
White, R.D., 131, *134*
White, S., 158, *160*
Whittaker, J.R., 190, *192*
Widdowson, G.M., *16*
Wiest, L., 288, *294*
Wiestler, O., 288, *294*
Wigle, D.T., 315, *324,* 330, 331, *338*
Wigler, M., *311*
Wilcox, A.J., *354*
Wilcox, B., *17*
Wild, C.P., *256*
Wilkie, N.M., 306, *311*
Wille, J.J., Jr., 299, *311*
Willey, J.C., **273-285**, 275, 276, 279, *282,* 283, **299-314**, 300, 302, 303, 306, *311*
Williams, P.T., *337*
Williams, R.R., 329, 330, 331, 332, *338,* 367, *372*
Williams, S.A., 289, 290, *293*
Williams, T.B., 144, *146*
Wilson, J., *323*
Wilson, L.W., *160*
Wilson, R.A., 164, *177*
Winkelstein, W., Jr., 44, 147, 195, **329-341**, 329, 330, 332, 333, *338,* 339, 340, 341, 357, 359, 360, 394, 402
Winn, D.M., 46, *60,* 102, 106, *109,* 204, *212,* 213, **361-375**, 362, 364, 366, 368, *370, 372,* 373, 374, 402
Wise, M.B., **151-162**, 160, 161, 262, 400
Wise, R.W., 319, *324*
Wolf, H., *176,* 320, *324*

Wolff, R.K., *43*
Wong, K.-Y., 217, *228*
Wong, T.K., 265, *269*
Wood, L.W., *18*
Woutersen, R.A., 216, *225, 226,* 228
Wright, N.H., 330, 331, 334, *338*
Wright, S.T., *322*
Wu, A.H., 344, 347, *355*
Wu, C.H., *211*
Wu, S.-M., *267*
Wynder, E.L., **3-19**, 4, 8, *17, 18, 42,* 82, *83,* 102, 103, *109, 118,* 131, *134,* 153, 158, *160, 268,* 274, 279, *283,* 302, *309, 311,* 315, *324, 338,* 344, 347, 351, *354, 355,* 367, 369, *372,* 384, 390, *393*

Yagi, H., *269*
Yahagi, T., *133, 134*
Yamaguchi, K., *134*
Yamamoto, F., *310*
Yamasaki, E., 121, *123,* 132, *134,* 332, *338*
Yamazoe, Y., 316, 319, *322, 324*
Yang, L.L., *282*
Yarosh, D.B., 274, *283,* 288, 289, 291, *292, 294*
Yeats, D., *337*
Yee, M.C., *18*
Yoakum, G., 119, 212, 213, 243, 271, *282,* **299-314**, 305, 306, *311, 312,* 312, 313, 314, 373, 373
Young, J.F., 316, 317, 319, *324*
Young, J.L., 368, 369, *373*
Young, S.K., 34, *43, 242*
Young, V.R., *146*
Yu, M.C., *193, 354, 355*
Yuasa, Y., 300, 305, *312*
Yunis, J.J., 106, *109*
Yuspa, S.H., *269,* 279, *283,* 299, 303, 308, *310, 312*

Zajdela, F., *269*
Zaridze, D.G., *101*
Zenser, T.V., *323, 324*
Ziegler, R.G., *109, 372*
Zinkgraf, S., *372*
Ziolkowski, C.H., *294*
Zlotogorski, C., 289, 290, *294*
Zollner, H., *282*
Zukowski, K., *324*
Zunzunegui, M.V., 335, 336, *338*
zur Hausen, H., 336, *339*
Zwelling, L.A., *282*

Subject Index

Abruptio placenta, association of with maternal smoking, 13
Acetaldehyde
   cross-link, hypothetical structure for, 229-230
   and decreased colony survival and clonal growth rates, 278
   and DPX formation, 222-224
   effects of on human bronchial fibroblasts, 247-277
   interaction of with NMU, 284-285
   in tobacco smoke, 215, 222-224
Acetylation
   N,O-acyltransferase, 324
   dual nature of in bladder tumor induction, 321
   hepatic, 319-321
   hydroxylamine, 324
Acetylator phenotype
   and bladder cancer, 75
   in smokers, 74-75
Acetyl coenzyme A-dependent acetyltransferases, catalyze hepatic N-acetylation, 319-321
N-Acetylcysteine, reaction of with 4(carbethoxynitrosamino)-1 (3-pyridyl)-1-butanone, 252-254
Acrolein
   causes DNA damage, 277
   and DPX formation, 221
   effects of on human bronchial fibroblasts, 274-277
   and reduced cell survival, 277
   in tobacco smoke, 215, 221-222
Additive vs. multiplicative models, 388-391
Adenoncarcinoma, induced by aldehydes in animal model, 215-216
Age of starting snuff, and influence on cancer risk, 373
AGT. See O^6-Alkylguanine-DNA-alkyltransferase.
Air pollution, as source of aniline o-toluidine, 82
Albumin, as dosimeter, 64
Alcohol
   and cotinine level, 19
   and increased risk of oral cancer, 362
   influence of on urinary excretion of NDMA, NPRO, 26, 28
   as promoter, 384
   and smoking, no evidence of synergistic effect of, 114-115

Aldehydes
   and carcinogenicity of tobacco smoke, 400-401
   effect of on colony-forming efficiency, 275
   and enhanced terminal differentiation of cells, 279, 281
   generated from metabolism of N-nitrosamines, 280-281
   growth, inhibitory effects of, 275-276
   and peroxide formation, 285
   in saliva of snuff dippers, 204
   in tobacco smoke, 401
   in tobacco smoke and formation of DNA-protein cross-links, 215-230
   tobacco smoke-related pathobiological effects of, 273-285
O^6-Alkylguanine
   no correlation of with tumorgenicity of nitroso compounds, 241
O^6-Alkylguanine-DNA-alkytransferase (AGT)
   activity, inhibitors of, 289-290
   activity, in human cell lines, 289
   assay for, 287-297
   cellular distribution of 288-289
   factors affecting, 287-297
   mechanics of action, 296-297
   purpose of, 295-296
   reaction, specificity of, 290-291
   and reduced toxicity of NMU, 290
Alkyltransferase DNA repair enzyme, factors that increase or decrease level of, 297
Alpha-beta ketones, quantification of in tobacco, 177
Alpha-humulene, in clove oil, 152
d,l-alpha-tocopherol. See Vitamin E.
Aluminum industry, and exposure to PAHs, 34
Aluminum workers
   lung cancer rates in smokers and non-smokers, 44
   PAH exposure level in 36-40
4-Aminobiophenyl (4-ABP)
   activation of, 65
   amount of in smoke of one cigarette, 74
   average daily exposure to, 68-69
   exposure to monitored via quantification of Hb binding, 65-66
   hemoglobin adduct level in smokers/non-smokers, 66-68

417

[4-Aminobiophenyl (4-ABP)]
  as hepato- or mammary gland carcinogen, 65
  quantification of adduct to Hb, 66
  sources of in environment, 71-72
  in tobacco smoke, 64-66
2-Amino-α-carbolines, amount of in smoke of one cigarette, 74
Amplification, as mechanism in neoplastic transformation, 100-101
Aniline
  analysis of in human urine, 77-84
  in nonsmoker's urine, 83
  scheme for analysis of, 78
  sources of, 83-84
Areca alkaloids
  in betal quid chewers' saliva, 205-206
  in betal quid, smokeless tobacco, 197
Areca nut-specific nitrosamines (ASNA), 46
Arecaidine, 208
  nitrosation of, 46
Arecoline, 208
  nitrosation of, 46
Aroma, tobacco, isoprenoids as component of, 163-178
Aromatic amines. *See also* aniline o-toluidine.
  acetylation of, 321
  analysis of in urine, 78
  as cause of bladder cancer, 77
  excretion of in cigarette smokers, 398
  and induction of urinary bladder cancer, 315-326
  metabolic activation of, 402
  tobacco-related, hemoglobin adducts, 63-75
Asbestos
  effect of on NHBE cells, 304-305
  and smoking and lung cancer, 379-380
  and uptake and metabolism of B(a)P in hamsters tracheal cells, 266
Ascorbic acid. *See also* Vitamin C.
  as inhibitors of nitosation, 53
  protective effect of, 56
Assay
  AGT, 287-297
  ^{32}P-postlabeling for DNA adducts, 86-88
  for urinary nitrosamines, 22
Azo-dyes
  potential precursor of aniline, o-toluidine, 83

Beer intake, and NPRO formation, 143
Benza(a)anthracene
  induced DNA adducts, PEI cellulose maps of, 90

[Benz(a)anthracene]
  in urine of smokers, 41
Benzfluoranthenes, metabolism of, 260
Benzo(a)pyrene (B[a]P)
  binding of to human bronchial DNA, 265
  binding levels of to DNA, 261
  binding variation in, 270
  DNA adduct patterns and genetic factors, 270
  DNA adducts, relative distribution of in human cells, tissue, 264
  induced DNA adducts, PEI cellulose map of, 89, 90
  interindividual variation in binding to DNA, 262
  metabolism of, 260
  metabolites, relative distribution of in human tissue, cells, 263
  possible role of in oral cancer, 147-213
  as transplacental carcinogen, 180
  in urine of smokers, 41
  water soluble metabolites of, 262
Beta-carotene
  measurement of in MEC, 109-110
  and reduction of MEC in oral mucosa of snuff dippers, 103-104
Beta-caryophyllene, in clove oil, 152
Betel quid
  correlation of with oral cancer, 46
  genotoxic agents in, 206-208
  level of nitrosamines in before and after nitrosation, 52
  MEC frequency associated with, 102
  synthetic nitro musks in, 208
  tannins and polyphenols in act as nitrosation catalysts, 55
  with tobacco saliva analysis of, 207
Betel quid chewers, formation of NOC in oral cavity of, 52-56
Betel quid chewing, and N-nitrosamines, 205-206
Bicylodamascenone A, formation of, 167
14,15-bisnor-B(17)-labden-13-one, UV-irradiation of, 175
Black tea, aniline, o-toluidine in, 83
Black tobacco
  association of with bladder cancer, 73
  and higher risk of bladder cancer, 56
Bladder cancer. *See also* Urinary bladder cancer.
  aromatic amines as causative agent, 77
  and association with black tobacco, 73
  cigarette smoking as contributing factor for, 131
  hamster experimental model for, 72-73
  increased risk of in cigarette smokers, 55-56

Subject Index / 419

[Bladder cancer. *See also* Urinary bladder cancer.]
  increased risk of in individuals with urinary infection history, 55-56
  and relationship to rate of acetylation, 75
  risk, 4-ABP as predictive of, 72
  SMR by occupation and smoking habit, 382
  and snuff dipping, 212
Bladder tumor
  formation and urinary pH, 135
  induction, dual nature of acetylation in, 321
Brain cancer
  low-dose effect on passive smoking, 352
Broiled foods, anilines in, 83
Bronchi, labeled DNA digests from in smokers, 92-93
Bronchial carcinoma, induced by NNK, 241
Bronchial epithelial cells. *See also* Normal human bronchial epithelial cells.
  effects of aldehydes on, 273-285
  human carcinogenesis studies of 299-314
  O^6-n-butylguanine, and inhibition of AGT activity, 289-290
Buccal mucosa, cancer, animal model for, 213
Buccal mucosa cells, micronucleus test on, 113-114

Cancer. *See also* specific types.
  of buccal mucosa, animal model for, 213
  deaths associated with tobacco, xi
  and passive smoking, 343-360
4-(Carbethoxynitrosamino)-1-(3-pyridyl)-1-butanone
  reaction of with N-acetycysteine, 252-254
  reactions of deoxyguanosine with, 251
Carboxyhemoglobin
  and higher nicotine yield cigarette, 9
  and lower nicotine yield cigarette, 9
Carcinogen formation, modifiers of, 45-61
Carcinogen
  activation of by fetal enzyme system, 180
  in tobacco smoke, 300
Carcinogenesis
  multistage, in human lung, 301
  possible role of passive smoking in, 348-349
Carcinogenicity, comparative, NNK and NDMA, 247
Carotenoids
  degradation of, 164-165
  metabolism of, 165
  structure of, 164

Caryophyllene-expoxide, in clove bud oil, 160
Cell proliferation, effect of aldehydes on, 225
Cembranoids
  biological transformation of, 166-172
  structure of, 164
Cervical aspirates, nicotine and cotinine content of, 341
Cervical cancer
  casual association of cigarette smoke with, 117
  risk, and husband's smoking habits, 336
  risk, male influences, 335-336
  viral etiology of, 119
Cervical dysplasia, role of nicotine and cotinine in, 117
Cervical fluids, smokers', cotinine and nicotine in, 147
Cervical neoplasia and dysplasia, relative risk for by cigarette smoking history, 334
Cervical smears, micronucleus test on, 114
Chewing tobacco, carcinogenicity of, 204
Chromatid breaks, indicated by micronuclei, 106
Chrysene-induced DNA adducts, PEI-cellulose map of, 90
Chrysene, metabolism of, 260
Cigarette smoke, *See also* Tobacco smoke; Sidestream smoke.
  aromatic amines in and bladder cancer risk, 77
  causal association with cervical cancer, 117
  tumor-enhancing substances in, xi
  tumor initiators in, xi
  undetectable effect on MEC frequency, 103
Cigarette smoke absorption, biochemical measurement of, 10
Cigarette smoke condensation
  assay of DNA adduct induced by, 88-92
  in baboons, 129-130
  effects of on NHBE cells in vitro, 300-303
  induced DNA adducts PEI-cellulose maps of, 91
Cigarette smoke, particulate phase, PAH in, 259-271
Cigarette smoked, number, and micronucleus level, 115-116
Cigarette smokers
  analysis of saliva of, 207
  mutagens in urine of, 121-136
  as passive smokers also, 358-359
Cigarette smoking
  developmental effects of, 179-195
  influence of on hormone metabolism, 340

[Cigarette smoking]
  transplacental exposure and fetal uptake, 13-15
  and uterine cervix cancer, 329-341
Cigarette smoking baboon animal model, 121-136
  mutagenic urine in, 126-130
Cigarette smoking behavior, compensation and nicotine tolerance, 6-8
C^{15} and C^{16} labdanoids, biogenesis, 175
C^{20} labdanoids, structure of, 173
Clara cells, malignant transformation of, 194-195
Clonal growth assay, human bronchial epithelial cells, 283
Clove cigarette
  gas-phase profile of, 154-155
  high eugenol delivery of, 158
  whole-smoke profile, 155
Clove cigarette smoke
  characteristics of, 153-154
  chemical analysis of, 151-162
  symptoms linked to, 151-152
Clove-containing cigarettes, 400
Clove extract, analysis of, 152
Clove oil, analysis of, 152
C^{13} methyl ketones, as precursors of tobacco aroma constituents, 164
Cocarcinogenesis, tobacco, and herpes virus, 212-213
Cocarcinogens, in tobacco smoke, 300
Coffee intake, and NPRO formation, 143
Colony-forming efficiency, human bronchial fibroblasts, effects of aldehydes on, 275
Cotinine
  biochemical measurement of in urine as good indicator of passive smoking, 12
  in cervical aspirates, 341
  in cervical mucus of smokers, 147
  distribution of in saliva and plasma of smokers, nonsmokers, 5
  elimination of from urine of newborn infants, 14-15
  elimination time of in smokers, nonsmokers, 15
  level of in urine of smokers, nonsmokers, 124-126
  levels of as predictor of nicotine compensation, 18-19
  metabolism of in smokers vs. nonsmokers, 19
  presence of in cervical mucus of smokers, 117
  quantitation of as measure of smoke absorption, 3

[Cotinine]
  quantitation, value of in validating smoking behavior, 15
  saliva and plasma levels of to validate cigarette use, 4
  urinary concentration and number of cigarettes smoked, 13
  in urine and saliva of infants, 12
Cotinine:creatinine ratios, in urine of exposed and nonexposed babies, 14
Cotinine (plasma)
  and higher nicotine yield cigarettes, 9
Creatinine, urinary excretion of, 43
CSC. See cigarette smoke condensate.
Cytochrome P-450
  associated mixed-function oxidose, and PAH metabolism, 259
  catalyzes hepatic N-oxidation, 317
  increased levels of in active cigarette smokers, 359

Damascones, as tobacco flavorants, 166
Dentition status, as cofactor for oral/pharynx cancer, 364-365
Deoxyguanosine, reaction of with 4-(3-pyrdyl)-4-oxobutyldiazohydrozide, 251
Detoxification, metabolic pathways of in heavy smokers, 19
Development, affected by cigarette smoking, 179-195
Dibenzo[a,1]pyrene, in urine of smokers, 41
Diet
  as cofactor for oral/pharynx cancer, 364
  effect of on excretion of mutagens in urine of smokers, 121-136
  effect of on mutagens in urine, 122-126
  interaction of with smoking, 377-395
  and lung cancer, and smoking interaction, 384-388
  and mutagenic activity of smokers' urine, 399
Dimethylamine, concentrations of in body, 31
Diozabicyclo (3.3.1)nonane, formation of, 172
Dioxabicyclo (3.2.1)octane, formation of, 172
Diphenylhydantoin, and continine levels, 19
Diterpenoids. See also Cembranoids; Labdanoids.
  as tobacco aroma constituents, 166-175
DNA, B[a]P binding to, 261, 262

Subject Index / 421

DNA adducts
  assay for, 86–88
  bladder epithelial arise from PHS-mediated peroxidation, 319
  cigarette smoke condensate-induced, assay of, 88–92
  as key element in initiation of chemical carcinogenesis, 85
  smoking-related, ^{32}P-postlabeling test for, 85–98
  in tissues of smokers, ^{32}P-postlabeling assay of, 92–93
DNA binding,
  and B[a]P, 259–271
DNA methylation
  and carcinogenicity of NNK, 233
  comparative, NNK and NDMA, 247
  NNK, immunochemical measurement of, 247
  in snuff dippers, 205
DNA-protein cross-links (DPX)
  caused by aldehydes, cigarette smoke condensate, 276–277
  formation of by aldehydes present in tobacco smoke, 215–230
  increased by thiol depletion, 229
DNA repair, mechanism of inhibition by formaldehyde, 280–281
DNA repair enzyme, O^6-alkylquanine-DNA-alkyltransferase, 401
DNA single-strand breaks, caused by aldehydes, cigarette smoke condensate, 276–277
Dosimeter
  albumin as, 64
  hemoglobin as, 64
  NNK, NNN as, 246
Dosimetry, and metabolic activation of tobacco-specific nitrosamines, 245–257
DPX. *See* DNA-protein cross-links.

Endogenous carcinogen formation, modifiers of, 45–61
Enhanced terminal differentiation of cells, and aldehydes, 279, 281
Epoxide formation, increased with aging of cigarette, 160
Esophageal cancer, role of alcohol in, 384
Estrogens
  adducts of, 97
  lower urinary excretion of during luteal phase in smokers, 340
Ethanol. *See also* Alcohol.
  effects of on N-nitrosamine metabolism, 194

[Ethanol. *See also* Alcohol.]
  and metabolic activation of TSNA, 56
Eugenol, 208
  anesthetic properties of, 58–59, 161
  in clove oil, 152
  contact phenomenon with lung tissue, 162
  toxicity of, 161
Exposure levels, 4-ABP, 68–69
Eye melanin, fetal, NNK distribution in, 181

Fetus, exposure of to maternal smoking, 13–15
Flavonoids, as mutagen in food products, 131
Formaldehyde
  amount covalently bound in DNA of respiratory mucosa, 219–221
  causes DNA damage, 277
  and decreased clonal growth rate, 277–278
  effect of on O^6-mG repair, 277
  effects of on human bronchial fibroblasts, 274–277
  enhances mutagenicity of NMU, 279
  GSH-dependent oxidation of, 224
  and mechanism of formation of DPX, 217–219
  metabolic incorporation of, 219–221
  in tobacco smoke, 215, 219–221
Fruit consumption, and decreased lung cancer risk, 387

Gas chromatography
  aromatic amine fraction in smokers' urine, 79
  high resolution mass spectrometry assay, for quantifying NDMA, 21
  use of in nitrosation test, 46
Genetic factors, and B[a]P-DNA binding patterns, 270
Genome reshuffling, indicated by micronuclei, frequency, 107
Glass fibers, effects of on NHBE cells, 304–305
Glucuronidation, 315–317
Glutathione (GSH)
  conjugation with as cellular defense against toxic compounds, 279
  -dependent oxidation, and formaldehyde, 224
  effects of aldehydes on, 274–277
  level of in rat respiratory mucosa, 229
  protective effect of, 274

Hair samplings, measurement of cotinine, nicotine in to validate smoking, 6
HBE cells, v-Ha-*ras* transfected phenotypic properties of, 307
Heavy smokers, metabolic pathways of deoxification in, 19
Hematopoietic cancers, increased risk of in children of smokers, 194
Hemoglobin, as dosimeter, 64
Hemoglobin adducts
  of tobacco-related aromatic amines, 63–75, 398
Hemoglobin dosimeter, 4-ABP, accuracy of, 70
Hepatic oxidation, 315–317
Hepatocytes, as site of highest AGT activity, 291
Herpes virus type II, and cervical cancer, 336
High-performance liquid chromatography (HPLC), and PAH analysis, 35–40
Hormone metabolism, influence of cigarette smoking on, 340
Hydrazines, as transplacental carcinogen, 180
Hydroperoxydiols, 169
4-Hydroxyalkenals, 283
Hydroxylation, vs. methylation, 256

Infants, nicotine and cotinine concentrations in urine and saliva of, 12
Isoprenoids
  as alpha-beta ketones that react with DNA, 177
  as flavor components of tobacco, 163–178

Khaini tobacco, MEC frequency associated with, 102
Kidney, fetal, NNK distribution in, 181
Kreteks. *See* Clove cigarette smoke.

Labdanoids
  biogenesis of, 172–175
  structure of, 164
Larynx cancer
  association of with black tobacco, 73
  and smoking and alcohol, 386
Leukoplakia, association with oral cancer and snuff habit, 369
Liver
  cytochrome P-450 activity in, 317
  high AGT level in, 288
Low-yield cigarettes, and compensation for reduced nicotine yield, 6–8
Lung, human, multistage carcinogenesis in, 301
Lung cancer
  decreased risk of with fruit consumption, 387–388
  histologic types of, 351–352
  increased risk of in workers exposed to coal tar pitch volatiles, 33–34
  low-dose effect of passive smoking, 352
  mechanisms of, 34
  and occupation and smoking, 379–383
  rates of in smoking vs. nonsmoking aluminum workers, 44

Mainstream smoke
  aromatic amine concentration in, 77
  aromatic amines, 65
  constituents of, 350
Material metal workers, and smoking and lung cancer, 381
Maternal smoking
  toxic effects of on fetus, 400
  transplacental exposure and fetal uptake, 13–15
Meat diet, and mutagens in urine of smokers, nonsmokers, 122–126
MEC. *See* Micronuclei in exfoliated cells.
Megastigmatrienones, and tobacco aroma, 164
Methemoglobin formation, by aromatic amines, 65
5-Methylchrysene, metabolism of, 260
O^6-Methyldeoxyguanosine,
  levels of in tissues after NNK, NDMA treatment, 249–250
O^6-Methylguanine (O^6-mG)
  in DNA of animals treated with NNK, 190
  effects of aldehydes on, 274–277
  effects of formaldehyde on, 277
  in fetal nose and liver after NNK injection, 186
  and inhibition of AGT activity, 289–290
  localization of in MNNG- and NNK-treated tissues, 238–239
  mediates tumorigenic properties of NNK, 254
  as promutagenic DNA lesion, 281
  in target tissue exposed to NNK, 233
7-Methylguanine, in fetal nose and liver after NNK injection, 186
4-(Methylnitrosamine)-1-(3-pyridyl)-1-butanone (NNK)
  and appearance of O^6-methylguanine in DNA of treated animals, 190
  as carcinogenic in snuff, 205
  carcinogenicity of, 233

Subject Index / 423

[4-(Methylnitrosamine)-1-(3-pyridyl)-1-butanone (NNK)]
  comparative carcinogenicity of with NDMA, 247
  comparative DNA methylation by with NDMA, 247
  comparison of effects of with MNNG, 233-244
  DNA pyridyloxobutylation, 245
  dosimetry, hemoglobin adducts, 255
  effect of on pancreatic epithelium, 237-238
  effect of on respiratory epithelium explants, 234-236
  and induction of bronchogenic carcinoma, 241
  metabolic transformations of, 186
  metabolism and biological effects of, 233-244
  metabolites of in fetal tissue, 184
  as potential dosimeter for tobacco carcinogenesis, 246
  role of in induction of pancreatic cancer, 241
  tissue distribution of fetal mice, hamsters, 181-186
  tumorigenic properties of mediated by O^6-mG, 254
  tumor induction by, 248
N-Methyl-N-nitrosoguanidine (MNNG)
  comparison of effects of with NNK, 233-244
  effect of on pancreatic epithelium explants, 237-238
  effect of on respiratory epithelium explants, 234-236
N-Methyl-N-nitrosourea (MNU)
  additive effect of with formaldehyde on O^6-mG repair, 277
  AGT inactivated by, 289
  mutagenicity enhanced by formaldehyde, 279
Micronucleated cells
  frequency of in passive smokers, 116
  higher frequency of in oral mucosa of tobacco user, 102-103
Micronuclei
  frequency, indicates period of genome reshuffling, 107
  increase of in early stages of carcinogenesis, 100
  induction of by various tobacco brands and mixtures, 104-105
  use of in tracing genotoxic damage in oral mucosa of tobacco users, 99-111
Micronuclei in exfoliated cells (MEC)

[Micronuclei in exfoliated cells (MEC)]
  correlation of frequency of with oral cancer risk, 106
  frequency, factors modulating, 103
  measurement of beta-carotene in, 109-110
  significance of in neoplastic transformation, 106-107
Micronuclei formation, 399
  in radiotherapy patients, 110-111
Micronucleus test
  advantages of, 101
  restrictions of, 101-102
  to validate smoking history, 113-119
MNNG. See N-Methyl-N-nitroguanidine
Molecular epidemiology, 63-75
Monoclonal antibody, for localization of O^6-mG, 234, 238-239
Mouth cancer, role of alcohol in, 384
Multiple-factor studies, 377
Musk additives, synthetic, in smokeless tobacco, 197
Mutagenic urine, in nonsmokers, 122
Mutagens, in urine of cigarette smokers, 121-136

N-Acetylation, rapid and slow phenotypes for, 320-321
β-Naphthylamine, in tobacco smoke, 71
Nasal cancer
  induced by inhaled aldehydes in rodents, 215-219
  low-dose effect of passive smoking, 352
Nass, MEC frequency associated with, 102
NDEA. See N-Nitrosoamine-N-nitrosodiethylamine.
NDMA. See Nitrosodimethylamine.
Neonates, cotinine:creatinine ratios in urine of, 14
Neoplastic transformation, significance of MEC in, 106-107
NHBE. See Normal human bronchial epithelial cells.
Nickel sulfate, effects of on NHBE cells, 303-304
Nicotine
  in cervical aspirates, 341
  in cervical mucus of smokers, 147
  compensation, biochemical predictors of, 18-19
  dioxides, 16
  effect of on fetal weight, 195
  metabolites, measurement of to quantitate smokeless tobacco use, 16
  N'-oxides, 16

[N'-oxides]
  presence of in cervical mucus of smokers, 117
  quantitation of as measure of smoke absorption, 3
  quantitation of as measure of smoke uptake, 16
  short biological half-life of, 4
  tolerance, and compensation, 6–8
  in urine and saliva of infants, 12
Nitrate
  -reducing bacteria in urinary infections, 56
  urinary excretion of in smokers, nonsmokers, 140, 142
Nitrobenzenes, as potential precursor for aniline, o-toluidine, 83
Nitro musks, 208
N-Nitrosamines. *See also* specific names.
  and betel quid chewing, 205–206
  levels in dry vs. moist snuff, 375
  metabolism of, 280
  perinatal disposition and metabolism of in mice and hamsters, 179–195
  in saliva of snuff dippers, 204
  in smokeless tobacco, 198–203
  tobacco-specific, 401
  tobacco-specific, metabolic activation of, 245–257
  as transplacental carcinogen, 180
  urinary, assays for, 22
N-Nitrosamine-N-nitrosodiethylamine (NDEA)
  CO_2 formation by tissues of animals treated with, 189
  fetal metabolism of, 187
  induction of tumors by in offspring of treated mothers, 187
Nitrosation
  inhibition of with vitamin C, 52–56
  by NO_2, 146–147
  in oral cavity of betel quid chewers, 55
  in saliva of betel quid chewers with tobacco, 53
  in saliva of betel quid chewers without tobacco, 54
  in tobacco users, 45–61
  urinary bladder as site of, 55–56
N-Nitrosamino acids (NAA)
  increased urinary excretion of in smokers, 47
  measurement of in urine as indicator of NOC exposure, 47
  in saliva of tobacco users, 49
  synthesis of in human urine, 48
  urinary excretion of in Indian tobacco users, 51
  in urine of smokers, nonsmokers, 50

N-Nitrosoanatabine (NAT)
  in saliva of betel quid chewers with and without tobacco, 52
N-Nitrosodiethanolamine (NDELA)
  decrease of in tobacco, 202
  in snuff, 198
N-Nitrosguvacine (NGCI), in saliva of betel quid chewers with or without tobacco, 52
N-Nitroguvacoline (NGCO), in saliva of betel quid chewers with or without tobacco, 52
N-Nitrosohydroxyproline, excretion of, 60
N-Nitrosomorpholine (NMOR), in snuff, 198
N-Nitroso compounds (NOC)
  effects of tobacco smoking on formation of, 398
  formation of in oral cavity of betel quid chewers, 52–56
  human exposure to in tobacco products, 45–46
  as initiators of pancreas carcinoma, 240–242
  quantification of, 21–35
Nitrosodimethylamine (NDMA)
  comparative carcinogenicity of with NNK, 247
  comparative DNA methylation by with NNK, 247
  as DNA methylating agent, 245
  effect of smoking, alcohol on urinary excretion of, 26, 28
  effect of vitamins C and E on, 23–25
  increase in urinary excretion of in smokers, drinkers, 29
  metabolism of, 246
  tumor induction by, 248
  urinary excretion of, 23–28
4-(N-Nitroso-N-methylamino) butyric acid (NMBA), in saliva of tobacco users, 49
3-(N-Nitroso-N-methylamino) propionic acid (NMPA), in saliva of tobacco users, 49
N-Nitroso-N-methylpropionaldehyde, formation of by nitrosation of arecoline, 46
N-Nitroso-N-methylpropionitrile, formation of by nitrosation arecoline, 46
N-Nitroso-2-methylthiazolidine-4-carboxylic acid (NMTCA), source of in human urine, 47–48
N'-Nitrosonornicotine (NNN)
  as carcinogenic factor in snuff, 205
  dosimetry, hemoglobin adducts, 255
  fetal distribution of, 186–187

[*N'*-Nitrosonornicotine (NNN)]
  as potential dosimeter for tobacco carcinogenesis, 246
  tissue-specific metabolism of in treated animals, 190
Nitrosoproline (NPRO)
  effect of vitamins C and E on, 23–25
  endogenous formation of in smokers, nonsmokers, 137–148
  excretion, correlation of with urine volume, 143
  excretion of in urine of smokers, 47
  formation, inhibition of by ascorbic acid, 54
  urinary excretion of in smokers, nonsmokers, 140, 142
  in urine, detection limit for, 146
  in urine of smokers, chewers of betel quid, 49, 51
  urinary excretion of, 21–35
N-Nitrosothiazolidine 4-carboxylic acid (NTCA), source of in human urine, 47–48
NNK. *See* 4-(Methylnitrosamino)-1-(3-pyridyl)-1-butanone.
NNN. *See N'*-Nitrosonornicotine.
NO_2
  atmospheric, influence of on urinary excretion of NDMA, 23
  atmospheric, and variations in urinary excretion of NDMA, 29
  sources of, 31
NOC. *See N*-Nitroso compounds.
Nonsmokers
  4-ABP-Hb adduct levels in, 66–68
  aniline, *o*-toluidine in urine of, 82
  endogenous NPRO formation by, 137–148
  and exposure to sidestream smoke, 8–12
  increasing salivary nicotine concentrations in, 12
  mutagenic urine in, 122
Normal human bronchial epithelial cells (NHBE)
  effects of nickel sulfate on, 303–304
  malignant transformation of by transfected, v-Ha-*ras*, 305–308
  phenotypic properties of, 307
  tumor promoters for, 302–303
Norsolanadione
  structure, 171
  as tobacco flavor constituent, 170
NPRO. *See* Nitrosoproline.

Occupation, interaction of with smoking, 377–395

Occupational exposure to industrial carcinogens, and relative risk for lung cancer by cigarette smoking, 383
Oncogenes
  activation of by tobacco smoke, 300
  activation, in tobacco-related carcinogenesis experiments, 312–313
  transfection into human bronchial epithelial cells, 401–402
  transposition as mechanism in neoplastic transformation, 100–101
Oral cancer
  correlation of with chewing of betel quid, 46
  increased risk in alcohol drinkers, 362
  need for registry of cases, 374
  role of alcohol in, 384
  and smokeless tobacco, 197–213
  synergistic effect of cigarette smoke and alcohol in induction of, 103
  risk of correlated with MEC frequency, 106
Oral hygiene, as cofactor for oral/pharynx cancer, 364
Oral mucosa
  reduction of MEC in with beta-carotene, 1–3
  tracing genotoxic damage in with micronuclei, 99–111
Oral/pharynx cancer
  cofactors for, 362–366
  and smokeless tobacco, 361–375
  in white women in southeastern U.S., 361–362
Oxidation, hepatic, 315–317

PAH. *See* Polycyclic aromatic hydrocarbons.
Pancreas cancer
  high risk of in snuff dippers, 212
  role of tobacco in, 241
Pancreas carcinogenesis
  in vitro model system for, 401
  nitroso compounds as initiators of, 240–242
Pancreatic epithelium explants, effects on MNNG and NNK on, 237–238
Papilloma viruses, and cervical cancer, 335, 336
Particulate phase, cigarette smoke, PAHs in, 259–271
Passive smokers, frequency of micronucleated cells in, 116
Passive smoking, 8–12
  biochemical measurement of by cotinine levels in urine, 12

[Passive smoking]
  and cancer, 343-360, 402
  and cancer, biologic plausibility of, 348-349
  data confounded by active smoking, 349
  epidemiology, 343-348
  and exposure to aromatic amines, 64-66
  low-dose effect in, 351
  and low-dose effect in lung, nasal cavity, and brain cancers, 352
  and measurement of uptake and absorption of sidestream smoke, 8
  and NPRO formation, 143-145
Pentafluoropropionamide, in smokers' urine, 80, 81
Perinatal death, association of with maternal smoking, 13
p21 expression, in v-Ha-*ras* transfected NHBE cells, 313
Phenobarbital, and cotinine levels, 19
Phenols, as nitrosation modifier, 53
Phorone, reaction of with DNA, 229
Placenta, labeled DNA digests from in smokers, 92-93
Placenta previa, association of with maternal smoking, 13
Plasma, cotinine and thiocyanate distribution in smokers, nonsmokers, 5
Polycyclic aromatic hydrocarbons (PAH), 397
  environmental monitoring of, 397
  exposure to determined by urine analysis, 33-44
  exposure levels of in aluminum workers, 36-40
  HPLC analysis of, 35-40
  HPLC method to determine, 397
  level of occupational exposure, 41
  levels of in occupationally nonexposed workers, 37
  levels of in urine of smoking workers, 44
  metabolic pathways of, 401
  metabolism of, 34, 259-271
  metabolites, reduction of, 35
  particulate, in aluminum plant, 38
  route of exposure, 44
  types of exposure to, 33-34
  in urine with and without reduction of metabolites, 35
  in workers' urine and in work atmosphere, 39
Polyphenols, as nitrosation modifiers, 53
Polonium-210, possible role of in oral cancer, 197-213
[32]P-Postlabeling nucleotide, chromatography, 399

[32]P-Postlabeling test, for smoking-related DNA adducts, 85-98
Procarcinogens, PAHs, 259
Proline, as basis of nitrosation test, 46

Race, as cofactor for oral/pharynx cancer, 362-363
α-Radiation, emitted from Po-210 in smokeless tobacco, 197
Radiation patients, elevated levels of micronucleated cells in, 114
Radiotherapy patients, micronucleus formation in, 110-111
Rapid acetylator phenotype, N-acetylation, 320-321
Relative risks, smoking and cervical cancer, 331
Respiratory epithelium explants, MNNG and NNK treatment of, 234-236
Rhabdomyosarcoma, increase risk of in offspring of smokers, 194

Saliva
  betel quid chewers, agents in, 205-206
  betel quid chewers, analysis of, 207
  cigarette smokers, analysis of, 207
  cotinine and thiocyanate distribution in smokers, nonsmokers, 5
  snuff dippers, alkaloids and N-nitrosamines in, 204
  tobacco chewers, genotoxicity of, 104
Salmonella typhimurium, as mutagenicity assay, 123
Sexual partners, number, and relative risks for smoking and cervical cancer, 332
Sidestream smoke, 8-12
  4-ABP in, 64-66
  aromatic amines in, 65
  aromatic amine concentration in, 77
  constituents of, 350
  evaluation of by measurement of nicotine and cotinine, 4
  higher concentration of toxic and carcinogenic substances in, 348-349
Sidestream and mainstream smoke, difference in chemistries of, 356
Singlet oxygen
  oxidation, in labdanoids, 172, 174
  proneness of cembratrienediol double bonds to react with, 168
Slow-acetylator phenotype
  and bladder cancer, 320
  Danish bladder cancer study, 325-326
  N-acetylation, 320-321
Smoke, tobacco. *See* Tobacco smoke.

Smokeless tobacco, 400. *See also* Snuff; Snuff dippers.
  damage to oral mucosa by, 99-111
  nitrosamines in, 198-203
  nonvolatile nitrosamines in, 201
  and oral cancer, 197-213
  and oral/pharynx cancer, 361-375
  popularity of, 367
  risk factor for oral cancer, 402
  TSNA in, 203
  use of quantitated by measurement of nicotine metabolites, 16
  use, high cotinine levels in, 6
  volatile nitrosamines in, 200
Smokers
  4-ABP-Hb adduct levels in, 66-68
  aniline, o-toluidine in urine of, 81
  aromatic amine fraction in urine of, 79
  endogenous NPRO formation in, 137-148
  increased excretion of urinary N-nitrosamino acids, 47-51
  PAH levels in, 37, 40
  rate of acetylation in, 74-75
Smoking
  additive models, 378
  and alcohol, no evidence for synergistic effect of, 114-115
  animal vs. human models, 135-136
  behavior, self-reported, validation of, 4-6
  and cervical cancer, relative risks, 331
  effect of on NDMA, NPRO urinary excretion, 26, 28
  and enhanced urinary NPRO excretion, mechanisms of, 144
  habits, age-adjusted, 392
  history, validation of with micronucleus test, 113-119
  influence of on urinary excretion of NDMA, NPRO, 26, 28
  interaction of with occupation, diet, 402
  interactions with other exposures, 377-395
  multiplicative models, 378
  as source of PAH exposure, 41
  status, potential for misclassification of, 225-256
  status, validation of, 351
Snuff
  B[a]P in, 204
  carcinogenic nature of, 198
  and gum and buccal mucosa cancer, 362
  MEC frequency associated with, 102
  polonium in, 204
Snuff dippers
  alkaloids and N-nitrosamines in saliva of, 204
  bladder cancer in, 212

[Snuff dippers]
  DNA methylation in, 205
  effect of beta-carotene on MEC in oral mucosa of, 103
  and high risk of pancreas cancer, 212
  levels of nitrite, nitrate, and nicotine ingested, 55
Solanone
  degradation of, 171
  quantification of in Virginia tobacco, 177
  structure, 171
  as tobacco flavor constituent, 170
Sputum, micronucleus test on, 114
Squamous cell carcinoma
  induced by aldehydes in animal models, 215-216
  as large percentage of oral cancers in smokeless tobacco users, 366
  and smoking and alcohol, 385
Squamous cell type, and relative risk of cancers for smokers, 322
Synergistic effect, smoking and alcohol, no evidence for, 114-115

Testosterone, lower plasma levels of in smokers, 340
12-O-Tetradecanoylphorbol-13-acetate, role of, with NNK, in development of anaplastic carcinoma, 241
Thermal energy analyzer (TEA), use of in nitrosation test, 46
Thiocyanate
  distribution of in plasma and saliva of smokers, nonsmokers, 5
  and higher nicotine yield cigarettes, 9
  and lower nicotine yield cigarettes, 9
  quantitation of as measure of smoke absorption, 3
  use of to validate cigarette use, 4-6
Thiol depletion, and increased DPX, 229
Tobacco aroma constituents. *See also* Carotenoids; Cembranoids; Labdanoids.
  isoprenoids, 163-178
Tobacco brands, induction of micronuclei by various, 105
Tobacco chewers
  genotoxicity of saliva of, 104
  levels of nitrate, nitrite, and nicotine ingested, 55
Tobacco cigarette
  gas-phase profile, 154
  whole-smoke profile, 156
Tobacco nitrate content, as primary determinant for aromatic amines, 71
Tobacco postharvest treatment, 163

Tobacco smoke
 4-ABP in, 64–66
 absorption, measures of, 3–4
 aldehydes present in and formation of DPX, 215–230
 aroma, 400
 carcinogens in, 300
 high concentration of TSNA in, 46
 N-nitroso compounds in, 21
 particulate phase, cocarcinogens and tumor promoters in, 216
 pathobiological effects of aldehydes in, 273–285
 quantification of absorption of, 3–4
 relation of to transplacental carcinogenesis, 180
 uptake of components of, 3–19
Tobacco-specific nitrosamines (TSNA)
 formation of, 199, 202
 high concentrations of in tobacco smoke, 46
Tobacco type, and relative risk for oral/pharynx cancer, 364
Tobacco users
 genotoxic damage in oral mucosa of, 99–111
 increased frequency of MEC in oral mucosa of, 102–103
 in vivo nitrosation in, 45–61
o-Toluidine
 analysis of in human urine, 77–84
 in nonsmokers' urine, 82
 scheme for analysis of, 78
Total particulate matter (TPM), average delivery per cigarette, 157
TPA. See 12-O-Tetradecanoylphorbol-13-acetate.
Transformation, NHBE cells by transfected v-Ha-ras, 305–308
Transplacental carcinogenesis, relation of tobacco smoke inhalation to, 180
Tumor induction, by NNK, NDMA, 248
Tumor promoters, for NHBE, 302–303

Underground mining, and smoking and lung cancer, 380
Urinary arylamines, N-oxidation of in bladder epithelium, 319
Urinary bladder
 as nitrosation site, 55–56
 NNK distribution in, 181
Urinary bladder cancer, induction of by aromatic amines, 315–326
Urinary pH, 317–319
 and bladder tumor induction, 135
Urine

[Urine]
 analysis and indicators of tobacco-specific uptake, 10–11
 analysis of aniline in, 77–84
 analysis of o-toluidine in, 77–84
 analysis of to determine PAH exposure, 33–44
 aniline in that of smoker, 81
 aromatic amine fraction in, 79
 excretion of creatinine in, 44
 excretion of NDMA in, 23–28
 excretion of NPRO in, 23–28
 levels of NAA in, 50
 measurement of PAHs in, 35
 mutagenic, in cigarette-smoking baboons, 126–130
 mutagenic, in nonsmokers, 122
 mutagenic activity of in smokers, 131–132
 mutagenicity, value of, 136
 mutagens in of smokers, 121–136
 o-toluidine in that of smoker, 81
 volume, higher in smokers than in nonsmokers, 139
Urotheliol prostaglandin H synthase, 319
Uterine cervix cancer
 and cigarette smoking, 329–341
 and smoking, 402

Vegan diet, and mutagens in urine of smokers, nonsmokers, 122, 126
Verrucous carcinoma, in smokeless tobacco users, 369
v-Ha-ras
 transfection of into human bronchial epithelial cells and transformation, 299
 -transformed NHBE cells resistant to TPA-induced differentiation, 308
Virginia tobacco, quantification of solanone in, 177
Vitamin C
 effect of on NPRO, NDMA urinary excretion, 29
 as nitrosation inhibitor, 52–56
 and urinary excretion of NDMA, NPRO, 23–25
Vitamin E
 effect of on NPRO, NDMA urinary excretion, 29
 and urinary excretion of NDMA, NPRO, 23–25

Woodworking and smoking, and lung cancer risk, 380

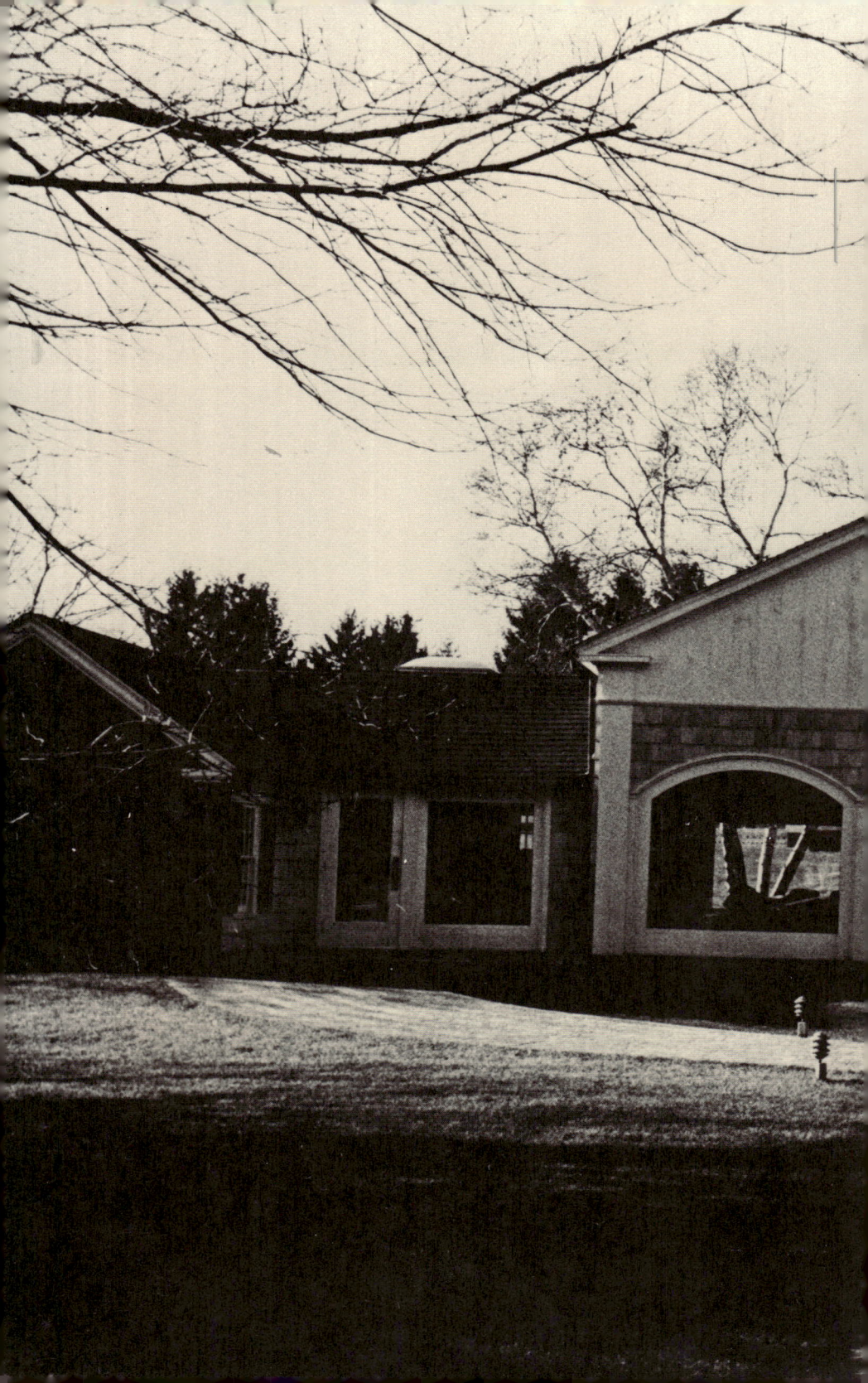